KiNG WEST X-RAY &
ULTRASOUND
1178 KING ST. W.
TORONTO, ONT.
M6K 1E6

Introduction to
Vascular Ultrasonography
Second Edition

Edited By

William J. Zwiebel, M.D.
Associate Professor of Radiology
University of Utah School of Medicine
Chief of Ultrasound and Body CT
Veterans Administration Medical Center
Salt Lake City, Utah

W. B. SAUNDERS COMPANY
Harcourt Brace Jovanovich, Inc.

Philadelphia   London   Toronto
Montreal   Sydney   Tokyo

Library of Congress Cataloging-in-Publication Data
Main entry under title:

Introduction to vascular ultrasonography.

Includes bibliographies and index.
1. Diagnosis, Ultrasonic. 2. Blood-vessels—Diseases
—Diagnosis. I. Zwiebel, William J. [DNLM: 1. Ultra-
sonic Diagnosis. 2. Vascular Diseases-diagnosis.
WG 500 I636]
RC691.6.U47I57   1986   616.1'307543   85-30230
ISBN 0-8089-1781-1

Library of Congress Catalog Number 85-30230
International Standard Book Number 0-8089-1781-1

Printed in the United States of America
        88 89 10 9 8 7 6 5 4

Contents

SECTION I—BASICS

SECTION II—CEREBROVASCULAR DIAGNOSIS

SECTION III—EXTREMITY VASCULAR DIAGNOSIS

SECTION IV—ABDOMINAL VASCULAR DIAGNOSIS

SECTION V—INTRAOPERATIVE AND POSTOPERATIVE VASCULAR ASSESSMENT

Preface to the Second Edition

Advances in instrumentation and methodology, particularly in the area of cerebrovascular diagnosis, have made necessary the publication of a second edition of *Introduction to Vascular Ultrasonography,* even though the original textbook is only three years old. When the first edition was published, "pure" Doppler methods were the predominant mode for cerebrovascular examination, but these techniques have been superseded through widespread application of duplex devices that combine B-mode imaging and Doppler flow assessment. Doppler methods also have made tentative inroads into the fields of abdominal and extremity vascular diagnosis, and increasing utilization of duplex instrumentation is anticipated in these areas, especially for the diagnosis of extremity venous occlusive disease.

Increasingly widespread application of duplex instrumentation has mandated the addition of several new chapters and thorough revision of the material on cerebrovascular diagnosis. Portions of the second edition, especially those concerned with extremity vascular diagnosis, are reprinted from the first edition without substantial change, since well established diagnostic methods are used in these areas. It should be noted, however, that the entire textbook has been revised and brought up-to-date.

The second edition also has been reformatted to provide a greater sense of cohesion of related subjects. Chapters have been arranged in five sections dealing with: (1) basic information, (2) the cerebrovascular system, (3) the extremity vasculature, (4) abdominal vessels and (5) postoperative vascular evaluation.

The editor sincerely hopes that modifications included in the second edition will enhance the educational value of this work. Our goal is unchanged: We wish to provide technologists and physicians with a solid foundation of basic information upon which to develop diagnostic skills.

The dramatic progress in ultrasound vascular diagnosis that has occurred in recent years is gratifying to everyone working in this field. Especially pleasing is the burgeoning clinical application of vascular ultrasound techniques which indicates that the value of ultrasonograpy is increasingly appreciated by clinical practitioners. A case that is close to the editor's heart illustrates the breadth of clinical application of vascular ultrasonography. Recently, the editor's step-mother, who resides in a rural Pennsylvania community of 2000 population, was noted to have a carotid bruit. Mrs. Zwiebel was referred to the local community hospital (60 beds) for a duplex carotid examination. A high-grade stenosis was found on the duplex study and Mrs. Zwiebel was sent to a regional medical center where arteriography confirmed the presence of an 80 percent (diameter reduction) internal carotid stenosis. Carotid endarterectomy was performed without complication and Mrs. Zwiebel has done well. The availability of vascular ultrasonography in a 60 bed hospital is quite a statement about the widespread application of this technique. In Mrs. Zwiebel's case, access to carotid ultrasonography may have weighed heavily on the clinician's decision to further evaluate her carotid bruit. Perhaps her physician would not have sought further evaluation of this bruit if the only recourse were arteriography, and perhaps Mrs. Zwiebel subsequently would have suffered a debilitating or fatal cerebral infarct.

Acknowledgments

The editor is greatly indebted to the numerous authors who have contributed chapters to this textbook. The depth of the contributors' knowledge is indicated by the thorough yet succinct treatment of the material contained within this textbook. The efficient and diligent assistance of the editor's secretary, Mrs. Deborah Hofmann, is also greatly acknowledged. The difficult task of organizing and editing this work would have been an unbearable drudgery without Mrs. Hofmann's willing assistance.

Contributors

Robert W. Barnes, M.D.
Davis Hume Professor Surgery
Medical College of Virginia
Richmond Veterans Administration
   Hospital
Box 221
MCV Station
Richmond, VA 23298

Eugene F. Bernstein, M.D., Ph.D.
Division of Vascular and Thoracic Surgery
Scripps Clinical and Research Foundation
10666 North Torrey Pines Road
LaJolla, CA 92037

Stefan A. Carter, M.D., M.SC., F.R.C.P.(C)
Professor of Medicine and Physiology
Faculty of Medicine
University of Manitoba Medical College
750 Bannatyne
Winnipeg, Manitoba
CANADA ROE OW3

Andrew B. Crummy, M.D.
Professor of Radiology
University of Wisconsin
   School of Medicine
600 Highland Avenue
Madison, WI 53792

Edward B. Diethrich, M.D.
Medical Director
Arizona Heart Institute
Post Office Box 10,000
Phoenix AZ 85064

D. Preston Flanigan, M.D.
Associate Professor of Surgery
Chief, Division of Vascular Surgery
University of Illinois at Chicago
Post Office Box 6998
Chicago, IL 60680

Gretchen A. W. Gooding, M.D.
Associate Professor of Radiology
University of California, San Francisco
Veterans Administration Medical Center
4150 Clement Street
San Francisco, CA 94121

Junji Machi, M.D., Ph.D.
First Department of Surgery
Kurme University School of Medicine
Kurme, JAPAN

William H. Pearce, M.D.
Assistant Professor of Surgery
University of Colorado Sciences Center
   and Veterans Administration Center
1055 Fairmont Street
Denver, CO 80220

Jean-Baptiste Ricco, M.D.
#2 BisRue Ste. Opportune
Poitiers
FRANCE

James J. Schuler, M.D.
Assistant Professor of Surgery
Division of Vascular Surgery
University of Illinois at Chicago
Post Office 6998
Chicago, IL 60680

Bernard Sigel, M.D.
Professor and Chairman
Department of Surgery
The Medical College of Pennsylvania
3300 Henry Avenue
Philadelphia, PA 19129

Merrill P. Spencer, M.D.
Institute of Applied Physiology
  and Medicine
701 Sixteenth Avenue
Seattle, WA 98112

Michael F. Stieghorst, M.D.
Department of Medical Imaging (Radiology)
St. Mary's Hospital Medical Center
707 South Mills Street
Madison, WI 53715

D. Eugene Strandness, Jr., M.D.
Professor of Surgery
Department of Surgery
University of Washington School
  of Medicine
FR 25
Seattle, WA 98195

David S. Sumner, M.D.
Professor of Surgery
Chief, Section of
  Peripheral Vascular Surgery
Southern Illinois University
  School of Medicine
Post Office Box 3926
Springfield, IL 62708

Steven R. Talbot, R.V.T.
Periphral Vascular Laboratory
LDS Hospital
8th Avenue and C Streets
Salt Lake City, UT 84143

Denis N. White, M.D., F.R.C.P.
Professor Emeritus Queens University
230 Alwington Place
Kingston, Ontario
CANADA K7L 4P8

James S. T. Yao, M.D., Ph.D.
Professor of Surgery
Director of Blood Flow Laboratory
Northwestern University
303 East Chicago Avenue
Chicago, IL 60611

James A. Zagzebski, Ph.D.
Professor of Medical Physics
University of Wisconsin School of Medicine
1300 University Avenue
Madison, WI 53706

R. Eugene Zierler, M.D.
Assistant Professor of Surgery
University of Washington
  School of Medicine
  and Chief, Vascular Surgery Section
Seattle Veterans Administration
  Medical Center
Seattle, WA 98101

William J. Zwiebel, M.D.
Associate Professor of Radiology
University of Utah School of Medicine
Chief of Ultrasound and Body CT
Veterans Administration Medical Center
500 Foothill Drive
Salt Lake City, UT 84148

Color Plate 1. Flow patterns in the normal carotid bifurcation. Red indicates cephalad flow and blue caudad flow. Lighter shades correspond to higher velocities and darker shades to lower velocities. First, note the region of blue shades in the proximal internal carotid (lower branch). The blue color represents a zone reversed flow present in virtually all normal carotid bifurcations. The location and size of the reverse-flow zone varies with the configuration of the bifurcation. Second, note the region of dark red shades in the distal common carotid artery that corresponds to decreased flow in the bulbous portion of the bifurcation. Third, observe the area of darker red colors along the walls of the common and internal carotid arteries as well as lighter shades in the center of these vessels. This appearance indicates a laminar flow pattern with slower velocities near the vessel walls and higher velocities near the center of the lumen. (Color reproduction courtesy of Quantum Medical Systems, Issaquah, Washington. With permission.)

Color Plate 2. Color frequency spectral display of Doppler signals associated with stenosis at the origin of the internal carotid artery. (A) In the stenotic zone, f_{max} reaches 10 kHz. The smooth spectrum with high energies concentrated in a narrow upper band indicates a blunt flow profile. The continuous wave Doppler image of this carotid bifurcation is shown in the lower right hand corner. The mandible is indicated by the diagonal streak, and the position of the probe is indicated by the black dot and white arrow. (B) The probe position has been moved very slightly downstream from (A) into the poststenotic zone. High frequencies still persist in the jet expelled from the stenotic lumen, but strong turbulent qualities and the Doppler bruit are also apparent. The normal systolic spectral window seen in panel A is filled in by low frequency turbulent energies. The Doppler bruit is evidenced by the bright, high energy pattern seen above and below the baseline in late systole and early diastole. (Color reproduction of Sonocolor spectra courtesy of Carolina Medical Electronics, King, North Carolina. With permission.)

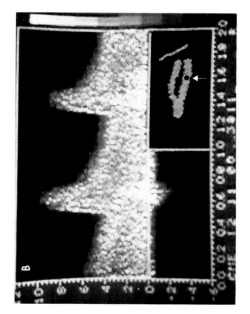

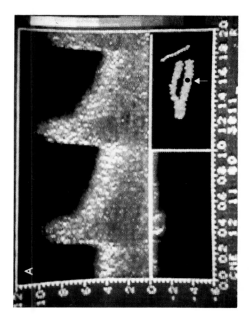

Color Plate 2

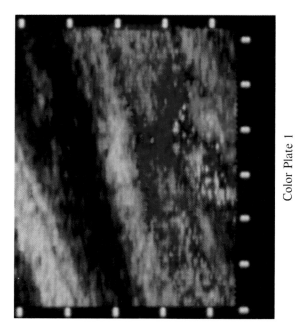

Color Plate 1

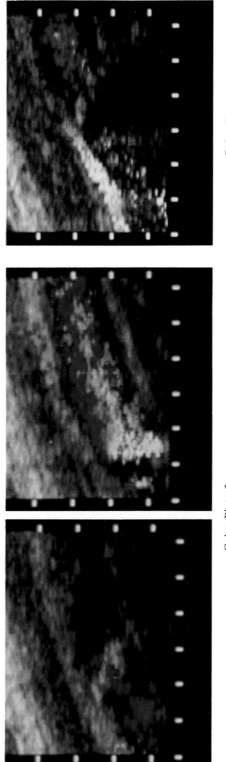

Color Plate 3

Color Plate 4

Color Plate 3. Flow abnormalities resulting from severe stenosis (90 percent diameter reduction) of the proximal internal carotid. (A) A color-coded flow image obtained in diastole demonstrates only a trickle of flow (red zone) through the stenosis (gray band across vessel). Note that flow in the remainder of the vessel is so slow that no Doppler shift is recorded (black areas of lumen). This appearance corresponds to the high resistance flow pattern seen on Doppler sonograms obtained proximal to severe lesions. (B) During systole, a high velocity jet (white region) crosses the stenosis and strikes the distal wall of the vessel. Wall vibrations from such jets cause a "moaning" or "segal" sound in the audible Doppler signal, and described in Chapter 2. Note also the exaggerated laminar flow pattern evident proximal to the stenosis. The black layer adjacent to the vessel wall represents virtually stationary blood, while high velocities (lighter shades) are seen in the center of the vessel. (Color reproduction courtesy of Quantum Medical Systems, Issaquah, Washington. With permission.)

Color Plate 4. Poststenotic turbulence. The zone of acoustic shadowing crossing the vessel results from a large, calcified plaque that results in a high grade, common carotid stenosis. Distal to the stenosis (left side of image, mixed blue and red shades are present in the vessel due to severe turbulence and associated swirling of blood. The jugular vein is represented by the blue/white stripe seen above the turbulent zone. (Color reproduction courtesy of Quantum Medical Systems, Issaquah, Washington. With permission.)

SECTION I

BASICS

Accurate ultrasound vascular diagnosis requires knowledge of hemodynamics and instrumentation. Accordingly we will begin with a section that provides this fundamental information. In Chapter 1, Dr. Carter condenses the complex subject of arterial and venous hemodynamics into a small volume of concentrated information. The same is true in Chapter 2, for Dr. Zagzebski's rendering of ultrasound physics and instrumentation. In Chapter 3, Dr. Spencer thoroughly reviews the principles of frequency spectrum analysis, as applied to vascular ultrasonography. Specific applications of spectral analysis are included elsewhere in the text, but only in this chapter may the reader learn the underlying principles of this important technology.

Stefan A. Carter, M.D., M.Sc., F.R.C.P.(C)

1

Hemodynamic Considerations in Peripheral and Cerebrovascular Disease

The circulatory system is extremely complex in both its structure and function, and blood flow is influenced by a great number of factors, including cardiac function, elasticity of the vessel walls (compliance), the tone of vascular smooth muscle and the various patterns, dimensions and interconnections of millions of branching vessels. Some of these factors can be measured and described in reasonably simple terms, but many others cannot be described succinctly because they are difficult to quantify and in general are not well understood.

With these limitations in mind, this chapter deals in basic terms with the dynamics of blood circulation, the many factors that influence blood flow and the hemodynamic consequences of occlusive disease. These basic considerations are of help in understanding the normal physiology of blood circulation and the abnormalities that can result in the presence of vascular obstruction.

PHYSIOLOGICAL FACTORS GOVERNING BLOOD FLOW AND ITS CHARACTERISTICS

Energy and Pressure

For blood flow to occur between any two points in the circulatory system there has to be a difference in the energy level between these two points. Usually, the difference in energy level is reflected by a difference in pressure, and the circulatory system in general consists of a high-pressure high-energy arterial reservior and a venous pool with low pressure and energy. These reservoirs are

Acknowledgments. The author held grants-in-aid of research from the Manitoba Heart and the St. Boniface Hospital Research Foundations, which supported studies the results of which are discussed in this chapter. He is also grateful to Dr. William J. Zwiebel for valuable exchange of ideas and assistance, and the excellent secretarial work of Mrs. Constance Twomey.

1

connected by a system of distributing vessels (smaller arteries) and by the resistance vessels of the microcirculation, which consists of arterioles, capillaries, and venules.

During flow, energy is continuously lost from the blood because of the friction between its layers and particles, with the result that both pressure and energy levels fall from the arterial to the venous end. The energy necessary for flow is continuously restored by the pumping action of the heart, which forces blood from the venous into the arterial end, thus maintaining the arterial pressure and the energy difference needed for flow to occur.

The high arterial energy level is due to the large volume of blood in the arterial reservoir. The function of the heart and blood vessels is normally regulated to maintain volume and pressure in the arteries within limits required for smooth function. This is achieved by maintaining a balance between the amount of blood that enters and leaves the arterial reservoir. The amount that enters the arteries is the cardiac output. The amount that leaves depends on the arterial pressure and on the total peripheral resistance, which, in turn, is controlled by the amount of vasoconstriction in the microcirculation.

Under normal conditions, flow to all the tissues of the body is adjusted according to the tissues' particular needs at a given time. This adjustment is accomplished by alterations in the level of vasoconstriction of the arterioles within the organs supplied. Maintenance of the normal volume and pressure in the arteries thus allows for both adjustment of blood flow to all parts of the body and regulation of cardiac output (which equals the sum of blood flow to all the vascular beds).

The Forms of Energy Present in the Blood and its Dissipation During Flow

This section considers the forms in which energy exists in the circulation and the important factors that govern the dissipation of energy during flow, including friction, resistance, and the influence of laminar and turbulent flow. Poiseuille's law and the equation which summarizes the basic relationship of flow, pressure and resistance are discussed, as well as the effect of connections of vascular resistance in parallel and in series.

Potential and kinetic energy.   The main form of energy present in flowing blood is the pressure distending the vessels (a form of potential energy), which is created by the pumping action of the heart. Some of the energy of the blood is kinetic, however, namely, the ability of flowing blood to do work as a result of its velocity. Usually, the kinetic energy component is small compared with the pressure energy, and under normal resting conditions is equivalent to only a few millimeters of Hg or less. The kinetic energy of blood is proportional to its density (which is stable in normal circumstances) and the square of its velocity. There-fore, important increases in kinetic energy occur in the systemic circulation when flow is high, e.g., during exercise, and in stenotic lesions, where luminal narrowing leads to high velocities. Kinetic energy is converted back into pressure when velocity is decreased, e.g., in a normal segment of the artery distal to a stenosis.

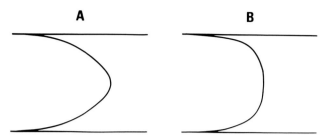

Figure 1-1. Flow velocity profiles across a normal arterial lumen: (A) parabolic profile of laminar flow, (B) flattened profile with a central core of relatively uniform velocity encountered in the proximal portion (inlet length) of arterial branches or with turbulent flow.

Energy differences related to differences in the level of body parts. There is also variation in the energy of the blood associated with differences in the level of the body part. For example, the pressure in the vessels in the dependent parts of the body, such as the lower portions of the legs, is increased by an amount that depends on the weight of the column of blood resting on the blood in the legs. This hydrostatic pressure increases the transmural pressure and the distension of the vessels. Gravitational potential energy (potential for doing work related to the effect of gravity on a free-falling body), however, is reduced in the dependent parts of the body by the same amount as the increase due to hydrostatic pressure. For this reason, differences in the level of the body parts usually do not lead to changes in the driving pressure along the vascular tree unless the column of blood is interrupted, as may be the case when the venous valves close. Changes in energy and pressure associated with differences in level are important under certain conditions, such as with changes in posture or when the venous pump is activated because of muscular action during walking.

Dissipation of energy during laminar flow. In the majority of vessels, blood moves in concentric layers, or laminae; hence, the flow is said to be *laminar*. Each infinitesimal layer flows with a different velocity and, theoretically, a thin layer of blood is held stationary next to the vessel wall at zero velocity because of an adhesive force between the blood and the inner surface of the vessel. The next layer flows with a certain velocity, but is delayed by the stationary layer because of the viscous properties of the fluid and the resulting friction between the layers. The second layer, in turn, delays the next layer, which flows at a greater velocity. The layers in the middle of the vessel flow with the highest velocity, and the *mean velocity across the vessel is one-half the maximal velocity*. Since the rate of change of velocity is greatest near the walls and decreases toward the center of the vessel, a velocity profile with the shape of a parabola exists along the vessel diameter (Fig. 1-1A).

Loss of energy during blood flow occurs because of friction, and the amount of friction and energy loss is determined by the dimensions of the vessels. In small vessels, especially in the microcirculation, even the layers in the middle of the lumen are relatively close to the wall and thus are delayed considerably, resulting in a significant opposition or resistance to flow. In large vessels, by contrast, a large central core of blood is far from the walls and the frictional energy losses are minimal. As indicated below, friction and energy losses are increased if laminar flow is disturbed.

Poiseuille's law and equation. In a cylindrical tube model, the mean linear velocity of laminar flow is directly proportional to the energy difference between the ends of the tube and the square of the radius, and is inversely proportional to the length of the tube and the viscosity of the fluid. In the circulatory system, however, volume flow is of more interest than velocity. Volume flow is proportional to the fourth power of the vessel radius, since it is equal to the product of mean linear velocity and the cross-sectional area of the tube. These important considerations are helpful in understanding Poiseuille's law as expressed in Poiseuille's equation:

$$Q = \frac{\pi(P_1 - P_2)r^4}{8L\eta} \tag{1-1}$$

where Q = volume flow; P_1, P_2 = pressures at the proximal and distal ends of the tube; r, L = radius and length of the tube; and η = viscosity of the fluid.

Since volume flow is proportional to the fourth power of the radius, even small changes in radius can result in large changes in flow. For example, a decrease in radius of 10 percent would decrease flow in a tube model by about 35 percent, and a decrease of 50 percent would lead to a 95 percent decrease in flow. *Since the length of the vessels and the viscosity do not change much in the cardiovascular system, alterations in blood flow occur mainly as a result of changes in the radius of the vessels and the pressure of energy level available for flow.*

Poiseuille's equation can be rewritten as follows:

$$\frac{8L\eta}{\pi r^4} = \frac{P_1 - P_2}{Q} \tag{1-2}$$

$$R = \frac{8L\eta}{\pi r^4} \tag{1-3}$$

$$R = \frac{P_1 - P_2}{Q} \tag{1-4}$$

The resistance term (R) depends on the viscous properties of the blood and the dimensions of the vessels. Although these parameters cannot be measured in a complex system, the pressure difference ($P_1 - P_2$) and the blood flow (Q) can be measured, and thus the resistance can be calculated. Since resistance is equal to the pressure difference divided by the volume flow (the pressure difference per unit flow), it can be thought of as the pressure difference necessary to cause 1 unit of flow and, therefore, as an index of the difficulty in forcing blood through the vessels.

Vessel interconnection and energy dissipation. Poiseuille's law applies precisely only to constant laminar flow of a simple fluid such as water, in a rigid tube of a uniform bore. In blood circulation, these conditions are not met. Instead the resistance is influenced by the presence of numerous interconnected vessels with a combined effect similar to that observed in electrical resistances. In the case of vessels in series, the overall resistance is equal to the sum of the resistances of the individual vessels; whereas, in the case of parallel vessels, the reciprocal of the total resistance equals the sum of the reciprocals of the individual vessel resistances. Thus, *the contribution of any single vessel to the total resistance of a vascular bed, or the effect of a change in the dimension of a vessel, will depend on the presence and relative size of the other vessels linked in series or in parallel.*

Deviations from the conditions to which Poiseuille's law applies also occur in relation to changes in blood viscosity, which is affected by hematocrit, temperature, vessel diameter and rate of flow.

Dissipation of energy in nonlaminar flow. Various degrees of deviation from orderly laminar flow occur in the circulation under both normal and abnormal conditions. The factors responsible for these deviations include (1) the flow velocity, which changes throughout the cardiac cycle as a result of acceleration during systole and deceleration in diastole, (2) alteration of the lines of flow, which occurs whenever a vessel changes dimensions, including variations in diameter associated with each pulse, (3) the lines of flow, which are distorted at curves, at bifurcations and in branches that take off at various angles. For example, the parabolic velocity profile is often not re-established in branches for a considerable distance beyond their origin. Instead, the parabola is flattened so that there is a relatively large central core of blood that flows with relatively uniform speed (Fig. 1-1B).

Because of these and other factors, laminar flow may be disturbed or flow may be fully turbulent, even in a uniform tube. The elements that affect development of turbulence are expressed by the dimensionless Reynolds number (*Re*):

$$Re = \frac{vq2r}{\eta} \tag{1-5}$$

where v = velocity, q = density of the fluid, r = radius of the tube and η = viscosity of the fluid. Since the density (q) and viscosity (η) of the blood are relatively constant, *the development of turbulence depends mainly on the size of the vessels and the velocity of flow.* In a tube model, laminar flow tends to be disturbed if the Reynolds number exceeds 2000, but in the circulatory system, disturbances, as well as various degrees of turbulence, are likely to occur at lower values because of body movements, the pulsatile nature of blood flow, changes in vessel dimensions, roughness of the endothelial surface and other factors. Turbulence develops more readily in large vessels under conditions of high flow and can be detected clinically by the finding of bruits or thrills. Bruits may at times be heard over the ascending aorta during systolic acceleration in normal individuals at rest, and frequently are heard in states of high cardiac output and blood flow, even in more distal arteries such as the femoral.[1] Distortion of laminar flow velocity profiles can be assessed using ultrasound flow detectors and such assessments can be applied for diagnostic purposes. For example, in arteries with severe stenosis, pronounced turbulence is a diagnostic feature observed in the poststenotic zone. Turbulence occurs because the jet of blood with high velocity and high kinetic energy suddenly encounters the normal diameter lumen or a lumen of increased diameter (due to poststenotic dilatation) where both the velocity and energy level are lower than in the stenotic region or in the vessel segment proximal to the stenosis.

During turbulent flow, the loss of pressure energy between two points in a vessel is greater than that which would be expected from the factors included in Poiseuille's equation, and the parabolic velocity profile is flattened.[2]

Pulsatile Pressure and Flow Changes in the Arterial System

With each heartbeat, a stroke volume of blood is ejected into the arterial system, and results in a pressure wave that travels throughout the arterial tree. The speed of propagation, the amplitude (strength) and the shape of the pressure wave change as it traverses the arterial system. These alterations are influenced both by the elastic properties of the arteries being traversed and by the varying characteristics of the vessels in the peripheral circulation. The velocity and, in some parts of the circulation, the direction of flow, also vary with each heartbeat. Correct interpretation of noninvasive tests based on recordings of arterial pressure and velocity, and of the pressure and velocity wave forms requires understanding of the factors that influence these variables. This section considers these factors as they occur in various portions of the circulatory system.

Pressure changes from cardiac activity. As indicated previously, the pumping action of the heart maintains a high volume of blood in the arterial end of the circulation and thus provides the high pressure difference between the arterial and venous ends necessary to maintain flow. Because of the intermittent pumping action of the heart, pressure and flow vary in a pulsatile manner. During the rapid phase of venticular ejection, the volume of blood at the arterial end increases, raising the pressure to a systolic peak. During the latter part of systole, when cardiac ejection decreases, the outflow through the peripheral resistance vessels exceeds the volume being ejected by the heart and the pressure begins to decline. This decline continues throughout diastole as blood continues to flow from the arteries into the microcirculation. Part of the work of the heart leads directly to forward flow, but a large portion of the energy of each cardiac contraction results in distension of the arteries that serve as reservoirs to store both the blood volume and the energy supplied to the system. This storage of energy and blood volume provides for continuous flow to the tissues during diastole.

The arterial pressure wave. The pulsatile variation in blood volume and energy occurring with each cardiac cycle are manifested as a pressure wave that can be detected throughout the arterial system. The amplitude and shape of the arterial pressure wave depends on a complex interplay of factors, which include the stroke volume and time course of ventricular ejection, the peripheral resist-

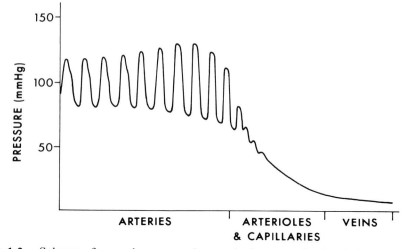

Figure 1-2.   Schema of normal pressure changes in the systemic circulation. From Carter SA: Peripheral artery disease: pressure measurements ease evaluation. Consultant 19(9):102–115, 1979. With permission.

ance and the stiffness of the arterial walls. In general, an increase in any of these factors results in an increase in the pulse amplitude, i.e., pulse pressure (difference between systolic and diastolic pressures), and frequently by concomitant increase in systolic pressure. For example, increased stiffness of the arteries with age tends to increase both the systolic and pulse pressures.

The arterial pressure wave is propagated along the arterial tree distally from the heart. The speed of propagation, or pulse wave velocity, increases with stiffness of the arterial walls (the elastic modulus of the material of which the walls are composed) and with the ratio of the wall thickness to diameter. In the mammalian circulation, arteries get progressively stiffer from the aorta towards the periphery. Therefore, the speed of propagation of the wave increases as it moves peripherally. Also, the gradual increase in stiffness tends to decrease wave reflection (discussed below) and has a beneficial effect in that the pulse and systolic pressures in the aorta and proximal arteries are relatively lower than in peripheral vessels. The pressure against which the heart ejects the stroke volume and the associated cardiac work are accordingly reduced.[3]

Pressure changes throughout the circulation.   Figure 1-2 shows changes in pressure in the systemic circulation from large arteries through the resistance vessels to the veins. Because there is little loss of pressure energy due to friction in large and distributing arteries, they offer relatively little resistance to flow, and the mean pressure falls little between the aorta and the small arteries of the limbs, such as the radial or the dorsalis pedis.[4,5] The diastolic pressure also shows only minor changes. The amplitude of the pressure wave and the systolic pressure actually increase, however, as the wave travels distally (systolic amplification), because of increasing stiffness of the walls toward the periphery and the presence of reflected waves. The latter arise at sites where the vessels change diameter and

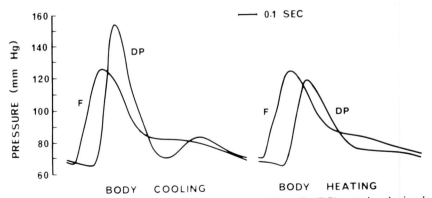

Figure 1-3. Pressure waves from the femoral (F) and dorsalis (DP) arteries during heating and cooling. Note that the pulse pressure of the dorsalis pedis artery is greater with vasoconstriction (body cooling) and falls dramatically with vasodilatation (body heating). From Carter SA: Effect of age, cardiovascular disease, and vasomotor changes on transmission of arterial pressure waves through the lower extremities. Angiology 29:601–616, 1978. With permission.

stiffness, divide or branch, and are superadded to the oncoming primary pulse wave.[3,4] The reflected waves, at least in the extremities, are strongly enhanced by increase in the peripheral resistance.[4] Direct measurements of pressure in small arteries in experimental animals and in man, and indirect measurements of systolic pressure in human digits, indicate that pulse amplitude and systolic pressure decrease in smaller vessels such as the digital vessels of the human extremities.[6-9] Some pulsatile changes in pressure and flow may remain evident even in minute arteries and capillaries, however, at least under conditions of peripheral vasodilatation, and can be recorded by various methods including plethysmography. The effect of peripheral vasoconstriction on pulsatility in the microcirculation is opposite to that seen in the proximal small- or medium-sized arteries of the extremities. *Pulsatile changes in minute arteries, arterioles and capillaries are reduced by vasoconstriction and enhanced by vasodilatation. In medium- and small-sized arteries of the limbs, however, pulsatile changes are increased by vasoconstriction as a result of enhanced wave reflection, and are decreased by vasodilatation.* Figure 1-3 shows arterial pressure pulses recorded directly from the femoral and dorsalis pedis arteries during peripheral vasoconstriction and vasodilatation induced, respectively, by body cooling and heating.

There is practically complete disappearance of amplification in the dorsalis pedis artery in response to vasodilitation induced by body heating. Similar changes in the distal pressure waves result from other factors that alter peripheral resistance, e.g., reactive hyperemia and exercise. Exercise, by decreasing resistance in the working muscle, would be expected to decrease reflection in the exercising extremity. Because of vasoconstriction in other parts of the body during exercise (the result of cardiovascular reflexes that regulate blood pressure and circulation), however, the reflection may be increased and lead to a high degree of amplification. For example, it has been shown that during walking the

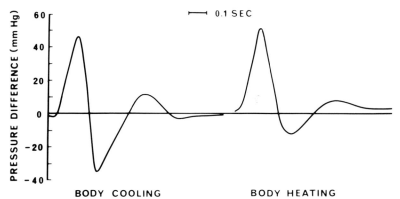

Figure 1-4. Pressure differences between the femoral and dorsalis pedis arteries obtained from the waves shown in Figure 1-3. Note the effect of vasodilatation (body heating) on the negative (reverse flow) component.

pulse pressure in the radial arteries can exceed that in the aorta by perhaps 100%.[10]

These considerations are important for correct interpretation of pressure measurements in peripheral arterial obstruction. For example, as indicated in Chapter 13, brachial systolic pressure corresponds well to aortic or femoral systolic pressure and is used as a standard against which ankle pressures is compared. The systolic pressure at the ankle usually exceeds brachial pressure in normal subjects; therefore, the finding of ankle systolic pressure that are even slightly lower than brachial systolic pressure indicates a high likelihood of the presence of a proximal stenotic lesion. On the other hand, systolic pressure in human digits is usually lower than systolic pressures proximal to the wrist or the ankle. This observation has to be taken into account when measurements of digital systolic pressures are used as an index of distal arterial obstruction. In such instances, the appropriate norms for the differences between the proximal and digital systolic pressure have to be applied.[11]

Pulsatile flow patterns. Pulsatile changes in pressure are associated with corresponding acceleration of blood flow with systole and deceleration in diastole. Although the energy stored in the arterial walls maintains a positive arteriovenous pressure gradient and overall forward flow in the microcirculation during diastole, temporary cessation of forward flow or even diastolic reversal occurs frequently in portions of the human arterial system. How these phenomena occur may be clarified by consideration of pulsatile pressure changes at two points along the arterial tree. Figure 1-3 shows arterial pressure pulses in the femoral and dorsalis pedis arteries. The corresponding pressure gradient between the two arteries, shown in Figure 1-4, varies during the cardiac cycle not only because of differences in the shape and magnitude of the original pressure waves but, more importantly, because the wave arrives later at the dorsalis pedis. The pressure gradient is greatest during the first half of systole, at which time, the peak of the wave arrives at the femoral site. Thereafter, the gradient decreases, and by the time the peak arrives at the dorsalis pedis, the femoral pressure has fallen and a negative pressure gradient appears. Such negative gradients related to different arrival times of the pressure wave at various sites in the arterial system are commonly observed along human arteries and are conducive to the reversal of blood flow. Despite the reversal of the pressure gradient, however, the direction of flow may not be reversed if there is a large forward mean flow component.[12]

The presence of reversed flow during diastole can also be understood if one imagines a major arterial segment with a certain diastolic pressure that has several branch vessels leading to areas with different levels of resistance. If one of the proximal branches leads to an area with low peripheral resistance, flow during diastole in the main vessel will occur toward this branch and flow will reverse in the distal portion of the main vessel if distal branches supply areas with higher peripheral resistance. Such situations of transient flow reversal may exist in the limb during cooling (Fig. 1-4); however, during body heating, when peripheral resistance in the distal cutaneous circulation is reduced to a low level, reversed flow is decreased or may be abolished. Diastolic flow reversal is generally present or is greatest in vessels that supply vascular beds with high peripheral resistance. It tends to be absent in low-resistance vascular beds or when peripheral resistance is reduced by peripheral dilation, such as occurs in the skin with body heating or in working muscle during exercise or reactive hyperemia. These principles are important in assessing blood flow in arteries supplying various regions including the cranial circulation. For example, flow reversal can be observed in the external carotid because extracranial resistance is relatively high; it is absent, however, in the internal carotid since the cerebrovascular resistance is low.

THE EFFECTS OF ARTERIAL OBSTRUCTION

Arterial obstruction can result in reduced pressure and flow distal to the site of blockage, but the effects on pressure and flow are vastly influenced by a number of factors proximal and especially distal to the lesion. One must be familiar with these factors when interpreting noninvasive studies, since they affect the pressure and velocity wave forms observed both proximal and distal to the obstructive lesion. In this section of the chapter, the concept of the critical stenosis will be considered, as well as the pressure, velocity and flow manifestation of arterial obstructive disease.

Critical Stenosis

Encroachment on the lumen of an artery by an arteriosclerotic plaque can result in diminished pressure and flow distal to the lesion, but this encroachment on the lumen has to be relatively extensive before changes in the hemodynamics are manifested, since arteries offer relatively little resistance to flow compared with the resistance vessels with which they are in series. Studies in man and animals indicate that about 90 percent of the cross-sectional area of the aorta has to be encroached upon before there is a change in the distal pressure and flow; whereas, in smaller vessels, such as the iliac, carotid, renal and femoral arteries, the "critical stenosis" varies from 70 to 90 percent.[13,14] It is important to differentiate between percentage decrease in cross-sectional area and diameter.

For example, a decrease in diameter of 50 percent corresponds to 75 percent decrease in cross-sectional area, and a diameter narrowing of 66 percent is equivalent to about 90 percent reduction in area.

Whether or not a hemodynamic abnormality results from a stenosis, and how severe it may be, depends on several factors including: (1) the length and diameter of the narrowed segment, (2) the roughness of the endothelial surface, (3) the degree of irregularity of the narrowing and its shape (i.e., whether the narrowing is abrupt or gradual), (4) the ratio of the cross-sectional area of the narrowed segment to that of the normal vessel, (5) the rate of flow, (6) the arteriovenous pressure gradient, and (7) the peripheral resistance beyond the stenosis.

The concept of "critical stenosis," i.e., a stenosis that causes a reduction in flow and pressure, has been treated extensively in the literature. This concept has been accepted because generally there is little or no change in hemodynamics when an artery is first narrowed by disease, but a relatively rapid decrease in pressure and flow occurs as greater degrees of narrowing take place. Therefore, graphs that relate changes in pressure or flow to the degree of stenosis tend to show a fairly sudden drop in both parameters when the point of critical narrowing is approached. The concept is of practical significance because lesser degrees of narrowing of human arteries often do not produce significant changes in hemo-dynamics or clinical manifestations. It must be recognized, however, that the concept of the "critical stenosis" in a gross simplification of a very complex interplay of numerous circulatory factors. In particular, changes in peripheral resistance, such as those occurring with exercise, may profoundly alter the effect of a given stenotic lesion. These considerations dictate that the hemodynamic and clinical significance of stenotic lesions be assessed, whenever possible, by physiologic measurements; otherwise, erroneous conclusions might be reached.[12] In evaluating the hemodynamic effect of stenotic lesions, it is also important to recognize that two or more stenotic lesions that occur in series have a more pronounced effect on distal pressure and flow than a single lesion of equal total length. This difference is due to large losses of energy at the entrance, and particularly at the exit, of the lesion resulting from grossly disturbed flow patterns, including jet effects, turbulence and eddy formation. Thus, the resulting energy losses far exceed those that result from frictional resistance in the stenotic lumen as represented in Poiseuille's equation.

Pressure Changes

Experiments with graded stenosis in animals indicate that whereas the diastolic pressure does not fall until the stenosis is very severe, a decrease in systolic pressure is a sensitive index of reduction in both the mean pressure and the amplitude of the pressure wave distal to a relatively minor stenosis (Fig. 1-5)[15,16] Also, damping of the wave form, increased time to peak and greater width of the wave at half amplitude can be detected distal to an arterial stenosis or occlusion.[17,18]

These abnormal features of the pulse wave correlate well with the results of measurement of systolic pressure and can be demonstrated by noninvasive techniques employing pulse waveform recording by various types of plethysmography (Fig. 1-6). In the case of very mild stenotic lesions, however, little or no pressure or pulse abnormality may be evident distal to the lesion when

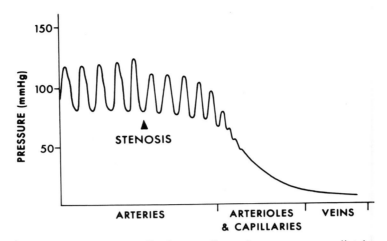

Figure 1-5. Decrease in pulse amplitude, systolic, and mean pressures distal to a stenosis. In minimal stenosis, alterations in pulse pressure such as this may be evident only during high volume flow induced by exercise or hyperemia. From Carter SA: Peripheral artery disease: pressure measurements ease evaluation. Consultant 19(9):102–115, 1979. With permission.

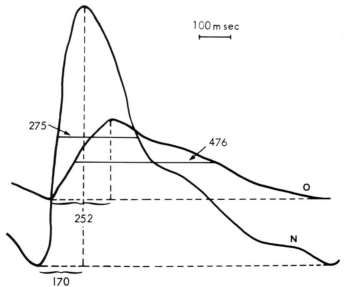

Figure 1-6. Dorsalis pedis pulse waves from a normal limb (N) and a limb with a proximal occlusion (O). The wave from the limb with occlusion shows a prolonged time to peak (252 msec) and increased width at half of the amplitude (476 msec). From Carter SA: Investigation and treatment of arterial occlusive disease of the extremities. Clin Med I 79(5):13–24, 1972; Clin Med II 79(6):15–22, 1972. With permission.

the patient is at rest. The presence of such lesions may be demonstrated by increasing flow with exercise or through induction of hyperemia. Enhanced flow through the stenosis results in increased loss of energy, which can be detected by a decrease in pressure distal to the lesion.[15,19]

Flow Changes

At rest, the total blood flow to an extremity may be normal in the presence of a severe stenosis or even a complete obstruction of the main artery because of the development of collateral circulation, as well as a compensatory decrease in the peripheral resistance. In such circumstances, measurement of systolic pressure, as discussed above, is a much better method of assessing the presence and severity of the occlusive or stenotic process than measurement of blood flow.[12,17] Resting blood flow is reduced only when the occlusion is acute and the collateral circulation has not had a change to develop or, in the case of a chronic arterial obstruction, when the occlusive process is very extensive and consists of two or more lesions in series. Although single lesions might not be associated with symptoms or significant changes in blood flow at rest, such lesions can significantly affect the blood supply when need is increased during exercise. In such cases, the sum of the resistances of the obstructions (stenosis, collateral resistance, or both) and of the peripheral resistance may prevent normal increase in flow and symptoms of intermittent claudication will develop.

Arterial obstruction can lead to changes in the distribution of the available blood flow to "neighboring" regions or vascular beds depending on the relative resistance and anatomic arrangement of these areas. For example, flow during exercise can increase in the skeletal muscle of an extremity distal to an arterial obstruction, but because the distal pressure is reduced during exercise, the muscle "steals" blood from the skin and the blood supply to the skin of the foot is diminished. Such reduction in flow to the skin may be manifested clinically by numbness of the foot, a common symptom in patients with claudication. In lower extremities with extensive large vessel occlusion and additional obstruction in small distal branches, vasodilator drugs or sympathectomy may divert flow from the critically ischemic distal areas by decreasing resistance in less ischemic regions.[20] Obstruction of the subclavian artery is known to cause cerebral symptoms in some patients due to reversal of flow in the vertebral arteries (the subclavian steal syndrome); likewise, obstructive lesions of the internal carotid may lead to reversal of flow in the opthalmic vessels, which communicate with external carotid branches on the face and scalp.

Velocity Changes

Recall that in normal arteries, flow velocity increases rapidly to a peak during early systole and decreases during diastole, when flow reversal can occur. The shape of the resulting pulse velocity wave resembles the pressure gradient shown in Figure 1-4. The character of this velocity profile can be quantified from analog velocity recordings by calculating various indices of "pulsatility" and damping.[12,21] The characteristics of the wave form can also be appreciated by listening to the arterial flow sounds emitted by Doppler flow detectors.[12] Over normal peripheral arteries, double or triple sounds are heard, the second sound representing the diastolic flow reversal and the third sound the second forward component. Whether the sounds are double or triple is probably not of clinically practical significance and is likely related to a complex interplay of several factors, such as the basal heart rate frequency and the shape of the pressure and flow waves which, as discussed earlier, depends on the degree of peripheral vasoconstriction and elastic properties of the arteries.

Distal to an arterial stenosis, however, the pulse velocity wave is more damped and is similar in pattern to the pressure wave seen in Figure 1-6. Also, flow reversal disappears distal to an arterial stenosis. The calculated wave indices thus are altered and the audible Doppler signals have a single component rather than the double or triple components usually heard.[12,21] The disappearance of reversed flow distal to a stenosis probably results from a combination of several factors including (1) the maintenance of a relatively high level of forward flow throughout the cardiac cycle (because of the pressure gradient across the stenosis), (2) resistance to reverse flow created by the stenotic lesion, (3) a decrease in peripheral resistance as a result of relative ischemia, and (4) damping of the pressure wave by the lesion, resulting in attenuated pressure pulses, which are less subject to the reflections and amplification which normally contributes to diastolic flow reversal.

Recordings of flow velocities at and distal to arterial obstructions are useful in the assessment of occlusive processes. The recent introduction of on-line frequency spectrum analysis allows better detection and quantification of flow abnormalities resulting from stenotic lesions. This subject is considered in further detail in Chapter 3, but it is of interest to comment on the physiological principles illustrated by frequency spectra in normal and abnormal vessels. As noted previously, the velocity pattern across a vessel is flattened by such factors as the effect of branching (Fig. 1-1B). As a result, the particles in the central core of normal arteries flow with relatively uniform and high velocities during systole. This can be demonstrated by spectrum analysis of the arterial velocity Doppler signals that show a narrow band of velocities near the maximum velocity.[22] Stenotic lesions result in marked disturbance of flow with the occurrence of abnormally high velocities, jet effects, irregular travel of particles in various directions and at different velocities, and eddy formation. The change in the direction of particle movement with respect to the axis of the vessel alters the observed Doppler shifts and also contributes to the occurrence of a large range of flow velocities registered with frequency spectral analysis. These effects af arterial stenosis are manifest as widening or dispersal of the band of systolic velocity (spectral broadening) or complete "filling in" of the spectral tracing, as discussed in Chapter 3.

VENOUS HEMODYNAMICS

As shown in Figure 1-2, the pressure remaining in the veins after the blood has traversed the arterioles and capillaries is low when the subject is in the supine position. Because of their relatively large diameters, medium-sized and large veins offer little resistance to flow, and blood moves readily from the small veins to the right atrium, where the pressure is close to atmospheric pressure. Although the effects of arterial pressure and flow waves are rarely transmitted to the

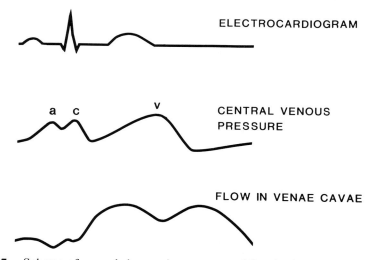

Figure 1-7.   Schema of normal changes in pressure and flow in the central veins associated with the cardiac cycle.

systemic veins, phasic changes in venous pressure and flow do occur in response to cardiac activity and because of alterations of intrathoracic pressure with respiration. Knowledge of these changes is necessary for correct assessment of peripheral veins by noninvasive laboratory studies which are described in Chapter 14.

The final section of this chapter discusses changes in pressure and flow in various portions of the venous system that are associated with cardiac and respiratory cycles. Also considered are alterations in lower extremity veins that occur with changes in posture, the important consequences of competence or incompetence of venous valves and the effects of venous obstruction.

Flow and Pressure Changes During the Cardiac Cycle

Figure 1-7 shows changes in pressure and flow in large veins such as the venae cavae that occur during phases of the cardiac cycle. Such oscillations in pressure and flow may, at times, be transmitted to more peripheral vessels. Characteristically, three positive pressure waves (a,c,v) can be distinguished in central venous pressure and reflect corresponding changes in pressure in the atria. The a-wave is caused by atrial contraction and relaxation. The upstroke of the c-wave is related to the increase in pressure when the atrioventricular valves are closed and bulge during isovolumetric ventricular contraction. The subsequent downstroke is due to the fall in pressure caused by pulling the atrioventricular valve rings toward the apex of the heart during ventricular contraction, thus tending to increase the atrial volume. The upstroke of the v-wave results from passive rise in atrial pressure during ventricular systole when the atrioventricular valves are closed and the atria fill with blood from the peripheral veins. The v-wave downstroke is due to the fall in pressure that occurs when the blood leaves the atria rapidly and fills the ventricles soon after the opening of the atrioventricular valves early in ventricular diastole.

The venous pressure events are associated with changes in flow. There are two periods of increased venous flow during each cardiac cycle. The first occurs during ventricular systole when shortening of the ventricular muscle pulls the atrioventricular valve rings towards the apex of the heart. This movement of the valve ring tends to increase atrial volume and decrease atrial pressure, thus increasing flow from the extracardiac veins into the atria. The second phase of increased venous flow occurs after the atrioventricular valves open and blood rushes into the ventricles from the atria. Venous flow is reduced in the intervening periods of the cardiac cycle as the atrial pressure rises during and soon after atrial contraction and in the later part of the ventricular systole. Since there are no valves at the junction of the right atrium and venae cavae, some backward flow may actually occur in the large thoracic veins during atrial contraction as blood moves in the reverse direction from the atrium into the venae cavae.

The changes in pressure and flow in the large central veins that are associated with the events of the cardiac cycle are not usually evident in the peripheral veins of the extremities. This is probably caused by damping related to 1) the high distensibility (compliance) of the veins, and 2) the compression of the veins by intra-abdominal pressure and as well as mechanical compression in the thoracic inlet. Since the effects of right heart contractions are more readily transmitted to the large veins of the arms, the pulsatile changes in venous velocity associated with the events of the cardiac cycle tend to be more obvious in the upper extremities than in the veins of the legs.

In abnormal conditions, such as congestive heart failure or tricuspid insufficiency, venous pressure is increased. This elevation of venous pressures may lead to the transmission of cardiac phasic changes in pressure and flow to the peripheral veins of the upper and lower limbs. Such phasic changes occasionally may be found in healthy well hydrated individuals, probably because a large blood volume distends the venous system.

The Venous Effects of Respiration

Respiration has profound effects on venous pressure and flow. During inspiration, the volume of the veins of the thorax increases and the pressure decreases in response to reduced intrathoracic pressure. Expiration leads to the opposite effect with decreased venous volume and increased pressure. The venous response to respiration is reversed in the abdomen, where the pressure increases during inspiration because of the descent of the diaphragm, and decreases during expiration as the diaphragm ascends. Increased abdominal pressure during inspiration decreases pressure gradients between peripheral veins in the lower extremities and the abdomen, thus reducing flow in the peripheral vessels. During expiration, when intra-abdominal pressure is reduced, the pressure gradient from the lower limbs to the abdomen is increased and flow in the peripheral veins rises correspondingly.

In the veins of the upper limbs the changes in flow with respiration are opposite to those in the lower extremities. Because of reduced intrathoracic pressure during inspiration the pressure gradient from the veins of the upper limbs to the right atrium increases and flow increases. During expiration flow decreases because of the resulting increase in intrathoracic pressure and the corresponding rise of the right atrial pressure. The respiratory changes in flow in the upper limbs may be influenced by changes in posture. With the upper parts of the body elevated venous flow tends to stop at the height of inspiration and resumes with expiration, probably because of the compression of the subclavian vein at the level of the first rib during contraction of the accessory muscles of respiration.

The respiratory effects are usually associated with clear phasic changes in venous flow in the extremities that can be detected with various instruments, including many forms of plethysmography and Doppler flow detectors. The respiratory changes in venous velocity may be exaggerated by respiratory maneuvers, such as the Valsalva maneuver, which increases intrathoracic and abdominal pressure, and decreases, abolishes or may even reverse flow in some peripheral veins. Also, the respiratory effects on venous flow may be diminished in the lower limbs in individuals who are "chest" or shallow breathers and whose diaphragm may not descend sufficiently to elevate intra-abdominal pressure. Venous flow then tends to be more continuous.

Venous Flow and Peripheral Resistance

Blood flow and flow velocity in the peripheral veins, particularly in the extremities, are profoundly influenced by local blood flow, which is in turn largely determined by the peripheral resistance or the state of vasoconstriction or vasodilatation. When limb blood flow is markedly increased as a result of peripheral vasodilatation, for example, secondary to infection or inflammation, the flow tends to be more continuous and the respiratory changes in flow are less evident. When there is increased vasoconstriction in the extremities, e.g., when there is need to conserve body heat and blood flow through the skin is decreased, venous flow is also markedly decreased and there may be no audible Doppler flow signals over a peripheral vein such as the posterior tibial. Also, severe arterial obstruction may decrease overall blood flow and velocity in the vessels of the extremities and lead to decreased velocity signals over the venous channels.

The Effect of Posture

In the upright position, the hydrostatic pressure is greatly increased in the dependent part of the body, and particularly in the lower portions of the lower extremities. This increase in hydrostatic pressure, as indicated earlier, is associated with high transmural pressures in the blood vessels and, in turn, leads to greater vascular distension. In the veins, which have low pressure to start with and are distensible, considerable pooling of the blood occurs in the lower parts of the legs. The resulting decrease in venous return to the right atrium is associated with diminished cardiac output. When the normal conpensatory reflexes that increase peripheral resistance are impaired, decreased cardiac output can lead to hypotension and fainting.

The movement of the skeletal muscles of the legs, such as occurs during walking, leads to decreased venous pressure because of the presence of one-way valves in the peripheral veins. Contraction of the voluntary muscle squeezes the veins and propels the blood toward the heart. Muscular contraction not only increases venous return and cardiac output, but it also interrupts the hydrostatic column of venous blood from the heart and thus decreases pressure in the peripheral veins, e.g., in the veins at the ankle. Activity of the skeletal muscles of the legs in the presence of competent venous valves therefore results in the lowering of pressure in the veins of the extremity, leading to decreased venous pooling, decreased capillary pressure, reduced filtration of fluid into the extracellular space than otherwise occurs, and increase in blood flow because of increased aterio-venous pressure difference.

The Effect of External Compression

Sudden pressure on the veins of the extremities, whether due to an active muscular contraction or external manual compression of the limb, increases venous flow and velocity towards the heart and stops the flow distal to the site of the compression in the presence of competent venous valves. The responses to sudden pressure changes are affected by venous obstruction and damage to the venous valves. The detection of such changes is important when assessing patients for the presence of venous disease and is discussed further below in Chapter 14.

Venous Obstruction

Venous obstruction can be acute or chronic. In the case of severe chronic obstruction, edema may occur. Also, the nutrition of the skin in the affected region may be impaired and characteristic trophic changes in the skin and venous stasis ulcers may result. Acute obstruction, usually associated with thrombosis, may lead to potentially fatal pulmonary embolism. Since the clinical diagnosis of acute deep vein thrombosis is unreliable, various noninvasive procedures have been developed over the past few years to enhance the accuracy of this diagnosis.[12] Various forms of plethysmography and Doppler flow detectors may be used for this purpose. The discussion that follows refers mainly to the Doppler signals that can be obtained easily by listening with an ultrasonic flow detector to peripheral veins of the lower extremities, but similar principles may be used in the examination of the upper extremities and are often applied in the methods that utilize plethysmography.

An audible Doppler signal should be present over peripheral veins and it can be easily distinguished from an arterial flow signal because of the absence of pulsatility synchronous with the heart. As indicated above, a signal may be absent in low flow states, especially when the limb is cold and auscultation is carried out over small peripheral veins. Squeezing of the limb distal to the site of examination should temporarily increase flow and result in an audible signal if the vein is patent. Spontaneous venous flow signals normally possess clear respiratory phases. However, if there is an obstruction between the heart and the examination site, the respiratory changes in venous velocity will be absent or attenuated. Over larger, more proximal veins, such as the popliteal and more proximal vessels, the absence of audible signals after an adequate search is indicative of an obstructed venous segment.

The presence or absence of obstruction is also gauged by increasing flow toward the examination site by squeezing the limb distally or by activating the *distal* muscle groups and thus increasing venous blood flow toward the flow-detecting probe. Absence of increased flow sounds or attenuation of increased flow is associated with obstruction between the probe location and the site from which the enhancement of venous flow is attempted.

Increase in flow is also elicited when manual compression of the limb proximal to the flow detecting probe is released, because of low filling and pressure in the proximal veins that have been emptied by the compression. If the proximal veins at or near the point of compression are occluded, the augmentation of flow after release of the compression is attenuated.

Venous Valvular Incompetence

When the valves are competent, flow in the peripheral veins is toward the heart. However, flow may be temporarily diminished or stopped soon after assumption of the upright posture, at the height of inspiration or during the Valsalva maneuver. The peripheral veins normally fill from the capillaries and the rate at which they fill depends on the peripheral resistance and blood flow as determined by the degree of peripheral vasoconstriction. When there are incompetent veins proximally, there may be retrograde filling of the peripheral veins, such as those in the ankle regions, from the more proximal veins, in addition to normal filling from the capillary beds.[12] This retrograde filling may have serious consequences because of resulting increase in hydrostatic pressure and filtration of fluid into the extravascular spaces in the upright position.

The presence or absence of the retrograde flow may be detected by listening with a Doppler flow detector and squeezing the limb proximally. Also, various plethysmographic methods can detect the rate of filling through measurement of venous volume, which changes with pressure, after the volume and pressure have been reduced by muscular action such a flexion-extension of the ankle in the upright position. After such exercise, the venous volume and pressure will increase more rapidly when the valves are incompetent because the peripheral veins fill as a result of retrograde flow from the more proximal parts of the limbs. The application of tourniquets or cuffs with appropriate pressures will compress the superficial veins and allow localization of the incompetent veins not only to the various segments of the limb, but also to the superficial veins as opposed to the perforating or deep veins.

SUMMARY

This chapter dealt with basic characteristics of pressure and flow and the effects of vascular obstruction. For more detailed treatment of these topics the reader is referred to other sources[2,23,24] and particularly to the excellent treatment of these subjects in the classic text by Strandness and Sumner.[12]

Stefan A. Carter, M.D, M.Sc., F.R.C.P.(C)
Professor of Medicine and Physiology
University of Manitoba
Director, Vascular Laboratory
St. Boniface General Hospital
409 Tache Avenue
Winnipeg, Manitoba
R2H 2A6
CANADA

REFERENCES

1. Carter SA: Arterial auscultation in peripheral vascular disease. JAMA 246:1682–1686, 1981
2. Kaufman W: Fluid Mechanics (2 Ed). New York, McGraw-Hill, 1963, pp 1–432
3. Taylor MG: Wave travel in arteries and the design of the cardiovascular system, in Attinger EO (ed): Pulsatile Blood Flow. New York, McGraw-Hill, 1964, pp 343–372
4. Carter SA: Effect of age, cardiovascular disease, and vasomotor changes on transmission of arterial pressure waves through the lower extremities. Angiology 29:601–616, 1978
5. Kroeker EJ, Wood EH: Comparison of simultaneously recorded central and peripheral arterial pressure pulses during rest, exercise and tilted position in man. Circ Res 3:623–632, 1955
6. Gaskell P, Krisman A: The brachial to digital blood pressure gradient in normal subjects and in patients with high blood pressure. Can J Biochem Physiol 36:889–893, 1958
7. Lezack JD, Carter SA: Systolic pressures in the extremities of man with special reference to the toes. Can J Physiol Pharmacol 48:469–474, 1970
8. Nielsen PE, Barras J-P, Holstein P: Systolic pressure amplification in the arteries of normal subjects. Scand J Clin Lab Invest 33:371–377, 1974
9. Sugiura T, Freis ED: Pressure pulse in small arteries. Circ Res 11:838–842, 1962
10. Rowell LB, Brengelmann GL, Blackmon JR, et al: Disparities between aortic and peripheral pulse pressure induced by upright exercise and vasomotor changes in man. Circulation 37:954–964, 1968
11. Carter SA: Role of pressure measurements in vascular disease, in Bernstein EF (ed): Noninvasive Diagnostic Techniques in Vascular Disease. St. Louis, CV Mosby, 1985, pp 513–544
12. Strandness DE Jr, Sumner DS: Hemodynamics for Surgeons. New York, Grune &

Stratton, 1975, pp 3–20; 73–120; 209–289; 396–511
13. May AG, Van de Berg L, DeWeese JA, et al: Critical arterial stenosis. Surgery 54:250–259, 1963
14. Schultz RD, Hokanson DE, Strandness DE Jr: Pressure-flow and stress-strain measurements of normal and diseased aortoiliac segments. Surg Gynecol Obstet 124:1267–1276, 1967
15. Carter SA: Peripheral artery disease: pressure measurements ease evaluation. Consultant 19(9):102–115, 1979
16. Widmer LK, Staub H: Blutdruck in stenosierten Arterien. Z Kreislaufforsch 51:975–979, 1962
17. Carter SA: Indirect systolic pressures and pulse waves in arterial occlusive disease of the lower extremities. Circulation 37:624–637, 1968
18. Carter SA: Investigation and treatment of arterial occlusive disease of the extremities. Clin Med I 79(5):13–24, 1972; Clin Med II 79(6):15–22, 1972
19. Carter SA: Response of ankle systolic pressure to leg exercise in mild or questionable arterial disease. N Engl J Med 287:578–582, 1972
20. Uhrenholdt A, Dam WH, Larsen OA, et al: Paradoxical effect on peripheral blood flow after sympathetic blockades in patients with gangrene due to arteriosclerosis obliterans. Vasc Surg 5:154–163, 1971
21. Johnston KW, Taraschuk I: Validation of the role of pulsatility index in quantitation of the severity of peripheral arterial occlusive disease. Am J Surg 131:295–297, 1976
22. Reneman RS, Hoeks A, Spencer MP: Doppler ultrasound in the evaluation of the peripheral arterial circulation. Angiology 30:526–538, 1979
23. Attinger EO (ed): Pulsatile Blood Flow. New York, McGraw-Hill, 1964, pp 1–462
24. McDonald DA: Blood Flow in Arteries. London, Edward Arnold, Ltd., 1960, pp 1–328

James A. Zagzebski, Ph.D.

2

Physics and Instrumentation in Doppler and B-Mode Ultrasonography

PRINCIPLES OF DOPPLER AND B-MODE ULTRASONOGRAPHY

This chapter presents an overview of the physical and technical aspects of vascular sonography. It begins with a brief review of relevant ultrasound-soft-tissue interactions. Pulse-echo principles and display techniques are outlined, followed by a description of the Doppler effect as it applies to echoes detected from moving reflectors and a discussion of continuous-wave and pulsed Doppler instrumentation. Finally, common techniques used for displaying Doppler-signal spectral information are presented.

SOUND PROPAGATION IN TISSUE

A sound wave can be produced in a medium by placing a vibrating source in contact with it, causing particles in the medium to vibrate. The resultant disturbance propagates away from the source and is attenuated, scattered and reflected by the medium. The disturbance corresponds to variations in pressure and is called a sound wave. The shape of the vibrating source in medical ultrasound is chosen so that the sound wave forms a beam with a well-defined direction. The reception of reflected and scattered echo signals provides information on the acoustic properties of the medium, makes possible the production of ultrasound images and allows detection of motion of structures in the medium.

Speed of Sound

The propagation speed for sound waves depends on the medium through which they are traveling. For soft tissues the average speed of sound has been found to be 1540 m/sec, and most diagnostic ultrasound instruments are calibrated

Table 2-1
Speeds of Sound for Biological Tissue

Tissue	Speed of Sound	Percent Change from 1540 m/sec
Fat	1450 m/sec	−5.8
Vitreous humor	1520 m/sec	−1.3
Liver	1550 m/sec	+ .6
Blood	1570 m/sec	+1.9
Muscle	1580 m/sec	+2.6
Lens of eye	1620 m/sec	+5.2

From Wells PNT: Propagation of ultrasonic waves through tissues, in Fullerton G, Zagzebski J (eds.): Medical Physics of CT and Ultrasound, New York, American Institute of Physics, p 381, 1980. With permission.

with the assumption that the sound beam propagates at this average speed. As Table 2-1 indicates, the speed of sound in specific soft tissues deviates only slightly from the assumed average.

Frequency and Wavelength

The number of oscillations per second of the source determines the frequency of the sound wave. Diagnostic ultrasound applications utilize frequencies in the 1 MHz (10^6 cycles per second) to 15 MHz frequency range.

The wavelength refers to the distance over which the acoustic disturbance repeats itself at any instant of time. It is defined by the following equation:

$$\lambda = c/f \tag{2-1}$$

where λ is the wavelength, c the speed of sound and f the frequency. If the frequency is 5 MHz, the wavelength in soft tissue is about 0.3 mm, and increases with decreasing frequency. Wavelength has particular relevance when describing dimensions of objects, such as reflectors in the body. The size of an object is most meaningfully expressed if given relative to the ultrasonic wavelength for the frequency of the sound beam.

Attenuation

As a sound beam propagates through tissue, its intensity or strength decreases as the distance of travel increases. This decrease in intensity with path length is called attenuation. Sources of attenuation include (1) reflection and scatter of the sound wave at boundaries between media having different densities or speeds of sound, and (2) absorption of ultrasonic energy by tissues.

The rate of attenuation is determined both by the the tissue(s) traversed and by the ultrasound frequency. Soft tissues differ in their attenuation rates, with attenuation quite high for muscle and skin, and much lower for fluid-filled vessels (Fig. 2-1).[1] An important characteristic of the attenuation of ultrasound in tissues is the frequency dependence of this process. For most soft tissues, the attenuation is nearly proportional to the frequency (Fig. 2-1). The proportionality between

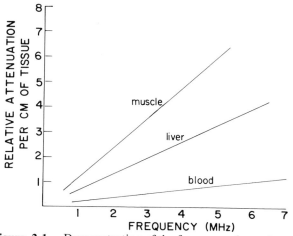

Figure 2-1. Demonstration of the frequency dependence of ultrasonic attenuation in soft tissues.

attenuation and frequency means that higher frequency sound waves are much more severely attenuated than lower frequency waves. Hence, diagnostic studies with higher frequency sound beams (7 MHz and above) are usually limited to superficial regions of the body. Lower frequencies (5 MHz and below) must be used for imaging large organs, such as the liver.

Reflection

Whenever an ultrasound beam strikes an interface formed by two tissues having different acoustic properties, part of the beam is reflected and part is transmitted. If the reflected wave travels back towards the ultrasound source, it may be detected as an echo. The amplitude or strength of the reflected wave is determined by the difference between the acoustic impedances of the materials forming the interface.

The acoustic impedance, Z, is the speed of sound in a material multiplied by its density. For perpendicular incidence of the ultrasound beam on a large, flat interface (Fig. 2-2), the ratio of the reflected to the incident amplitude, R, is given by

$$R = \frac{(Z_2 - Z_1)}{(Z_2 + Z_1)} \tag{2-2}$$

where the impedances Z_1 and Z_2 are those indicated in the figure. The larger the difference between Z_1 and Z_2, the more energy is reflected and the greater is the echo. Large differences in impedance are found at tissue-to-air or tissue-to-bone interfaces. In fact, such interfaces are nearly impenetrable to an ultrasound beam. Significantly weaker echoes originate at interfaces formed by any two soft tissues since, generally, there is not a large difference in impedance between soft tissues.

Large, smooth interfaces such as depicted in Figure 2-2 are called "specular

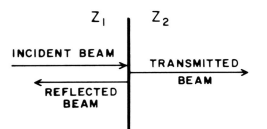

Figure 2-2. Specular reflection of an ultrasound beam at an interface between materials having impedances z_1 and z_2. The magnitude of the differences between z_1 and z_2 directly affects the strength of the reflected wave.

reflectors''. The direction the reflected wave travels after striking a specular reflector is highly dependent on the orientation of the interface with respect to the sound beam. The wave is reflected back toward the source only when the incident beam is perpendicular or nearly perpendicular to the reflector. The strength or amplitude of an echo from a specular reflector thus depends on the orientation of the reflector with respect to the sound beam direction.

Scattering

For acoustic interfaces whose dimensions are very small, "scattering" of the incident sound wave will take place. The scattered energy usually radiates in all directions, as suggested in Figure 2-3. In this textbook, we are most interested in scattering from blood. The scattering sites in this situation are the red blood cells, whose dimensions are much smaller than the ultrasonic wavelength. Such scatterers are called Rayleigh scatterers. The scattered intensity from a volumetric distribution of Rayleigh scatterers depends on (1) the dimensions of the scatterer, with an increasing scattered intensity as the size increases; (2) the number of scatterers present in the beam (for example, Shung and Reid demon-

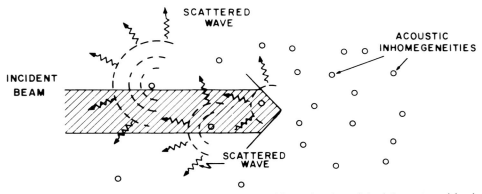

Figure 2-3. Scatter of sound by small inhomogeneities. The size of the inhomogeneities is the principal factor affecting reflection.

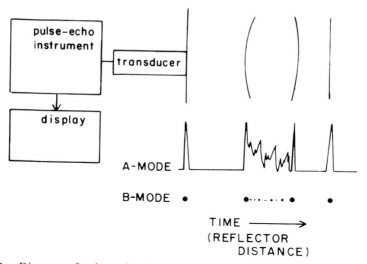

Figure 2-4. Diagram of pulse-echo ultrasound. A-mode and B-mode display characteristics are shown.

strated that when the hematocrit is low, scattering from blood is proportional to the hematocrit[2]); (3) the extent to which the density or elastic properties of the scatterer differ from those of the surrounding material; and (4) the ultrasonic frequency (for Rayleigh scatterers the scattered intensity is proportional to the frequency to the fourth power).

PULSE-ECHO ULTRASOUND

Ultrasound can be used to image interfaces and scatterers by using pulse-echo transmission, detection, and display techniques. An ultrasonic transducer is placed in direct contact with the skin or is coupled to the skin through a liquid path. The transducer repeatedly emits brief pulses of sound at a fixed repetition rate. After transmitting each pulse, the transducer serves as a detector for echoes originating from interfaces and scatterers in the sound beam. Echo signals picked up by the transducer are amplified and processed into a format suitable for display.

Two commonly used echo display techniques are illustrated in Figure 2-4. An A-mode (or amplitude-mode) display is a presentation of the echo signal amplitude in relation to the echo delay time following transmission of the pulse. Since the delay time is proportional to the distance from the transducer to the reflector, the A-mode display can also be thought of as a record of the echo amplitude compared with reflector distance. In the B-mode (or brightness-mode) display, used for most imaging applications, the reflected signal is converted to a series of dots on the display rather than spikes. Most modern systems utilizing the B-mode display employ "gray scale" processing, whereby the intensity or brightness of the displayed dots is proportional to the echo signal strength.

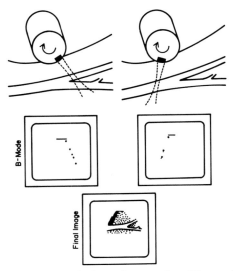

Figure 2-5. Ultrasonic B-mode scanning. The position and orientation of the incident ultrasound beam, along with the echo return time, are used to place echo signals in their representative anatomical positions on the display.

In B-mode scanning, the sound beam is swept through the region of interest and each echo signal is displayed on the B-mode display in a position that corresponds to its anatomical origin. The position and orientation of the ultrasound beam and the echo transit time are used to place echo signals in their proper position on the display. Steps in the generation of a B-mode image are illustrated in Figure 2-5. It is assumed in this illustration that the sound beam is swept by pivoting the ultrasound transducer, as suggested in the two panels on the top of the figure. The two diagrams in the middle show the resultant B-mode line on the display for each beam position. The B-mode image thus is built up line-by-line as the figure indicates (Fig. 2-5, bottom).

In peripheral vascular sonography, B-mode imaging is almost always performed with "real-time" ultrasound scanners. Real-time scanners sweep the sound beam over the imaged region automatically at a rapid rate. Three types of real-time transducer assemblies are illustrated in Figure 2-6.

Mechanical scanners. A single transducer or several transducers are oscillated within the scan head (transducer assembly), steering the sound beam over the region of interest. Alternatively, the beam from a stationary transducer may be swept by oscillating an acoustical mirror.

Sequential (linear) arrays. An array of perhaps 120 separate rectangular transducer elements is used to form an image. Scanning is done automatically by activating clusters of elements in the array, switching from one cluster to the next to produce individual acoustic lines.

Phased array scanners. The sound beam from an array of transducer

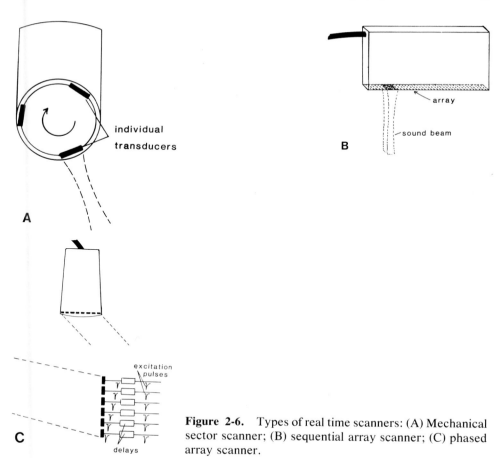

Figure 2-6. Types of real time scanners: (A) Mechanical sector scanner; (B) sequential array scanner; (C) phased array scanner.

elements is "steered" by introducing small time delays between sound pulses emitted by individual elements. The time delays are controlled electronically, sending the beam in different directions.

An image memory such as a "digital scan converter" or "freeze frame" is used in most instruments to retain images for review and photography and to convert the image display into a format suitable for television and video tape recording.

THE DOPPLER EFFECT

The Doppler effect is a change in the frequency of echo signals that occurs whenever there is relative motion between the sound source and the reflector.

Consider a stationary sound source producing an ultrasound beam whose frequency is f_o (Fig. 2-7). The beam is incident on a reflector that is moving toward the source with a velocity v. The frequency of the reflected echo signal, f_r, will be greater than f_o because of the Doppler shift. The Doppler frequency shift, f_D, is

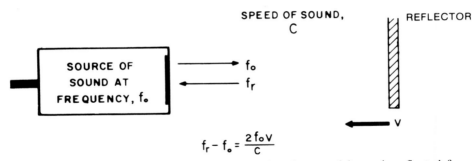

$$f_r - f_o = \frac{2 f_o v}{c}$$

Figure 2-7. Illustration of the Doppler effect. An ultrasound beam is reflected from a moving interface traveling toward the source with a velocity, v (f_o is transmitted frequency; f_r is the received frequency).

defined in this case as the difference between the received frequency and the transmitted frequency, and is related to the velocity of the reflector, v, by the following equations,

$$f_D = f_r - f_o \qquad (2\text{-}3)$$
$$= 2f_o v/c$$

where c is the speed of sound in the medium. This equation expresses the important fact that the frequency shift, f_D, is proportional to the velocity of the reflector relative to the source. If the direction of movement is toward the sound source, f_r will be greater than f_o. On the other hand, if the reflector is moving away from the source, f_r will be less than f_o.

Ultrasonic Doppler equipment can be employed for detecting motion of large structures, such as heart valves and fetal heart walls. This equipment is also commonly used for detecting and evaluating the characteristics of blood flow in arteries and veins. The usual vascular application is depicted schematically in Figure 2-8, where the sound source or ultrasonic transducer is placed in contact with the external skin surface and the ultrasound beam is directed toward the vessel of interest. The source of echo signals are the red blood cells flowing in the vessel. They represent small-sized inhomogeneities, which scatter ultrasound in the manner discussed earlier. In most instruments, the scattered echo signals are detected by the same ultrasonic transducer assembly used to produce the incident beam. The Doppler shift in this situation is given by

$$f_D = (2f_o v/c)\cos\theta. \qquad (2\text{-}4)$$

The difference in this expression in comparison to Equation 2-3 is the presence of the $\cos\theta$ term, where the angle θ is shown in Fig. 2-8. If the sound beam were propagating along the direction of blood flow, θ would be 0, $\cos\theta$ would be 1 and Equation 2-4 would simplify to the expression in Equation 2-3. For the sound beam incident at an angle other than $\theta = 0$, the detected Doppler frequency shift is reduced according to the $\cos\theta$ term. Notice that for perpendicular beam incidence, $\theta = 90°$ and $\cos\theta = 0$; therefore, there is no detected Doppler shift! In

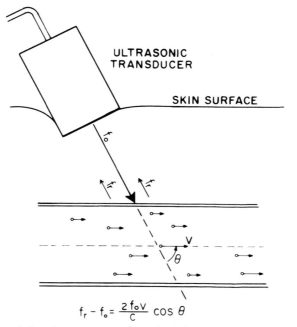

$$f_r - f_o = \frac{2 f_o V}{C} \cos \theta$$

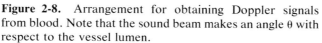

Figure 2-8. Arrangement for obtaining Doppler signals from blood. Note that the sound beam makes an angle θ with respect to the vessel lumen.

practice, the transducer beam is usually oriented to make a 30°-60° angle with the arterial lumen.

Continuous-Wave Ultrasonic Doppler Equipment

Continuous-wave Doppler instruments are the simplest and often the least expensive Doppler devices available. A simplified block diagram of such an instrument is presented in Figure 2-9. The transmitter continuously excites the ultrasonic transducer with a sinusoidal electrical signal of frequency, f_o. The transducer converts this electrical energy into ultrasonic energy, which propagates into the medium. Echo signals resulting from reflection and scattering return to the transducer, creating an electrical signal that is applied to the receiver amplifier. Within the amplifier, the signal is boosted in strength and applied to a detector and low-pass filter with the result that only low-frequency Doppler shift signals emerge in the output. The output of the device thus is a complex signal whose frequency is related to the velocity of all reflectors and scatterers within the sound beam.

It is possible to eliminate signals of certain frequency ranges from the output. This is done in instruments that have additional electrical filters in their circuitry. For example, when studying Doppler signals due to blood flow, relatively low frequency signals originating from movement of vessel walls may be eliminated from the output with a high-pass filter network. The lower cut-off frequency of the high-pass filter is usually operator selectable.

J.A. Zagzebski

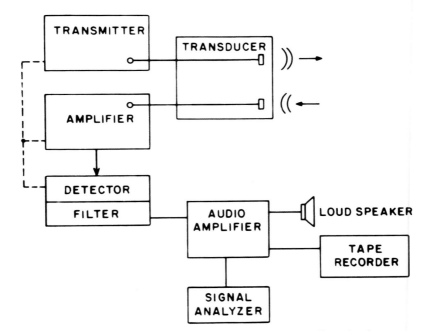

Figure 2-9. Schematic representation of a continuous-wave Doppler instrument. Note that one crystal transmits the ultrasound beam and the other receives the reflected echoes. The returning signal is compared with the transmitted signal in the detector to determine the Doppler frequency shift.

One can calculate the Doppler shift frequency, f_D, for typical operating characteristics encountered in the examination of blood flow. Suppose v = 10 cm/sec, the operating frequency, f_o = 5 MHz (5 × 10^6 cycles/sec) and the speed of sound, c = 1540 m/sec. Furthermore, let θ = 0° so that cosθ = 1. Using Equation 2-3, one finds

$$f_D = \frac{(2 \times 5 \times 10^6 \text{ cycles per second} \times 0.1 \text{ m/sec})}{1540 \text{ m/sec}} \tag{2-5}$$

$$= 600 \text{ cycles per second}$$

Thus it can be seen that for slowly moving structures and these operating conditions, *the Doppler signal is in the audible frequency range.*

The filtered-output Doppler signal usually is applied to a loudspeaker or headphones for interpretation. The signals also can be recorded on audio tape or applied to any of several spectral analysis systems, to be discussed below.

Pulsed Doppler

With continuous-wave Doppler instruments, reflectors and scatterers anywhere within the beam of the transducer can contribute to the instantaneous Doppler signal. Pulsed Doppler provides discrimination of Doppler signals from different depths, allowing for the detection of moving interfaces and scatterers

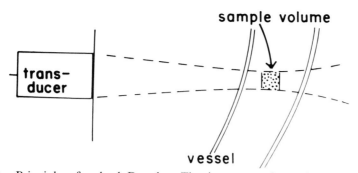

Figure 2-10. Principle of pulsed Doppler. The instrument is made sensitive only to Doppler signals originating within a sample volume. The distance (range) from the transducer to the sample volume can be adjusted. The size of the sample volume depends on the shape of the ultrasound transducer beam (dashed lines) and the pulse duration.

from within a well-defined "sample" volume (Fig. 2-10). The sample volume can be positioned anywhere along the axis of the ultrasound beam.

The principal components of a pulsed Doppler instrument are shown in Figure 2-11. In such devices, the ultrasonic transducer is excited with a short-duration burst from a pulsed oscillator. Scattered and reflected echo signals are detected by the same transducer, amplified in the receiver, and applied to detector circuits, where the Doppler shift frequency signal may be obtained. By "gating" (or turning on) the receiver for a short time interval at a specified time following each transmission of the burst, Doppler signals originating only from a particular depth are selected for display. As mentioned above the gate position can be adjusted by the operator to select Doppler signals from any distance.

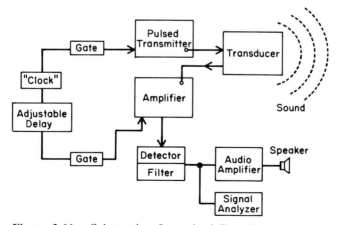

Figure 2-11. Schematic of a pulsed Doppler instrument. Note in comparison with Fig. 2-9, that a pulsing circuit has been added, consisting of a clock, range gates, and an adjustable delay for the length and location of the gates.

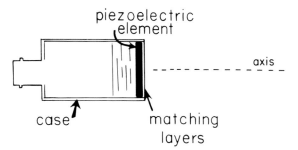

Figure 2-12. Schematic of a single-element, plane-disk ultrasonic transducer. The piezoelectric element is a thin, circular disk. The illustrated view cuts through the axis of symmetry of the transducer.

Duplex Ultrasound Instruments

A pulse-echo scanner and a Doppler instrument provide complementary information in that the scanner can best outline anatomical structures, whereas, a Doppler instrument yields information regarding flow and movement patterns. "Duplex" ultrasound instruments are real-time B-mode scanners with built-in Doppler capabilities. In typical applications, the pulse-echo B-mode image obtained with a duplex scanner is used to localize areas where flow will be examined using Doppler. The area to be studied in the Doppler mode may be identified on the B-mode image with a "sample volume indicator" or cursor. The cursor position is controlled by the operator, greatly facilitating positioning the Doppler sample volume over the region of interest. Many duplex instruments allow the operator to indicate the direction of blood flow (the flow vector) with respect to the ultrasound beam. The angle formed by the ultrasound beam and the flow vector (θ in Eq. 2-4); must be known to estimate flow velocity from the frequency of the Doppler signal.

Ultrasound Transducer Properties

An ultrasound transducer provides the communicating link between the Doppler or pulse-echo imaging instrument and the patient. Medical ultrasound transducers use piezoelectric ceramic materials to generate and detect sound waves. Piezoelectric materials convert pressure waves into electrical signals; because they also convert electrical signals into mechanical vibrations, they can be used as both generators and detectors of ultrasonic energy.

The internal components of a single element transducer, used in some scanners and pulsed Doppler systems, are shown in Figure 2-12. The illustration is of a plane circular piezoelectric disk, although other shapes have also been used. In the figure, the disk is seen from the side, and the ultrasound beam would be projected to the right. The thickness of the ceramic element governs the resonance frequency of the transducer. Quarter-wave matching layers between the piezoelectric element and a protective outer faceplate are used on some transducers. Analogous to special optical coatings on lenses and picture-frame glass, the matching layers are employed to improve the sound transmission

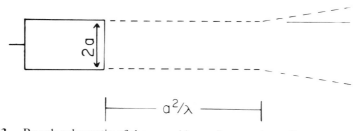

Figure 2-13. Rough schematic of the sound beam from a plane-disk transducer. The near field extends outward a distance of approximately a^2/λ. Within the near field the beam remains collimated; however, the intensity fluctuates from point to point. In the far field the beam diverges but intensity becomes uniform.

between the transducer and patient. This improves the sensitivity of the transducer. Backing material is often used in pulse-echo applications to dampen the piezoelectric element vibrations when the transducer is excited. Dampening shortens the duration of the transmitted pulse, improving the axial (or range) resolution. (Resolution refers to the minimum spacing between two reflectors which allows the reflectors to be distinguished on the display. Axial resolution applies to reflectors that are closely spaced along the sound beam axis. Lateral resolution applies to reflectors positioned on a line perpendicular to the sound beam axis.)

The sound beam emerging from a diagnostic transducer is very directional, that is, its direction of travel conforms to the axis of the transducer (Fig. 2-13). The beam may be thought of as having two components: a near field and a far field. The near field extends outward an axial distance of approximately a^2/λ, where a is the transducer radius, and λ the ultrasonic wavelength. For a transducer whose diameter is 13 mm and whose frequency is 3.5 MHz (3.5×10^6 cycles per second), the calculated near field length is 9.6 cm. Within the near field, the amplitude and intensity of the beam fluctuate from one spot to another. At points near the transition between the near field and far field the sound beam gradually becomes smooth. It remains smooth throughout the far field, not exhibiting the point-to-point intensity fluctuations found close to the transducer surface. Also, contrary to the near field where the beam remains collimated, in the far field the beam diverges with increasing distance from the transducer. The divergence angle is greater for lower frequency transducers than for higher frequency transducers of the same diameter. The width of the sound beam at any depth affects the lateral resolution of the ultrasound instrument at that depth.

Focusing of the sound beam is done in order to improve the lateral resolution. Focusing can be achieved using a lens or a curved piezoelectric element (Fig. 2-14). Focusing reduces the beam width over a volume called the focal region. The size of the focal region is determined by the lens or the degree of curvature of the element, as well as by the frequency and the transducer diameter. In general, higher frequency transducers yield narrower sound beams and better spatial resolution than lower frequency transducers.

With array transducer assemblies, focusing of the sound beam can be done electronically. Time delays of the appropriate sequence in the excitation pulses

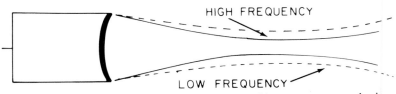

Figure 2-14. Principles of sound-beam focusing. In this case, a curved piezoelectric element is used. A higher-frequency element can be more sharply focused than a lower-frequency element for a given element diameter and curvature.

applied to individual elements in the array cause the wavefronts emerging from the array to converge (Fig. 2-15A). It is as though a focusing lens or a curved element were producing the beam. An advantage of the array, however, is that the focal region can be varied simply by selecting a different delay sequence for pulses applied to the elements.

Array transducers also allow focusing of the received echo signals, done by reversing the delay sequence among individual elements when echoes are picked up (Fig. 2-15 B). During reception the focal region may be changed dynamically, varying automatically with time (and consequently, with reflector depth) following the excitation of the transducer. Dynamic focus during reception of echoes improves the spatial resolution over the entire range of the image. This type of focusing is available on some instruments that use array transducer assemblies.

Most continuous-wave Doppler transducers employ separate transmitting and receiving elements. A typical design is shown in Figure 2-16, in which each of the elements is cut in the shape of a semicircle. Electrical connections are made with the front and back face of each element, and the elements vibrate in a direction perpendicular to their faces.

The sound beam emerging from the piezoelectric element and the receiving pattern of the receiver are very directional, as suggested by the dashed lines in Figure 2-16. To detect echo signals from scatterers, the beams from the transmitter and the receiver are caused to overlap as shown in the figure. This is done by inclining the transducer elements, or by using focusing lenses. The area of beam overlap defines the most sensitive region of the transducer.

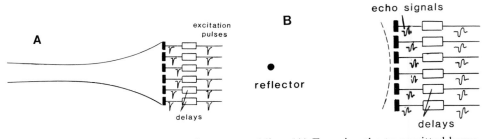

Figure 2-15. Focusing array transducer assemblies. (A) Focusing the transmitted beam. (B) Focusing during echo reception.

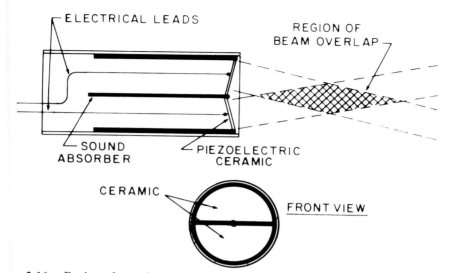

Figure 2-16.   Design of a typical ultrasonic transducer used in continuous-wave Doppler instruments. In most cases, either transducer element can be used as the transmitter or the receiver.

CHOICE OF ULTRASOUND FREQUENCY

Competing physical interactions govern the choice of the operating frequency, f_o, employed in an ultrasound instrument. For Doppler work, the choice is usually dictated by the need to obtain adequate signal strength for reliable interpretation of Doppler signals. For pulse-echo and some Doppler applications, spatial resolution requirements must also be considered.

Signal Strength

It was mentioned previously that the intensity of ultrasonic waves scattered from very small scatterers such as red blood cells increases with frequency, being proportional to the frequency raised to the fourth power. It thus would seem reasonable to use a high ultrasonic frequency to increase the intensity of scattered signals from blood. As the frequency increases, however, the rate of beam attenuation also increases (Fig. 2-1). In selecting the optimal frequency for detecting blood flow, these competing processes must be balanced, and the choice of operating frequency is often determined by the tissue depth of the vessel of interest.[3] For small, superficial vessels, where attenuation from overlying tissues is not significant, B-mode and Doppler probes operating at 8–10 MHz are commonly used. Doppler applications in the carotid artery usually employ somewhat lower frequencies in order to avoid significant attenuation losses, and frequencies of 4–5 MHz are typical. Frequencies as low as 2 MHz are used for detecting flow in deeper arteries and veins and for use in fetal monitoring devices.

Spatial Resolution

For B-mode imaging applications and some Doppler instruments, the spatial resolution requirements also play a role in dictating the operating frequency. Spatial resolution is limited by the lateral width of the sound beam (Fig. 2-14), as well as the axial length of the pulse if the beam is pulsed. The smaller these dimensions are, the better will be the resolution. Both the pulse duration, which governs the axial resolution, and the width of beam, which controls lateral resolution, can be made smaller if higher frequency transducers are used. Again, limitations are introduced by the increased tissue attenuation of higher ultrasonic frequencies. Transducer frequencies of 7.5 MHz are commonly used for imaging superficial structures; here resolution of better than 1 mm is obtainable. Attenuation losses dictate use of lower frequencies when imaging large areas such as the abdomen; the accompanying spatial resolution is not as good as that obtained for superficial structures.

An additional factor in the choice of the ultrasonic frequency in Doppler applications is the desire to avoid "aliasing" in the Doppler signal. This is discussed below.

DIRECTIONAL DOPPLER

Many basic Doppler instruments allow detection only of the magnitude of the Doppler frequency; that is, they provide no indication of whether the frequency shift is upward or downward from the transmitted frequency. Such information is necessary, of course, in order to be able to specify whether the flow direction is toward or away from the ultrasonic transducer.

Several techniques have been developed for producing directional-flow information using Doppler instruments. One that is commonly used is referred to as a quadrature detection.[4] This technique involves separation of the detected ultrasound signals into two channels in the receiver of the instrument. After suitable processing, the outputs of the separate channels have identical Doppler signals, except for small time lags between the two signals. The directional information is contained in these time (or phase) differences in the two quadrature output signals, and may be displayed after further processing.[4] Directional Doppler circuitry has been combined with real-time spectrum analyzers (see below), producing records that simultaneously indicate forward- and reverse-flow characteristics.[5]

DOPPLER SIGNAL ANALYSIS

We have indicated that for many structures of interest, the Doppler shift signal is in the audible frequency range. For some applications, adequate clinical interpretations can be made simply by listening to the signals. One then characterizes the movement that produced the Doppler shift according to the qualities of the audible signal.

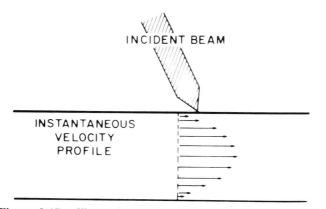

Figure 2-17. Illustration of the velocity profile of blood across the diameter of a vessel. Flow is slowest near the wall and highest near the center in this example. The lengths of the arrows schematically indicate the flow velocity at different distances from the center of the vessel.

Spectral Analysis

In applications involving blood flow, the Doppler signal may be fairly complex because of the complicated blood-velocity patterns found in most vessels. Usually, in a large blood vessel, the blood velocity is not the same at all points, but follows some type of profile, such as the parabolic flow pattern shown in Figure 2-17. The actual profile depends on a number of factors, including the size of the vessel, the blood pressure and the presence of obstructions. If the transducer sound beam and the sampled volume are large compared with the lumen diameter, scattered ultrasound signals will be received simultaneously from blood cells that are moving at different velocities. The resultant Doppler signal, therefore, will be rather complex.

A complex signal such as that shown in Figure 2-18A, may be shown to be composed of many single-frequency signals (Fig. 2-18B), each of these having a particular amplitude and phase, so that when added together, they form the original signal. Spectral analysis refers to separating a complicated signal into its individual frequency components so that the relative contribution of each frequency component to the original signal can be seen (Fig. 2-18C). Often the relative contribution is denoted by the signal power in a given frequency interval, and the spectrum is referred to as the power spectrum.

The power spectrum for Doppler signals depends on the flow characteristics within the vessel being studied. Figure 2-19 illustrates this for several hypothetical circumstances. We consider situations where the entire cross-section of the vessel is uniformly bathed by the sound beam. For simplicity, at this time we will consider only continuous flow within the vessel. If the flow profile is parabolic (Fig. 2-19A) velocities ranging from near zero at the vessel wall through the maximum value, v_{max}, are present. Corresponding Doppler signals, having

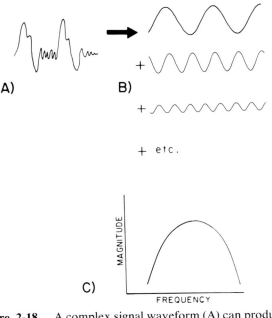

Figure 2-18. A complex signal waveform (A) can produced by an appropriate combination of single-frequency signals (B). Spectral analysis refers to seperating the complex signal into its single-frequency components and displaying the magnitude of each frequency component contributing to the signal (C).

frequencies ranging from nearly zero through the maximum ($f_{max} = 2[f_o v_{max}/c] \times \cos\theta$) are represented in the power spectrum (Fig. 2-19A). As a second example, some larger arteries are known to have blunt flow profiles. In these arteries, more of the flow occurs with the maximum velocity, and a Doppler signal frequency spectrum has the appearance shown in Fig. 2-18B. Notice that in this case the spectrum is more heavily weighted towards higher frequencies than the previous example. Finally, the flow distal to some stenotic regions may have a "jet" pattern. If only a small fraction of the blood flows with the extremely high velocities of the jet, the resultant Doppler Signal power spectrum has the appearance shown in Fig. 2-19C.

The appearance of the Doppler signal spectrum also depends on the size of the sample volume, that is, the volume contributing to the Doppler signal at any given time. A narrow sound beam that cuts through only a segment of the vessel lumen will generally result in a differently shaped spectrum than a sound beam that is broad enough to encompass the entire vessel. Similarly, a pulsed Doppler instrument, with its limited sample volume in the axial (or range) direction, will provide a considerably narrower spectrum than a continuous-wave device.

Another flow pattern that is of considerable interest in vascular studies is that produced by "turbulence" within the vessel. Turbulence, characterized, for example, by shedding of "vortices" and eddies as suggested in Figure 2-20, may

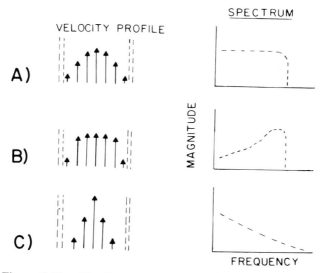

Figure 2-19. The frequency spectrum for Doppler signals depends on the characteristics of flow: (A) parabolic flow, (B) blunt flow profile, (C) jet profile (after Gill[15]). Continuous flow is illustrated. These are not the patterns seen with pulsatile flow.

occur distal to a stenotic region. In that case, the turbulence might result from the very high blood velocity present in the narrowed luminal opening. Small obstructions, such as kinks in a vessel or obstructions caused by atheromatous plaque formation, could also result in formation of vortices. The detection of turbulent flow is therefore of interest in evaluation of blood vessels.[17] Certain characteristics of the Doppler signal spectral display, such as "spectral broadening," provide indications of turbulent flow.

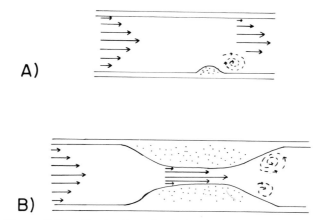

Figure 2-20. Production of turbulent flow by a small plaque (A) and by a stenosis (B).

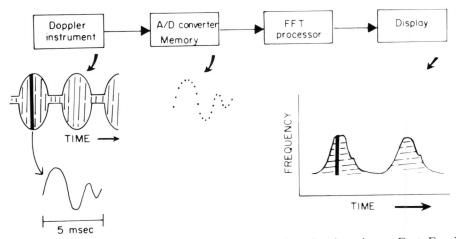

Figure 2-21. "Real-time" spectral analysis of Doppler signals using a Fast Fourier Transform (FFT) processor. The Doppler signal is analyzed in small time segments. The resultant display (lower right) shows frequency along the horizontal axis, time along the perpendicular axis and the amount of signal at a particular frequency and time as display brightness or color.

Pulsatile flow.   Several techniques have been used to display the Doppler frequency spectrum for pulsatile flow. Real-time, analysis of Doppler spectra can be carried out using sets of parallel electric filters.[7] More recently a digital technique involving fast Fourier transform (FFT) analysis has been used.[5] The latter technique is illustrated in Figure 2-21. The output Doppler signal (left side of Fig. 2-21) is applied to an analog-to-digital (A/D) converter, where it is digitized in segments and stored in the memory of a microcomputer. Each signal segment may be on the order of 5 msec in duration. An FFT analysis is carried out on the digitized signal segment, yielding the relative magnitude of each frequency component in the signal. The output of the FFT analyzer is sent to a screen, where the magnitude of the signal at each frequency is encoded in display brightness or in color. At this time another signal segment is available for analysis by the FFT instrument. The process goes on continuously, producing a display of the frequency spectrum of the signal in real-time.

The resultant spectral display of the FFT analyzer is in the format shown in Figure 2-22. The records depict Doppler frequency on the vertical axis, time on horizontal axis, and the relative amount of signal at a given frequency and time as a shade of gray. (Notice the different orientation of the frequency axis in comparison with Fig. 2-19.) For Doppler signals from the carotid artery, records are usually produced that represent 2–3 sec time intervals. Figure 2-22A shows a spectral analysis of the Doppler signal obtained from a normal carotid artery. A broad velocity spectrum in the artery, especially during the systolic portion of the cardiac cycle, is evident from these records. Figure 2-22B is the spectral analysis for a Doppler signal obtained from a segment of the internal carotid artery, immediately distal to a stenosis. The increased frequency resulting from the greater blood velocities through the stenotic region is demonstrated.

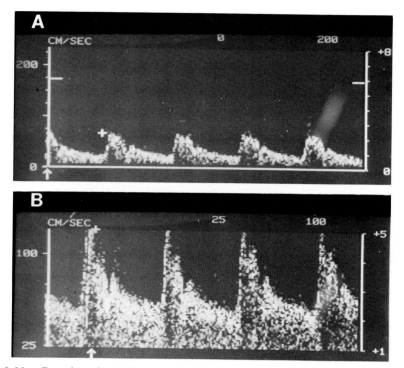

Figure 2-22. Doppler signal frequency spectra from the carotid artery. (A) Normal carotid artery, (B) spectrum from a stenotic artery.

When combined with directional detection equipment commercially available FFT analyzers provide combined forward- and reversed-flow spectral analysis. With some units, the frequency scale is replaced by a velocity scale. Velocity is otained by solving the Doppler equation (Eq. 2-4) for v when factors including the speed of sound, the ultrasound frequency and the Doppler angle (θ) are known.

Zero Crossing Detectors

A simple device commonly used to indicate the output Doppler frequency is the zero crossing detector. Its operation[8] is outlined in Figure 2-23. The Doppler signal voltage waveform is depicted in the top portion of the diagram as a waveform oscillating about the zero-volts line. Each time the signal waveform passes through zero in a given direction, a single, rectangular pulse is generated. The zero crossing detector simply counts the number of rectangular pulses produced in a small time interval, τ, and indicates this value on a display (see lower portion of Fig. 1-23). In actual practice, the rectangular pulse that is generated is not triggered precisely at the zero-voltage level, but is triggered whenever the Doppler signal rises above some threshold level. This is to prevent low-level noise signals from triggering the display.

The zero crossing detector responds to variations in the Doppler signal

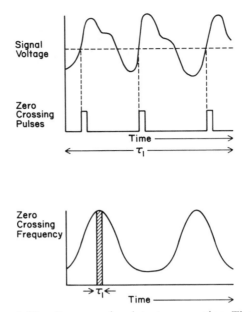

Figure 2-23. Zero crossing detector operation. The original Doppler signal (A) triggers a rectangular pulse (B) whenever the voltage crosses zero in one direction. The instrument counts the number of rectangular pulses per second to obtain the zero crossing frequency.

frequency during the normal cardiac cycle as well as variations associated with certain abnormal flow conditions. Thus, it may be used as a rough indicator of the Doppler signal frequency characteristics. In the presence of a spectrum of Doppler frequencies, however, the output of the zero crossing detector indicates a frequency that is neither the maximum instantaneous frequency (often of clinical interest in the detection of stenosis)[9,10] nor the mean frequency.[8] (The zero crossing detector output is proportional to the "root mean square" Doppler frequency.[8]) Another disadvantage of the zero crossing detector is that it cannot follow fast changes in the flow pattern, such as those that occur during pulsatile flow. The zero crossing detector has also been found to be susceptible to electrical noise.[11] Some of these limitations have been overcome by employing somewhat more sophisticated Doppler signal processing, such as that used in an offset frequency zero crosser.[12]

An inexpensive method that has been used to plot Doppler signal spectral characteristics is a time-interval histogram analyzer.[12] This device uses the trigger pulses produced by the zero crossing detector, producing a dot on the display for each zero crossing pulse. The vertical position of each dot (Figure 2-24) is proportional to the time interval between successive pulses. If this display is recorded over a period of time using, for example, a fiber-optic strip chart recorder, the resultant display appears similar to an actual spectral analysis display. Both the Doppler frequency characteristics resulting from laminar flow and properties of turbulent flow can be studied with this device.

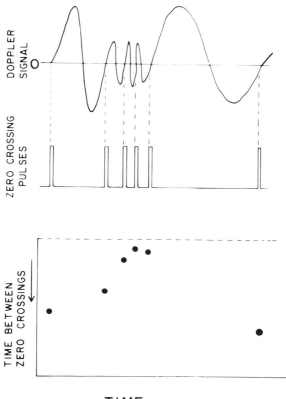

Figure 2-24. Derivation of the "time-interval histogram" (TIH) spectral display. Increasing frequency of the Doppler signal (decreasing time between zero crossings) is in the upward direction of this record.

LIMITATIONS OF PULSED DOPPLER

Aliasing

With a pulsed Doppler instrument a performance limitation occurs related to the pulse repetition frequency (PRF) of the instrument and the maximum frequency Doppler signal that can be successfully measured. The limitation referred to is called aliasing and, if present, it can lead to anomalies on Doppler signal spectral waveforms.

Consider the situation illustrated in Figure 2-25. We can think of a pulsed Doppler instrument as "building up" the Doppler output signal "piece by piece". Each burst of ultrasound emitted by the transducer and received from the sample volume contributes to the Doppler signal, as depicted by the arrows in the figure. The higher the PRF, the more pulses will be available per cycle of the Doppler signal and the better will be the rendition of that signal. It is not always practical,

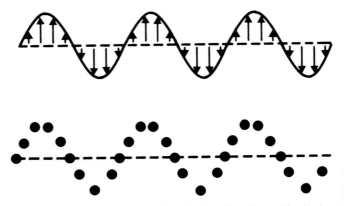

Figure 2-25. Illustration of technique for "sampling" the Doppler signal when a pulsed Doppler is used. The top waveform represents the Doppler signal and the arrows are successive "samples" of this signal by the instrument. The lower waveform represents the resulting sampled signal.

however, to have the pulse repetition frequency of the Doppler instrument significantly higher than the frequency of the Doppler signal. There are two reasons for this. First, as discussed in the next section, we must limit the PRF so there is sufficient time to collect all signals from one pulsing of the transducer prior to a subsequent pulsing. This restriction on the PRF is dependent on the depth of the sample volume. The greater the distance to the region of interest the longer it takes to pick up echoes from that region following pulse transmission. Secondly, higher PRFs are associated with greater acoustic power emitted by the transducer into the patient. Although the risk levels and the biological effects of diagnostic ultrasound are still not well quantified, prudence dictates that the lowest practical acoustic exposure level should be used in any diagnostic study.

The minimum repetition frequency that may be used in a pulsed Doppler instrument is equal to two times the frequency of the Doppler signal. If the pulse repetition frequency is lower than this, aliasing will occur. Aliasing refers to the generation of artifactual, lower frequency components in the signal spectrum when the pulse repetition frequency of the instrument is less than two times the Doppler signal frequency.

The production of aliasing is illustrated schematically in Figure 2-26. The actual Doppler signal (top) is sampled (arrows) at a rate less than two times each cycle of the signal. The resulting sampled waveform (lower part of Fig. 2-26) is one whose frequency is lower than that of the actual signal.

A common way aliasing is manifested on a Doppler spectral display is illustrated in Figure 2-27. This record was obtained using a Doppler phantom containing pulsatile flow, discussed later in this chapter. The top portion of the spectral envelope for each systolic pulse is clipped, or cut off. Doppler signals heard over the loudspeaker of the instrument were significantly lower in frequency than they were after the velocity scale (and presumably the PRF of the instrument) was increased (lower panel of Fig. 2-27). This change in instrument settings had the effect of no longer clipping the top portion of the waveform.

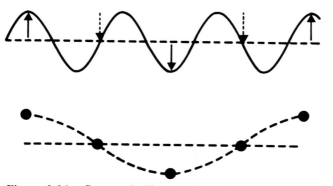

Figure 2-26. Same as in Figure 2-25, only now the Doppler signal (top) is sampled at a rate that is less than two times the frequency of the original signal. An artifactual signal (lower curve), whose frequency is less than that of the original signal, is produced.

Variations in tonal qualities of the audible Doppler signals between the two panels in Figure 2-27 were much more dramatic than the changes observed in the spectral display.

Sometimes aliasing is accompanied by a "wrapping around" of the Doppler signal spectral display (Fig. 2-28). However, it should be noted that display wrap around, as exhibited in Figure 2-28, can occur on some units even if aliasing is not present.

Errors due to aliasing must be avoided when attempting to measure velocity or flow with a pulsed Doppler instrument. Steps to avoid aliasing include using lower frequency transducers, resulting in a lower frequency Doppler signal (Eq. 2-3) for a given reflector velocity and using as high a PRF as practical in the instrument. Sometimes the examination conditions are such that aliasing cannot be avoided. In such circumstances a solution is to use continuous wave instruments when this occurs.

Maximum Velocity Detectable With Pulsed Doppler

Another limitation of current pulsed-Doppler systems is introduced by the finite travel time of sound pulses in tissue. As mentioned above, to unambiguously detect a Doppler signal (i.e., without aliasing) whose frequency is, f'_D, the pulse repetition frequency of the Doppler instrument must be at least twice this value, or $2 f'_D$. In equation form, this may be stated as

$$\text{PRF} \geq 2f'_D, \qquad (2\text{-}6a)$$

where $\geq$ means "greater than or equal to."

On the other hand, an upper limit on the pulse-repetition frequency is established by the time interval required for ultrasound pulses to propagate to the range of interest and return. Sufficient time must be allowed between successive pulses for the detection of all echoes down to the range of interest. If this is not

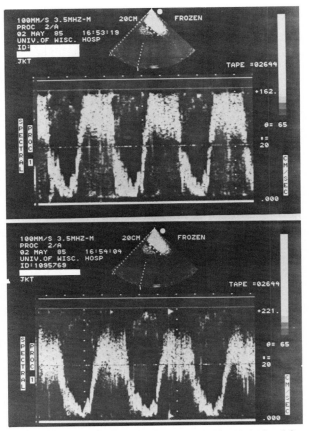

Figure 2-27. Exampling of aliasing in a signal derived from an internal carotid artery using a commercially available pulsed Doppler instrument. The incident Doppler frequency is 4.5 MHz.

done, range ambiguities arise in the position of reflectors. The time, T, for a pulse to travel a distance d and return to the transducer is given by

$$T = 2d/c, \tag{2-6b}$$

where c is the speed of sound in the medium. The inverse of T, $1/T$, is the maximum PRF allowable for detecting signals from reflectors at the depth d.

If we set the maximum permissible PRF for obtaining signal from a depth, d, equal to the minimum PRF implied in equation 2-5, and substitute for the Doppler signal frequency, f'_D using equation 2-3, we can compute the maximum velocity detectable from a reflector whose depth is d. We'll omit the steps (which are straightforward) and simply state the result:

$$v_{max} = \frac{c^2}{8f_0d} \tag{2-7}$$

where v_{max} is the maximum reflector velocity.

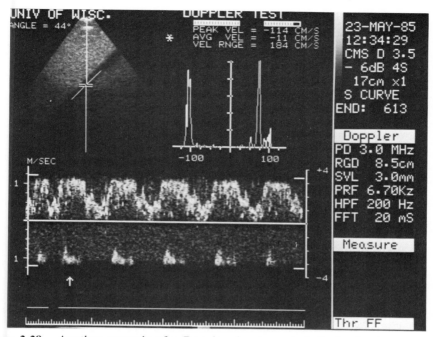

Figure 2-28. Another example of a Doppler signal spectral display in the presence of aliasing. Notice the "wrap around" of the spectral display.

Assuming a speed of sound of 1540 m/sec the plots in Figure 2-29 were generated using equation 2-7, relating the maximum reflector velocity which can be detected to reflector depth for 3 different ultrasound frequencies. (Notice that we have not considered angle effects; we're assuming an angle of 0° in Fig. 2-5). As the reflector depth increases the maximum detectable Doppler signal frequency, and hence the maximum reflector velocity that can be detected, decreases. At any depth lower ultrasound frequencies permit detection of greater velocities than higher frequencies.

MEASUREMENT OF VOLUME FLOW WITH DOPPLER INSTRUMENTS

The velocity information provided by a Doppler instrument could presumably be used in computing volume flow rates (in, for example, milliliters per minute) within a vessel. The volume flow rate may be defined as the mean velocity, averaged over the lumen of the vessel, multiplied by the vessel cross-sectional area. In order to measure volume flow with Doppler equipment, it is necessary to extract the mean velocity in the presence of whatever complex velocity profile exists in the vessel. In addition, geometric factors, including the vessel area and the angle of the vessel lumen relative to the ultrasound beam, must be known.

One approach to the problem of determining the mean velocity is to analyze the Doppler signal using mean frequency detection instruments. The mean

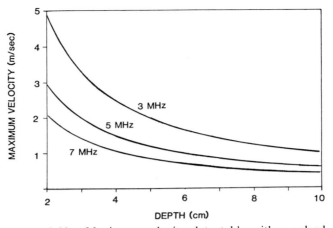

Figure 2-29. Maximum velocity detectable with a pulsed Doppler instrument *vs* reflector depth. Curves are shown for three operating frequencies.

frequency refers to the average Doppler frequency, weighted by the spectral density; that is, the relative intensity of the Doppler signal at each frequency.[13,14] Under conditions where a vessel is uniformly bathed by the ultrasound beam, mean frequency detection provides an indication of the mean blood velocity within the vessel, regardless of the velocity profile. Gill[15] has combined a mean frequency Doppler instrument with a pulse-echo ultrasound scanner for determining vessel geometric factors, to measure volume flow within vessels. The angle between the sound beam and the vessel lumen was known.

In principle, the mean frequency could be obtained using a pulsed Doppler instrument having a very small sample volume, and measuring the frequency at different positions of the sample volume across the vessel.[12] This technique has been used in a few cases, especially in superficial arteries. Another approach is to use the pulsed Doppler instrument to isolate the flow signals from a segment of a vessel. The mean frequency from this segment could be obtained using analog or digital methods. By assuming that flow within the vessel is symmetric about the vessel axis, and by using pulse-echo techniques to derive vessel geometric factors, volume flow may be estimated.

PHANTOM FOR EVALUATING ULTRASOUND DOPPLER EQUIPMENT

Many aspects of the performance of Doppler equipment may be evaluated using suitable flow phantoms. In medical physics, a phantom is any device that mimics the human body with respect to beam transmission properties of the modality of concern (i.e., x-ray, ultrasound, nuclear magnetic resonance, etc.). Ultrasound phantoms must have representative speeds of sound, ultrasound attenuation coefficients and scatter levels for the tissues being mimicked. For testing ultrasound Doppler equipment a phantom must also have vessels contain-

Doppler Ultrasound Phantom

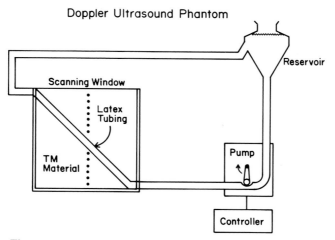

Figure 2-30. Phantom for evaluating Doppler ultrasound equipment.

ing flowing fluids. Besides their use for Doppler equipment evaluation, such phantoms are valuable for teaching and for equipment demonstrations.

Figure 2-30 shows a phantom for testing ultrasound Doppler equipment. It combines the following features: (1) a synthetic blood-mimicking material, housed in vessels and a 500 cc reservoir, (2) a variable flow-rate pumping system, and (3) phantom contents that mimic soft tissues. A 45° angle between the scanning surface and the vessel lumen allows for detection of Doppler signals over a range of 1 to 15 cm. The dots seen within the phantom represent 0.3 mm nylon line reflectors that may be used to test the range gate accuracy of the pulsed Doppler system.

The speed of sound, density and attenuation coefficient of the tissue mimicking material[16] are representative of parenchymal tissue; their values are 1560 m/sec, 1.05 g/cm^3, and 0.5 db/cm-MHz, respectively. The ultrasonic attenuation in the tissue mimicking material is proportional to the frequency. Vessels in the phantom are of latex tubing having an inside diameter of 5/8 in. and a 1/16-in. wall thickness.

Desirable features of a synthetic blood are that its backscattering should be the same as real blood, both in magnitude and in the Rayleigh-like frequency dependence. There needs to be a high enough particle concentration so that the echo signal characteristics, or the signal texture, look like those of actual blood. And the sedimentation rate of scattering particles should be low enough that excessive settling out of particles doesn't take place. The synthetic blood used in the phantom seen in Figure 2-30 consists of polystyrene spheres immersed in a glycerol-water mixture. The diameter of the spheres is 30 microns, which is small enough that Rayleigh scattering is assured throughout the ultrasonic frequencies of interest. The particle concentration required is determined by comparing signal levels from the synthetic blood mixture with that of fresh human blood. In the present phantom backscattered signals from the synthetic blood agreed with signals from human blood to within 2 db for frequencies from 2.2 MHz to 5 MHz.

The following tests may be carried out on Doppler phantom systems: Doppler system sensitivity, accuracy of range gate indicators, accuracy of velocity readouts, and directional discrimination capabilities.

SUMMARY

Ultrasonic echoes can be produced by specular reflectors, which are relatively large compared with the diameter of the sound beam, or by scatterers, which are much smaller than the sound beam. Pulse-echo techniques can be used to image the walls of vascular structures, whereas Doppler techniques are used for detecting and evaluating flow. The frequency, diameter, and focusing of the ultrasonic transducer influences the properties of the sound beam and the operating characteristics of the instrument. In particular, the frequency of the transducer must be chosen to allow adequate spatial resolution without sacrificing depth penetration. These principles apply both for B-mode imaging and Doppler techniques.

A Doppler instrument can continuously transmit an ultrasonic wave, in which case the term "continuous-wave Doppler" is applied. The Doppler sound beam can also be pulsed, permitting the sampling of Doppler signals from a discrete region along the course of the beam. The Doppler shift frequency is the difference between the frequencies of the transmitted sound beam and the returning echoes. The maximum Doppler shift frequency detectable may be limited when pulsed techniques are used to evaluate deep structures. Doppler instruments may be directional, that is, capable of determining the direction of blood flow relative to the transducer, or nondirectional, in which case flow can be detected but the direction is unknown.

The Doppler shift signal can be analyzed with zero crossing detectors. More sophisticated methods of analysis include frequency spectral analysis and time-interval histogram techniques. With duplex instrumentation, pulsed or continuous-wave Doppler is combined with B-mode imaging. Both the size (diameter or area) of the vessel and flow velocity characteristics are, therefore, known when such instruments are used. This information offers the potential for calculating volume flow within the vessel.

Aliasing is the generation of artifactual, lower frequency signals when the PRF of a pulsed Doppler instrument is less than two times the frequency of the Doppler signal. Because the PRF is also limited by the time it takes to pick up echo signals from the depth of the sample volume, there is an upper limit to the Doppler frequency (hence, reflector velocity) that can be detected at any depth with a pulsed Doppler instrument.

James A. Zagzebski, Ph.D.
Department of Medical Physics
University of Wisconsin Medical School
1300 University Avenue
Madison, WI 53706

REFERENCES

1. Wells PNT: Physical Principles of Ultrasonic Diagnosis. New York, Academic Press, 1969
2. Shung K, Reid J: Scattering of ultrasound by blood. IEEE Transactions on Biomedical Engineering, BME-23:260–467, 1967
3. Reid J: Challenges and opportunities in ultrasound, in Proceedings of the First International Seminar on Ultrasonic Tissue Characterization, NBS Special Publication 453, Washington, DC, US Government Printing Office, 1976
4. Wells PNT: Ultrasonic Doppler equipment, Fullerton G, Zagzebski J (eds), in Medical Physics of CT and Ultrasound, New York, American Institute of Physics, pp 343–366, 1980
5. Spencer M, Reid J, Hileman R, et al: On line dual-directional spectral display in Doppler diagnosis of stenotic and nonstenotic plaque. Proceedings of Abstracts 25th Annual Meeting of the American Institute of Ultrasound in Medicine, New Orleans, Louisiana, 1980
6. Gill RW: Pulsed Doppler with B-mode imaging for quantitative blood flow measurement. Ultrasound Med Biol 5:223–235, 1979
7. Light LH, Cross G, Hansen PL: Noninvasive measurement of blood velocity in the major thoracic vessels. Proc R Soc Med 67:142–144, 1974
8. Lunt MJ: Accuracy and limitations of the ultrasonic Doppler blood velocimeter and zero crossing detector. Ultrasound Med Biol 2:1–10, 1975
9. Keaghy BA, Pharr WF, Thomas P, et al: Evaluation of the peak frequency ratio (PFR) measurement in the detection of internal carotid stenosis. J Clin Ultrasoknd 10:109–112, 1982
10. Zweibel WJ, Zagzebski JA, Hirscher M, et al: Correlation of peak Doppler frequency with lumen narrowing in carotid stenosis. Stroke 13:386–391
11. Flax S, Webster J, Updike S: Statistical evaluation of the ultrasonic Doppler flowmeter. Biomed Sci Instrum 7:201–222, 1970
12. Baker DW, Forster FK, Daigle RE: Doppler principles and techniques in ultrasound: Its application in medicine and biology, in Fry FJ, (ed), Amsterdam, Elsevier, 1978, pp. 161–287
13. Arts M, Roevers J: On the instantaneous measurement of blood flow by ultrasonic means. Med Biol Eng 10:23–42, 1972
14. Reid J, Davis D, Ricketts H, et al: A new Doppler flowmeter system and its operation with catheter mounted transducer. Proceedings of an International Symposium on Cardiovascular Applications of Ultrasound, Beerse, Belgium. New York, Elsevier, 1974
15. Gill RW: Performance of the mean frequency Doppler modulator. Ultrasound Med Biol 5:237–247, 1979
16. Madsen EL, Zagzebski JA, Banjavic RA, et al: Tissue mimicking materials for ultrasound phantoms. Med Physics 5:391–394, 1978
17. D'Luna IJ, Newhouse VL: Vortex characterization and identification by ultrasound Doppler. Ultrason Imag 3:271–293, 1981
18. Waag R, Myklebust J, Rhoads W, et al: Instrumentation for noninvasive cardiac chamber flow rate measurement. Ultrasonic Symposium Proceedings, IEE Cat 72 CHO 708–850:74–80, 1972
19. Winsberg F: Real-time scanners: a review. Med Ultrasound 3:99, 1979
20. Woodcock JP: Development of the ultrasonic flowmeter. Ultrasound Med Biol 2:11–18, 1972

Merrill P. Spencer, M.D.

3

Frequency Spectrum Analysis in Doppler Diagnosis

The most appealing aspect of Doppler ultrasound in diagnosis of diseases of the cardiovascular system lies in its simple noninvasive capability to obtain physiologic information at a wide range of selected sites in audible form. The use of Doppler ultrasound by a skilled technician and interpreter provides a singularly cost-effective method of clinical diagnosis and quantitation. Because the human hearing mechanism lacks somewhat in objectivity, however, the availability of a spectral display of the underlying frequencies is desirable. Frequency spectral analysis of Doppler signals provides quantitative parameters for cardiovascular diagnosis as well as documentation for clinical records and research. The spectral display also assists in teaching how and where to recognize important diagnostic characteristics of the Doppler flow signal. The simultaneous viewing of the spectrum while listening to the signals, enhances the ability to recognize important features. Early in the use of Doppler, the audio spectrum was reduced to an analog tracing of the average frequency by means of zero-crossing meters. Difficulties of zero-crossing meters in the face of turbulent signals and the loss of complete spectral content (Chapter 2) have given impetus to the development of frequency spectral analysis devices.

Several methods of obtaining the frequency spectrum have been reviewed by Angelsen[1] and Hatle[2] who conclude that the faster Fourier transform (FFT) is the best available method for the power spectral display. The FFT is a method of breaking down the range and mixture of Doppler signals into individual components and displaying them as a function of time on a frequency scale from zero to any desired maximum, while also representing the relative amplitude of energy within such frequency band. The effect, as spread out in time, is that of passing the original Doppler signal through a bank of various bandpass filters. The "voice writes" of Bell Laboratories, developed in the 1940s, made such a display. Hileman[3] developed a microprocessor computer for the FFT to provide a

Acknowledgment: Much of the work underlying this chapter has been supported by the National Institutes of Health Grant #HL 19341.

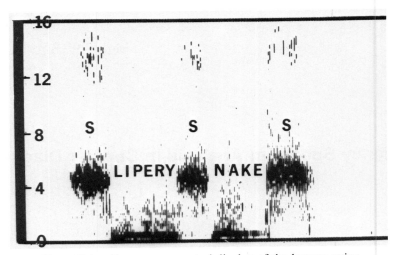

Figure 3-1. Frequency spectral display of the human voice announcing the words "slippery snakes." Note the high frequencies associated with the letter "s" compared to the low carrier frequencies of the vowels. Vertical scale in in kilohertz. (Recorded on the DOPPTECH spectral analyzer by Dr. Ray Gosling.

video-recordable directional display of the amplitude of various frequencies represented in a color-coded format. Figure 3-1 illustrates the representation of the human voice on the frequency spectrum.

Readers who are not familiar with commonly used methods of Doppler frequency analysis including FFT should review the material on this subject in Chapter 1 before proceeding with this chapter.

SPECTRAL FREQUENCIES OF NORMAL VASCULAR FLOW

Blood flow along a normal artery or vein is laminar, meaning that each layer of blood slides along the adjacent layers, slightly retarded by the viscous forces between them. These viscous forces cause the layers in the center of the stream to move with a higher velocity than the layers near the wall (Color plate 1). With steady flow, the velocity profile across the vessel diameter becomes parabolic, i.e., the change in velocity from the vessel wall to the center and on to the opposite wall follows a parabolic relationship. Figure 3-2, illustrates the parabolic laminar flow profile as well as the corresponding spectral distribution of frequencies that represents the distribution of velocities across the vessel. If the entire blood vessel cross-section is covered by the ultrasound beam, as with continuous wave Doppler, all velocities in the lumen are represented in the frequency spectrum, and a uniform distribution of frequencies is evident between the lowest

PARABOLIC PROFILE & DOPPLER SPECTRUM

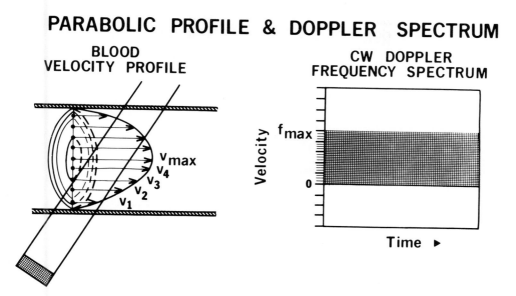

Figure 3-2. Relationship between the blood velocity profile and the Doppler spectrum produced by an ultrasound beam covering the entire cross section (left). In the case of the parabolic laminar blood flow, velocities and frequencies are represented with equally distributed amplitudes in the Doppler spectrum (right).

velocities near the wall and the highest ones, in the center of the stream (Fig. 3-2). The maximum frequency, termed f_{max}, represents the highest velocity detected within the ultrasound beam.

With range-gated pulse wave Doppler (PWD), only the velocities represented within the sample volume, generally around 1–2 mm^3, are represented in the frequency spectrum. With pulse Doppler we can study the velocity profile by moving the sample volume from point-to-point across the vessel lumen (Fig. 3-3) or by using a multigate pulsed Doppler as exemplified in Figure 9-10.

The continuous wave Doppler spectrum may also exhibit a narrow frequency range when the normal parabolic profile is converted into a more blunt (flattened) profile (Fig. 3-4), but the frequency range is never as narrow as that obtained with pulsed wave Doppler. A narrow frequency range may also occur with continuous wave Doppler when the beam is too narrow to sample all the velocities near the wall, when blood flow is accelerated or when blood flows into a narrow channel from a larger vessel. A concentration of frequencies near the upper edge of the spectrum (near f_{max}) also develops during systolic acceleration (Fig. 3-5). During deceleration, the velocity and frequency distribution spreads out into a more parabolic representation that generally persists throughout diastole. The concentration of flow energy near the maximum velocity is characteristic of normal vessels with laminar flow and may be recognized aurally as a smooth, whistling quality as opposed to the more noisy quality produced by a broader spectrum.

A
PW DOPPLER SPECTRUM OF LAMINAR FLOW

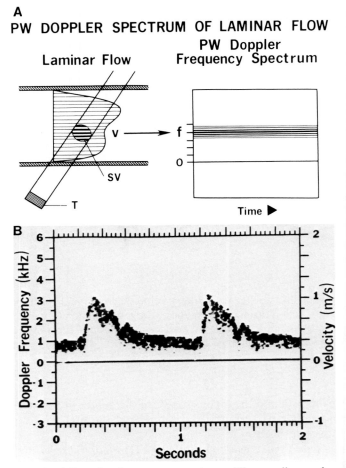

Figure 3-3. (A) Pulsed Doppler frequency spectrum. The small sample volume of the pulse wave Doppler positioned within the lumen of a blood vessel (left) produces a narrow frequency band (right) representing the velocity profile within only the sample volume. (B) The characteristic narrow waveform of a pulsed Doppler is illustrated in this spectrum obtained using a small sample volume positioned in the axial flow stream of a normal internal carotid. (Vingmed "Alfred" pulsed Doppler and SONOCOLOR spectral display. SONOCOLOR is the trademark of Carolina Medical Electronics, King, NC.)

NORMAL DOPPLER SIGNATURES OF VARIOUS VASCULAR CHANNELS

With training one can often recognize the source of Doppler signals without visual knowledge of the position of the Doppler probe on the body, by means of characteristic spectral qualities and the sound of the signals. The differentiation of signals from the external and internal carotid arteries is an important application of this ability (Fig. 3-6). The lower peripheral resistance represented in the internal carotid artery gives rise to higher frequency diastolic components than

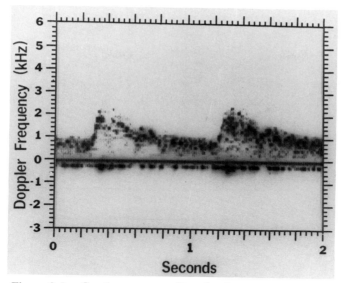

Figure 3-4. Continuous wave Doppler frequency spectrum of a normal internal carotid artery. Note the concentration of energies near the upper edge of the spectrum, indicating that laminar flow is present with a relatively blunt profile. The spectrum of frequencies is not as narrow as that seen with pulsed Doppler (Fig. 3B). Signals from an overlying vein are displayed below the baseline as low and relatively constant frequencies.

TEMPORAL ACCELERATION

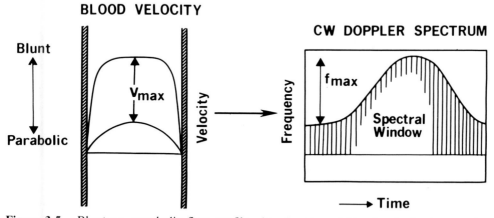

Figure 3-5. Blunt vs. parabolic flow profile. Acceleration of blood velocity in systole produces a blunt blood velocity profile (left) represented by a concentration of Doppler spectral energies near f_{max} and a clear spectral window (right). During deceleration, the spectrum broadens again as the flow profile becomes parabolic instead of blunt.

57

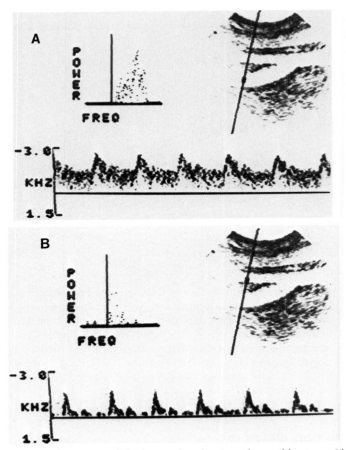

Figure 3-6. Doppler signatures of the internal and external carotid artery. (A) The pulsed Doppler frequency spectrum from the normal internal carotid artery is seen at the base of the display. The sample volume is placed just beyond the bifurcation as shown in the real-time B-mode image (upper right). The diastolic power frequency distribution is seen at the upper left. (B) The frequency spectrum of the normal external carotid artery is shown at the base of the display (same subject as [A]). Note that the sample volume is placed in the more superficial branch. Compare the higher pulsatility and lower diastolic components of the external carotid with the pulsatility features of the internal carotid shown in [A].

are present in the external carotid spectrum. The early systolic peaking and late systolic trough, characteristic of the external carotid, reflects predominance of radially directed blood flow due to compliance* of the blood vessel[4] and a relatively small proportion of axial flow through the peripheral resistance (Fig. 3-7). The opposite pattern is seen in the internal carotid where axial flow

---

* The term ''compliance'' refers to the ability of the vessel to distend in response to increased intraluminal pressure. A high compliance vessel distends readily; a low compliance vessel is rigid.

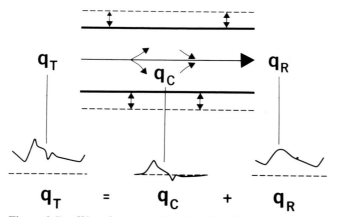

Figure 3-7. Waveform contribution of radial and axial flow. The radial (compliant) flow component (q_C) is superimposed upon the flow through component (q_R) of the peripheral resistance. The net waveform of total flow (q_T), as shown at the bottom left, is a combination of these two principle components. When peripheral resistance is low relative to the radial (compliant) component, the Doppler waveform is dominated by the q_R waveform (bottom right). When peripheral resistance is high, or obstruction exists downstream, only the q_C component (bottom center) may be represented in the local Doppler signal.

predominates over radial flow because of low peripheral resistance in the cerebral circulation.

The normal waveform in the ascending aorta, which is similar to the subclavian artery signal, is produced by left ventricular ejection (Fig. 3-8). Further distal in the brachial artery (Fig. 3-9A), reflected pulses from the periphery produce a stronger diastolic dip and a resultant brief backflow (reversed flow) phase. Flow reversal in extremity arteries does not occur in the presence of peripheral vasodilatation, which elevates the waveform above the baseline throughout diastole. Figure 3-9B illustrates the effect of vasodilation as induced by reactive hyperemia, following the application of an inflated blood pressure cuff to the arm.

Doppler spectral representations of the velocities in the normal superficial and deep (profunda) femoral arteries are represented in Figure 3-10. In the superficial femoral artery the early diastolic dip (dichrotic notch) is longer than in the femoral pulse. This difference results from the greater length (and flow resistance) in the superficial femoral channel as compared to the deep femoral artery. Readers are referred to Chapter 1 and to additional references for further understanding of the origin of the diastolic oscillations in peripheral arteries.[4]

Flow patterns from all vessels crossed by the ultrasound beam are superimposed in the frequency spectrum from a continuous wave Doppler. The superimposition of flow signals may complicate signal interpretation in some instances, but may actually aid interpretation in others, as illustrated in Figure 3-11. In this

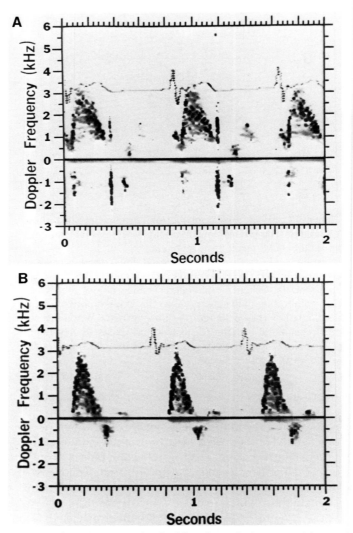

Figure 3-8. (A) Doppler spectrum of velocities through the normal human aortic valve. (Note superimposed ECG tracing.) Valve opening and closing transients are seen as vertical streaks on the spectrum immediately at the end of the QRS and the T waves of the ECG. Following valve opening, velocities rapidly accelerate to reach an early systolic peak. Relatively blunt velocity profiles are indicated during acceleration by the concentration of energies near the upper edge of the spectrum. (B) Subclavian artery spectrum (same normal subject as [A]). Note the slight difference between this waveform and that shown in [A]. Sagging is evident during late systole and a longer backflow component as well as a secondary forward rebound is seen in early diastole. A laminar and blunt flow profile is present as shown by the concentration of energies near f_{max}. Note also the phase delay in the relationship of the spectrum to the ECG tracing, as compared with the aortic ejection pulse (8A). Spencer MP, Fujioka K: Continuous Wave Doppler with spectral analysis in acquired valve disease. In Spencer MP (ed): Cardiac Doppler Diagnosis, Vol 1. The Netherlands, Martinus Nijhoff Publishers, 1984, p. 162. With permission.

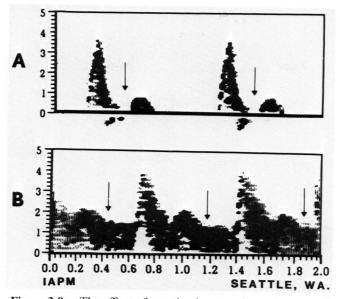

Figure 3-9. The effect of reactive hyperemia on the normal brachial artery spectrum (A) Brachial velocities during rest are shown. The arrow indicates a brief backflow phase and a relatively low frequency diastolic component. (B) The arrow indicates marked elevation of the diastolic component, the result of reactive hyperemia, following release of an ischemia-producing arm cuff. The vertical scale is in kilohertz and the horizontal scale is in seconds. From Spencer MP: Using carotid imaging and hand-held probing Doppler evaluation of the aortocranial circulation. In Reneman RS (ed): Doppler Ultrasound in the Diagnosis of Cerebrovascular Disease. The Netherlands, Research Studies Press, 1982, p. 182, with permission.

example, superimposition of flow signals from the internal and external carotid arteries simplifies the task of localizing the stenotic lesion. The waveform that has external carotid pulsatility is normal, while the waveform with internal carotid characteristics demonstrates systolic and diastolic frequency elevation consistent with stenosis.

An additional useful technique for identifying the blood vessel represented in a Doppler spectrum is that of finger vibration of immediately connecting arteries. Rapid finger vibration produces transmitted velocity oscillations, either retrograde or antegrade to flow, that are easily seen at the maximum edge of the spectrum (Fig. 3-12). Examples of the use of this technique are the following: (1) oscillation of the temporal artery to identify the external carotid artery and separate it from the internal carotid artery at the carotid bifurcation, (2) oscillation of the brachial artery to identify stenosis signals from the subclavian artery, (3) oscillation of the vertebral artery at the base of the skull to identify the vertebral artery lower in the neck near its origin, (4) compression or oscillation of the occipital artery at the base of the skull to identify it as a collateral to an occluded

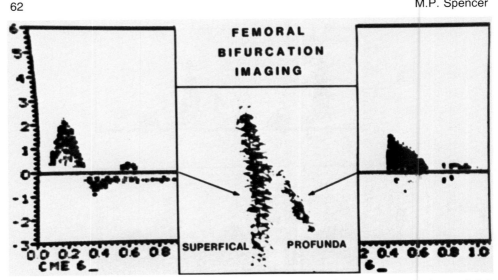

Figure 3-10. Normal pulsatility differences in the deep (profunda) femoral and superficial femoral branches of the common femoral artery. The center panel represents a continuous wave Doppler map of the femoral bifurcation. From Spencer MP, Reid JM, et al: Doppler Imaging. In Hegyeli RJ (ed): Atherosclerosis Reviews, Noninvasive Methods in Atherosclerosis Research. New York, Raven Press, 1983, p. 17. With permission.

internal carotid artery, and (5) diagnosis of iliac artery lesions by vibration of one of the femoral arteries. The finger vibration techniques may be used with both continuous wave and pulsed Doppler devices.

Normal venous flow characteristically produces a parabolic velocity profile because of low pulsatility, and the continuous wave Doppler frequency spectrum will, therefore, be evenly represented across the FFT display. This flow pattern is illustrated during the first second of Figure 3-13. Venous flow is easily influenced by external compression and deep respirations, however, producing corresponding changes in the venous Doppler spectrum also illustrated in Figure 3-13. With proximal venous compression or an increase in abdominal pressure (i.e., a Valsalva maneuver), flow decreases to zero but no flow reversal is seen if the venous valves are competent. If the values are incompetent, flow reverses when abdominal pressure is increased. After release of venous compression or abdominal pressure, there is rapid acceleration and recovery of the normal venous velocities if there is no obstruction to the venous channel under investigation.

NOMENCLATURE OF SPECTRAL FEATURES AND AUDIBLE QUALITIES

Doppler signals possess five features used in diagnosing cardiovascular disease: (1) the source or point of origin of the signal within the vessel being examined, (2) amplitude, strength or power of the signal, (3) frequency (velocity) and frequency distribution, (4) direction (approaching or receding from the transducer), and (5) pulsatility and waveform. These signal features may be modified by vascular pathophysiology, by pharmacological and physiological

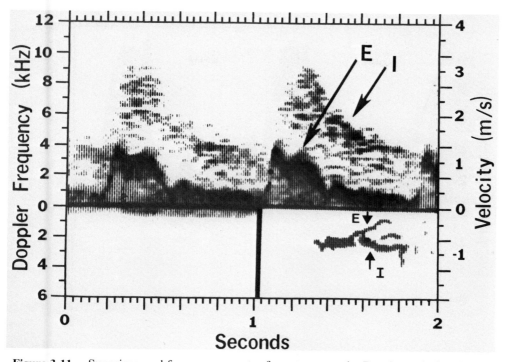

Figure 3-11. Superimposed frequency spectra from two vessels. Depth resolution limitations of continuous wave Doppler may be overcome by superimposing arterial spectra. In this patient with stenosis at the origin of the left internal carotid artery, the continuous wave ultrasound beam is passing through both the stenotic internal carotid artery and a nearby branch of the external carotid artery. Frequency spectra from the normal external carotid artery (E) and the stenosed internal carotid artery (I) may be clearly distinguished from one another through direct comparison of waveforms. The continuous wave Doppler map of the trifurcation of the common carotid artery is shown at the bottom right.

interventions, by external compression or by the technique of examination. All of these features of the signals are present in the spectrum and should be utilized diagnostically.

Source of Signal

Techniques for displaying the source of the Doppler spectrum from blood vessels or the heart are developing rapidly. The original and simplest display system is exemplified by continuous wave Doppler imaging of the carotid bifurcation. The Doppler probe is mounted in a mechanical arm and the position of the probe is continuously tracked by means of the *xy* coordinates of an oscilloscope or videoscreen[5] (see Fig. 6-11). This mapping method if useful for localizing pathology within the cervical carotid system. The duplex system for localization of Doppler signals is now in widespread clinical use. With duplex

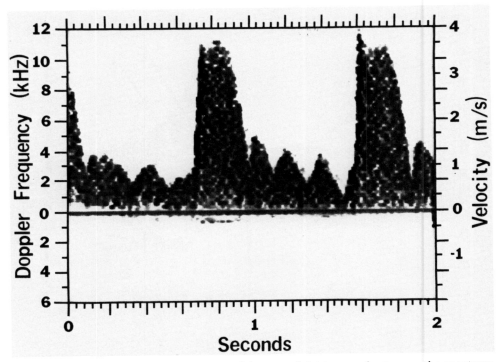

Figure 3-12. Effects of finger vibrations of the superficial temporal artery on the spectrum of the cervical external carotid near the carotid bifurcation. With the Doppler probe held just above the bifurcation, high frequencies reaching 11 kHz are noted that indicate severe stenosis. The response of the upper edge of the spectrum to finger oscillation of the temporal artery proves that the spectrum arises from the external branch and not the internal carotid artery. In this patient, the internal carotid spectrum (not shown) did not respond to temporal artery vibrations. Hence, one can be confident of the location of the stenosis.

instruments, the line of site of the Doppler transducer and the position of the Doppler range gate (if PWD is used), are superimposed on a B-mode image (Fig. 3-7). The future holds promise of even greater sophistication in Doppler localization techniques, such as the simultaneous, visual representation of flow and vessel anatomy as illustrated in color plates.

Amplitude

The overall amplitude or power of the Doppler signal is the least reliable diagnostic feature because it depends on many factors not related to blood velocity or blood flow, such as the depth of the vessel from the probe. The relative amplitude, however, is useful (1) when comparing one portion of a vessel with another area, (2) when comparing symmetry of the signal between opposite sides of the body and (3) in following changes within the same artery from one examination to the next. As the Doppler probe is moved along an artery, an abrupt

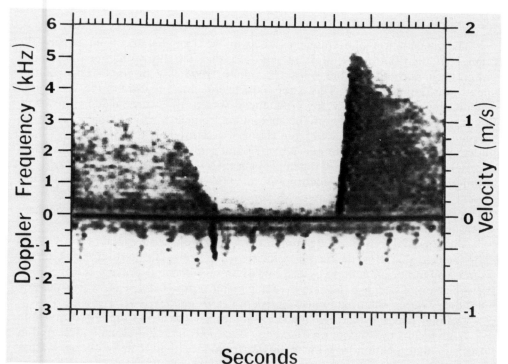

Figure 3-13. Normal femoral vein spectrum and changes caused by the Valsalva maneuver. Recording from left to right, a normal parabolic profile of venous flow, with maximum frequencies of 3 kHZ, is displayed on the spectrum during the first 3-sec (large division, horizontal axis). At 3 sec the Valsalva maneuver was begun, reducing vein flow to zero. At 7 sec, breath holding ceased. The flow velocity rapidly accelerated to 5 kHz and then returned gradually to the normal resting level. This normal response indicates competent venous valves because of the absence of reflux flow in response to the elevated intra-abdominal pressure of breath-holding. The flow spectrum of the adjacent femoral artery is seen below the baseline. Note that arterial flow persists throughout the respiratory maneuver.

decrease in amplitude suggests the presence of atheromatous involvement, which causes increased attenuation of the ultrasound beam.

In contrast to overall amplitude, the *distribution* of amplitudes across the frequency spectrum is of considerable diagnostic value. Color or gray scale spectral display of these relative amplitude provides much information, often not appreciated by the ear. Frequency distribution information is discarded in analog tracings. The thermal color spectrum developed by Hileman (color plate 2) represents the lowest amplitudes in red and the highest amplitudes in white, while ranges in between are represented by orange and yellow. Frequency spectrograms illustrated in this chapter were derived from color spectra of Hileman but, for economic reasons, these have been photographically reproduced in shades of gray. In these gray scale spectra, black represents the highest amplitude and white, zero amplitude.

Frequency Distribution

The distribution of frequencies seen in the Doppler spectrum is directly related to distribution of flow velocities within the ultrasonic beam sample volume. Of particular value is the maximum frequency or upper edge of the spectrum, designated f_{max}. This is the most useful single feature of the spectrum. The presence of high-energy, low frequencies such as those produced by turbulent flow may affect the clarity of the maximum frequency (f_{max}) (Fig. 3-3). Low frequencies may be eliminated from the spectrum by means of high pass (wall) filters. With a 5-MHz continuous wave Doppler, a wall filter cutting off frequencies below 1000 Hz is helpful for improving the quantitative accuracy of f_{max}. In addition, some instruments incorporate a "high boost" filter to accentuate the upper (f_{max}) edge of the spectrum. Maximum frequency estimators, such as those developed by Angelsen[1] are useful, but care must be taken with these devices when turbulence is present or when a signal-to-noise ratio is poor.

Mean spatial frequency, as computed using zero crossing meters, provides a simplified readout for the mean velocity waveform. The zero-crossing meter works well in normal blood vessels, but when turbulence is present the accuracy is compromised because the zero-crossing meter output is biased towards the low amplitudes rather than following the true mean frequency (Fig. 3-14).

Doppler spectral features and their auditory equivalents are listed in Table 3-1. *High* means the maximum frequency is greater than the normally detected in vessels at that location; *low* means lower frequency than usually obtained from that location. *Smooth* refers to the concentration of spectral frequencies near the maximum frequency throughout the cardiac cycle (Figs. 3-15A and 3-14 right). *Course* refers to spectral broadening not detectable normally at a specific arterial location (Fig. 3-15B). *Gruff* is a special quality of high-amplitude, low-frequency accentuation occurring only in systole, and is the Doppler representation of the audible bruit arising from a local site (Fig. 3-16A). A *whining* or *sea gull* quality refers to the spectral representation of periodic oscillation of the vessel wall (Fig. 3-16A). *Whipping* denotes a specific form of spiking that occurs at the peak of systole and probably represents disturbed flow (Fig. 3-17A). *Fluttering* means rapid fluctuation in the spectral distribution within each cardiac cycle (these fluctuations most obviously affect the f_{max} edge of the spectrum) (Fig. 3-17B). Disturbed flow may be regarded as an early form of turbulence which, if propagated or continued, produces a fluttering quality. The relevance of these findings to specific diagnostic situations is discussed below.

Pulsatile Waveform

The configuration of the f_{max} edge of the Doppler signal throughout each cardiac cycle carries a great deal of physiological information for the interpreter who understands underlying hemodynamics. Descriptive definitions of pulsatile waveforms include: *systolic only*, representing high pulsatility with low diastolic components and *continuous*, which indicates a low level of pulsatility with relatively high levels of diastolic flow as compared with f_{max} of the systolic peak. A continuous quality with low pulsatility is characteristic of flow in the arteries that supply organs or tissues with low peripheral resistance, such as the brain and kidneys. A systolic or high pulsatility spectrum is characteristic of the normal

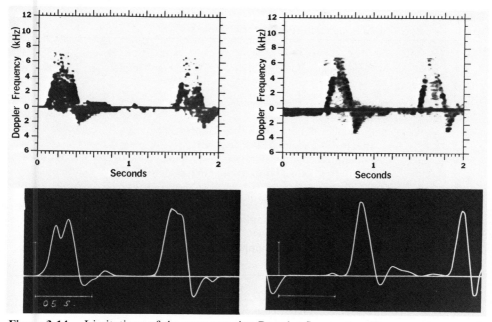

Figure 3-14. Limitations of the zero crossing Doppler flow meter. The upper two panels are frequency spectral displays of a subclavian artery stenosis (left) and a normal subclavian artery (right). Analog tracings from these same arteries are shown in the lower two panels. On the left, low frequency energies seen in the spectra produce distortions of the analog tracings. On the right, the smooth blunt profile of the normal subclavian artery is converted to a nondistorted analog tracing. Spectra and tracings were not made simultaneously. (Courtesy G. M. von Reutern, Freiburg, Germany.)

external carotid artery as compared to the internal carotid artery (Fig. 3-6). High pulsatility also is characteristic of the normal extremity vasculature during rest, as compared with the low pulsatility, hyperemic pattern found after exercise and following ischemia or other causes of peripheral vasodilatation (Fig. 3-9). The pulsatility indices of Pourcelot,[6,7] Gosling[8,9] and Mol[10] may be applied with equal validity to the f_{max} measurements of frequency spectral analysis or to the mean velocity analog tracings of a zero-crossing recorder.

Backflow refers to the reverse flow phase most frequently seen at the end of systole in extremity arteries. If two or more backflow phases are seen they are designated as triphasic or multiphasic because the diastolic oscillations pass through zero more than twice. *Rapid* or *slow* acceleration refer to the rate of change in velocity, particularly noted on the leading edge of the pulse in systole; slow acceleration refers to a lower rate of rise than normal and is sometimes termed "damped" if this feature is also associated with low velocities. *Phase lag* is a term applied to delay in the pulse, as compared with a reference signal, from another part of the circulation (an ECG, electrocardiogram, or a second Doppler signal may be used for reference). *Alternating flow* refers to the change in flow direction caused by the meeting of two pressure waves arising from different directions and out of phase with one another.

Table 3-1
Spectral Features and Nomenclature of Arterial Stenosis

PRIMARY

     A.   Increased local velocity-increased f_{max} or high frequency

SECONDARY

     A.   Downstream
           Turbulence, fluttering, gruff or Doppler bruit, dual directional,
              spectral broadening, low frequency
           Dampening, slow acceleration, low frequencies, decreased pulsatility
           Vasodilation, elevated diastolic component (HDq) or continuous

     B.   Upstream
           Decreased velocity
           Increased systolic pulsatility, diminished diastolic component, back
              flow, to-and-fro flow
           Waterhauser effect, thumping

TERTIARY

     A.   Adjacent to obstruction
           Increased Velocity as in A
           High amplitude or strong
           Decreased pulsatility HDq or Cn

     B.   Distant interconnecting collaterals
           Decreased velocity
           Alternating, tidal flow in bidirectional
           Reversed direction

Direction

Reliability of the indicated flow direction is occasionally compromised by the proximity of bony structures or calcium deposits that reflect the ultrasound beam and create a mirror image of the flow direction. Errors in determining flow direction may also occur in severely curved or looped arteries. Direction is defined in our laboratory in various ways: (1) *forward-moving* is the normal direction toward the perfused tissues; (2) *reversed* is opposite to the normal or toward the heart; and (3) *inverted* means the plus and minus polarities of the signal are exchanged but forward flow is documented in adjacent portions of the same vessel. Calcium deposits or proximity to bone can artifactually cause inversion of the signal, mimicking reversed flow. *Bidirectional* means the signals in a particular region exhibit both a positive and negative flow direction. *Monophasic* designates flow in one direction only, primarily during systole. Biphasic means the signal direction changes once only in early diastole (Fig. 3-18B), and triphasic designates two forward directions separated in sequence by a negative direction (Fig. 3-18A). Triphasic flow is typically seen in normal extremities of young people. *Dual direction* refers to flow streams within the ultrasound beam moving simultaneously in both directions, i.e., in turbulent flow (Fig. 3-18A).

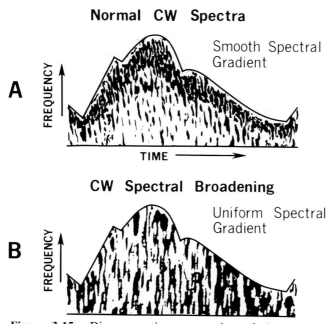

Figure 3-15. Diagrammatic presentation of the spectral appearances of the normal internal carotid artery. In panel A, a blunt profile is evident with flow energy concentrated near the upper edge of the spectrum. In panel B, spectral broadening proves that a parabolic profile is present.

SPECTRAL MANIFESTATIONS OF VASCULAR DISEASE

Diagnostic Features of Stenosis

Primary Effects

The primary hemodynamic effect of stenosis in vascular channel is localized increased velocity at the site of stricture.[11,12] This increase in velocity is produced by a diminished cross sectional area and an increased pressure gradient.[13] Local increases in velocity may reach 6 m/sec in the stenotic arteries of hypertensive patients. Such velocities produce Doppler frequency shifts of 19 kHz when a 5-MHz Doppler is used at a beam angle of 60°.

The effects of graded stenosis on the local Doppler frequency spectrum are illustrated by experimental compression of the normal human femoral artery (Fig. 3-18). In this experiment a 5-MHz continuous wave Doppler probe was held on the skin overlying the artery that was compressed by applying various degrees of pressure to the transducer, until total occlusion was produced. In the absence of compression, the normal femoral artery waveform is multiphasic with a smooth signal quality and a clear spectral window (Fig. 3-18A). As compression was applied, the first recognizable feature of stenosis was an increase in peak velocity accompanied by diminution of the backflow phases (Fig. 3-18B). At the same time, spectral broadening occurred in the form of increased lower frequency

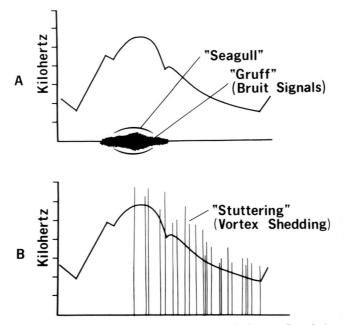

Figure 3-16. Two spectra of severe turbulence. Panel A represents a "sea gull" or harmonic bruit with an associated blowing quality. The symmetry around the zero line is characteristic of vessel wall vibrations. Panel B, "stuttering" is illustrated. This finding represents a violent form of turbulence in which vortices are marching past the ultrasound beam. The maximum power extends from beyond the peak to the baseline of the spectrum.

energies. With further compression, peak frequencies increased still higher while backflow and resonant wave features during diastole disappeared entirely. Eventually, the normal diastolic features were replaced by a continuous forward moving component (Fig. 3-18C).

In carotid artery stenosis, normal maximum systolic frequencies (1.5 to 3 kHZ) are increased, but the waveform is changed very little until the stenosis becomes very severe (Color plate 2,3). Hemodynamic significance in carotid stenoses generally implies approximately 70 percent reduction in cross sectional areas. With a 5-MHz Doppler probe, this level of carotid stenosis typically generates frequency shifts in excess of 10 kHz. A Doppler shift of this magnitude corresponds to a velocity of 3.2 m/sec and, in the carotid system, this flow rate represents a 40-mm pressure drop across the stenosis.

Secondary Effects

Secondary effects of arterial stenosis or occlusion are produced both upstream and downstream to the obstruction. In graded stenosis, the earliest secondary effect consists of downstream turbulence that can be detected with either pulsed[3] or continuous-wave[14] Doppler (Fig. 3-16, 3-17, and Color plate 4).

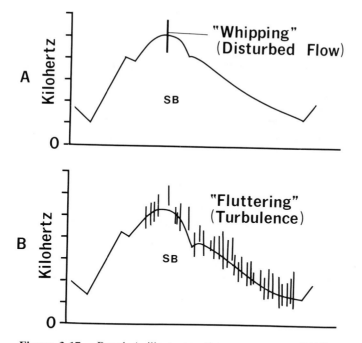

Figure 3-17. Panel A illustrates the appearance of "disturbed" flow often encountered in the normal bulbous origin of the internal carotid artery. In panel B, fluttering irregularity seen along the upper edge of the spectrum is produced by turbulent blood flow. This is usually accompanied by spectral broadening. Turbulence generally begins in midsystole, at peak velocities. Often, this sign of turbulence appears before a bruit can be heard over the artery.

Pulsed Doppler is reported to be more sensitive than continuous wave Doppler to low-grade arterial lesions.[15] Theoretically, detecting flow velocities only from the center of the stream may allow recognition of minimal turbulence causing spectral broadening. The specificity of low level spectral broadening as an indicator of stenosis is poor, however, since spectral broadening may be seen in normal arteries. For example, flow disturbances occurring in the normal bulbous portion of the internal carotid artery produce flow separations and helical flow streams[16] (Color plate 1), that are manifest as spectral broadening. Ironically, as atherosclerotic plaque begins to fill the bulb of the carotid, spectral broadening may disappear in the center stream, because flow disturbances are minimized. Spectral broadening in normal arteries will also be encountered if the pulsed sample volume is placed near the arterial wall due to the broad distribution of velocities normally present adjacent to the wall[17] (Fig. 3-19).

As a stenotic lesion further encroaches on the arterial lumen, turbulent flow develops and increases in intensity downstream to the obstruction (Color plate 4), and spectral broadening appears both on pulsed waves and continuous wave spectra. In moderate to severe stenoses, organized vortices form downstream to

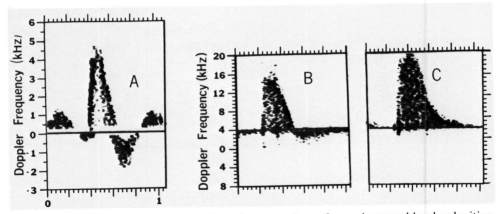

Figure 3-18. Effects of experimental graded stenosis on femoral artery blood velocities produced by compression of the femoral artery in a young subject. Panel A illustrates the normal femoral artery CW Doppler spectrum. In panel B, frequencies are elevated to 16 kHz by compression of the artery with the probe, and the diastolic components are altered. In panel C, further compression produces additional elevation of frequencies and further changes in waveform. (See text for full explanation.)

the stenotic zone and as these move through the Doppler sound beam, a stuttering quality is produced and represented by characteristic streaking across the entire spectrum (Fig. 3-16B). When turbulence is sufficiently severe to vibrate the arterial wall, a bruit is produced that can be heard with a stethoscope. These wall vibrations produce a gruff quality in the Doppler signal and track directly the frequencies heard with the stethoscope. Artery wall vibrations are recognized on the spectrum by low frequency energies shown with symmetrical displacement above and below the zero frequency line (Fig. 3-16A). The frequencies represented on the Doppler spectrum mimic directly those heard with a stethoscope and are independent of the incidental ultrasound frequency; this independence from the incident frequency results because the excursions of oscillations of the artery wall are less than one ultrasonic wave length. Generally, these Doppler "bruit" signals do not exceed 1 kHz.

Although continuous wave Doppler does not specify the location of various flow patterns as precisely as pulsed Doppler, it offers the advantage of displaying all of the flow features within the sound beam and across the entire lumen, including high velocities and secondary turbulent effects. With progressive luminal narrowing, increasing stenotic zone velocities produce higher and higher frequencies, but pulsed Doppler cannot follow the frequencies due to the aliasing effect resulting from the Nyquist limit (see Chapter 1). Consequently, the spectrum will "wrap around" and produce the appearance of spectral broadening when, in fact, the velocity profile within the stenosis is laminar.

Additional secondary effects seen downstream (distal) to severe stenoses include diminished velocities represented by diminished Doppler frequencies and a damped waveform consisting of low velocities overall, slowed acceleration of the systolic upstroke and relative elevation of diastolic velocities (Fig. 3-20). The

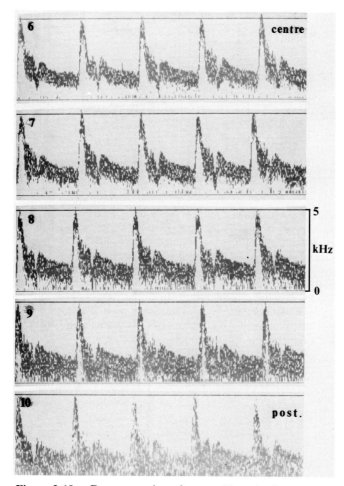

Figure 3-19. Demonstration of spectral broadening near the wall of a normal carotid artery. The pulsed Doppler sample volume (1.4 mm³) was moved from center stream (upper panel) to the posterior wall of the common carotid in four steps. The presence of a boundary zone with a large gradient of velocities near the wall is indicated by "filling in" of the spectral window in the lower two spectral panels. (Reproduced with permission from: Merode TV, Hick P, et al: Limitations of Doppler spectral broadening in the early detection of carotid artery disease due to the size of the sample volume. Ultrasound Med Biol 9(6):581–586, 1983. With permission.

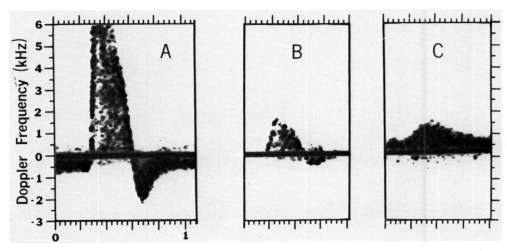

Figure 3-20. Pulsatility patterns upstream and downstream from a severe arterial stenosis. (A) A continuous wave Doppler spectrum just above a stenosis in the iliac artery demonstrates high pulsatility and a strong backflow phase. (B) A femoral artery spectrum from the same patient shows a moderately damped appearance. The biphasic flow pattern persists, but systolic accelerations are slower and frequencies are lower overall than those present in a normal individual. (C) The posterior tibial artery spectrum of the same patient is severely damped (very slow acceleration, low frequencies, and low pulsatility). The elevated diastolic flow component indicates vasodilatation. From these spectra, one can conclude that there are at least two significant arterial obstructions, one above the femoral artery and one between the femoral and popliteal arteries.

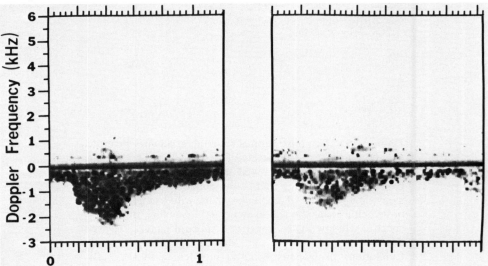

Figure 3-21. Doppler frequency spectra from the intracranial cavernous components of the internal carotid arteries detected through the orbits with pulsed Doppler. On the left, normal frequencies indicate absence of hemodynamically significant obstruction of the internal carotid. The right panel demonstrates lower velocities in the cavernous carotid artery, produced by hemodynamically significantly stenosis of the cervical portion of the right internal carotid artery.

74

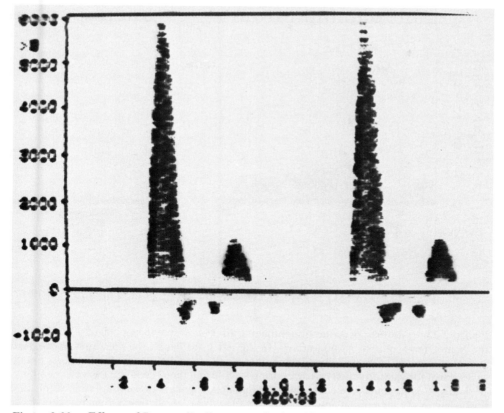

Figure 3-22. Effects of Raynaud's disease on the brachial artery spectrum. Seen are high pulsatility (f_{max} 6 kHz in systole), brief systolic phase and multi-phasic diastolic components characteristic of high peripheral resistance. (Doppler carrier frequency, 5 MHz.)

elevated diastolic velocities result from vasodilatation downstream to the obstruction that reduces peripheral resistance.

When low resistance is present, continuous flow is a normal situation, such as in the carotid arteries. Comparison of pulsatility patterns between the two sides of the body allows one to judge the significance of upstream (proximal) obstruction. As shown in Figure 3-21, proximal stenosis of the homolateral carotid artery produces diminished velocities and slow acceleration in the siphon segment of the internal carotid. The abnormal pattern on the obstructive side is easily recognized in comparison to the opposite carotid.[18]

Upstream (proximal) to a severe arterial obstruction, lower mean velocities and higher pulsatility ratios may be seen. This effect is especially helpful when assessing the common carotid arteries for significant obstruction of the internal carotid artery. If asymmetry in the diastolic component occurs, it may be concluded that the internal carotid is severely stenosed or occluded on the side manifesting little or no diastolic flow. Also, in Raynaud's phenomenon, where high peripheral resistance exists, the pulsatility increases upstream and a characteristic "snappy" quality occurs with multiple backflow phases (Fig. 3-22).

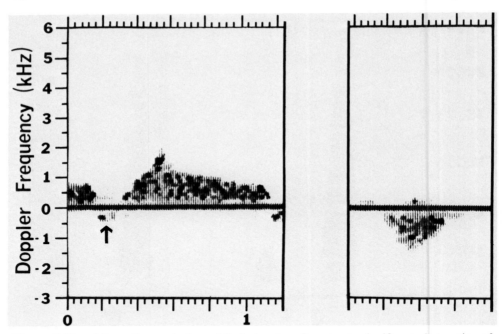

Figure 3-23. Alternating posterior ophthalmic artery flow due to significant obstruction of the homolateral internal carotid artery. In the left hand panel, the spectrum above zero indicates blood flow abnormally directed towards the Circle of Willis. Flow reverts briefly to a normal forward direction (arrow) during systole and then reconverts to reversed flow. In the right hand panel, the contralateral ophthalmic signal is present only in systole and flow is always in the normal anterior direction (downward deflections). Spectra were made with a 5-MHz probe placed over the closed eyelid.

Tertiary Effects

Tertiary manifestations of arterial stenosis occur within the collateral channels that bypass the obstructed region. In the major collateral channels immediately adjacent to the obstruction, there is a phase of diminished velocity as the obstruction worsens but before flow reversal occurs. An example of this phenomenon, as seen in ophthalmic artery collateralization, is illustrated in Fig. 3-23. In this case, a biphasic "balanced" velocity waveform results from to-and-fro motion of blood in the ophthalmic artery. This effect indicates that the pressure in the intracranial carotid is very nearly the same as in the periorbital arteries and only the phasic differences are manifest in the to-and-fro flow in the ophthalmic artery. When the pressure in the intracranial carotid is low, in comparison to the external carotid artery, a strong, high velocity reversal of ophthalmic artery flow is seen on the spectrum (Fig. 3-24).

Compression maneuvers are of great value in establishing the presence of tertiary effects during the study of the posterior orbital or periorbital arteries. For example, in the absence of significant internal carotid artery stenosis, compression of the temporal artery either has no effect or may augment blood flow in the periorbital arteries. However, compression of the temporal artery in the presence

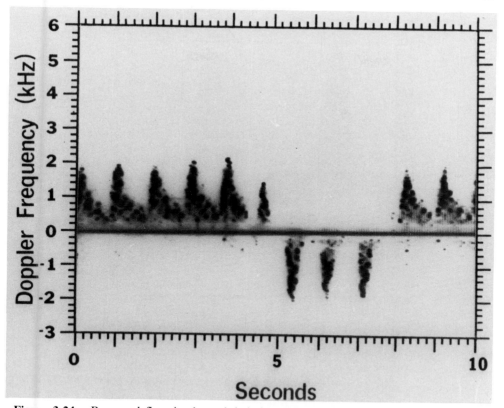

Figure 3-24. Reversed flow in the ophthalmic artery produced by homolateral carotid artery obstruction. At 1 sec, the reversed flow direction (upward spikes) is converted to a normal anterior direction by compression of the homolateral temporal artery for three cardiac cycles. These findings indicate that although strong collateral flow is available through the ophthalmic artery, intracranial collaterals also are significant enough to materially replace the temporal artery source.

of internal carotid obstruction may diminish the strength (amplitude) of the spectrum, obliterate the spectrum or produce flow reversal.

One of the most interesting examples of collateral effects is that of the vertebral artery-to-subclavian artery steal, occurring where there is obstruction of a subclavian or innominate artery (Fig. 3-25). Several abnormal patterns of vertebral flow are encountered with various degrees of obstruction of the innominate or subclavian arteries.[19] As the obstruction grows more severe and the pressure in the distal subclavian artery decreases, vertebral artery velocities diminish and acquire an alternating character. Eventually, they reverse in direction. Flow reversal may only occur during high flow states, and normally directed vertebral flow may exist with the patient at rest. In such instances, the reversal component may be brought out by producing reactive hyperemia in the arm.[19] The Doppler frequency spectrum provides documentation of an existing or potential steal.

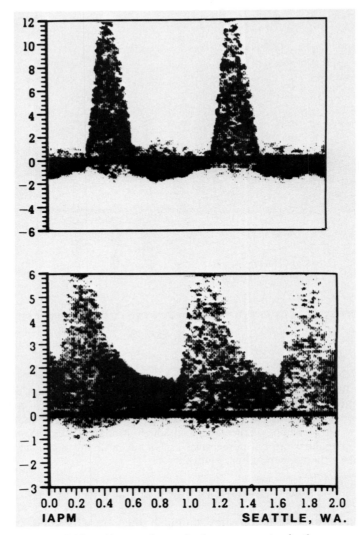

Figure 3-25. Abnormal vertebral artery spectra in the vertebral-subclavian artery steal. The top panel illustrates abnormal alternating flow (above and below the baseline) in the vertebral artery at the atlas loop during rest. The bottom panel is from the same position following deflation of the arm cuff and during reactive hyperemia response in the arm. The augmentation of the upward component of the spectrum proves that this component is in the direction of the brachial artery and that a partial steal has been converted to a continuous steal.

Diagnostic Features of Occlusion

The primary Doppler manifestation of arterial occlusion is the absence of flow signals in an area where blood flow is normally expected. Since negative information begs the question of adequate examination, there is great opportunity for error if occlusion is diagnosed solely on the absence of Doppler signal. The examiner must search for secondary and tertiary features that confirm the diagnosis of occlusion. Secondary findings, seen proximal to the occlusion, consist of overall decreased blood velocities, increased pulsatility and compliant, biphasic flow. The tertiary manifestations are the same as those found in stenosis.

CONCLUSIONS

All of the useful diagnostic features of the Doppler signal, other than the source, reside in the time-varying frequency-amplitude spectrum. Visual frequency spectral displays have advantages of precision and documentation over analog tracings. The spectral features of normal and disturbed vascular flow have been identified and defined both in terms of the audible and visual presentations. The spectral manifestations of the arterial disease may be divided into primary, secondary, and tertiary findings.

Merrill P. Spencer, M.D.
Institute of Applied Physiology and Medicine
701 Sixteenth Avenue
Seattle, WA 98122

REFERENCES

1. Angelsen BAJ: A theoretical study of the scattering of ultrasound from blood. IEEE Trans Bio Eng 27:61–67, 1980
2. Hatle L, Angelsen BAJ: Doppler ultrasound in cardiology: Physical principles and clinical applications. SINTEF Report STF 48A81028, The Federation of Scientific and Industrial Research, Trondheim, Norwegian Institute of Technology pp 197–235, 1981
3. Spencer MP, Hileman R, Reid JM: Visual vascular diagnosis with Doppler ultrasound using video display of dual direction spectrum and imaging. Proc. 26th Annual Meeting AIUM, p 110, 1981
4. Spencer MP, Denison AB: Pulsatile blood flow in the vascular system: In WF Hamilton (ed): Handbook of Physiology—Circulation II. Am Physiol Soc, 1963, pp 839–864
5. Reid JM, Spencer MP, Davis DL: Continuous-wave Doppler imaging of the carotid bifurcation. In Bernstein EF (ed): Noninvasive Diagnostic Techniques in Vascular Disease. St. Louis, C.V. Mosby Company, 1982, pp 248–257
6. Pourcelot L: Continuous wave Doppler techniques in cerebral vascular disturbances. In Reneman RS, Hoeks APG (eds): Doppler Ultrasound in the Diagnosis of Cerebrovascular Disease. New York, Research Studies Press (div. John Wiley), 1982, pp 103–128
7. Pourcelot L: Diagnostic ultrasound for cerebral vascular disease. In Donald I, Levi S (eds): Present and Future of Ultrasound, Rotterdam, Kooyker Scientific Publications, 1976, pp 141–147
8. Gosling RG, Beasley MG, Lewis RR: Noninvasive demonstration of disease at the carotid bifurcation by ultrasound. In Reneman RS, Hoeks APG (eds): Doppler Ultrasound in the Diagnostic of Cerebrovascular Disease. New York, Research Studies Press (div John Wiley), (1982), pp 215–253
9. Lewis R, Padayachee TS, Gosling RG:

Ultrasound screening for internal carotid disease. II Sensitivity and specificity of a single site periorbital artery test. Ultrasound Biol 10(1):17–25, 1984

10. Mol JMF: The clinical use of Doppler hematographic investigation in cerebral circulation disturbances. In Reneman RS, Hoeks APG (eds): Doppler Ultrasound in the Diagnosis of Cerebrovascular Disease. New York, Research Studies Press (div John Wiley) 1982, pp 129–156

11. Spencer MP: Hemodynamics of carotid artery stenosis. In Spencer MP, Reid JM (eds): Cerebrovascular Evaluation with Doppler Ultrasound. The Hague, Martinus Nijhoff Publishers, pp 113–116, 163–165, 1982

12. Spencer MP, Reid JM: Quantitation of carotid stenosis with continuous-wave (CW) Doppler ultrasound. Stroke 10(3):326–330. 1979

13. Spencer MP, Arts T: Hemodynamic principles for cardiac Doppler diagnosis. Cardiac Doppler Diagnosis 1:131–141, 1984

14. Reneman RS, Spencer MP: Local Doppler audio spectra in normal and stenosed carotid arteries in man. Ultrasound Med Biol 5(1):1–11, 1979

15. Knox RA, Phillips DJ, Breslau PJ, et al: Empirical findings relating sample volume size to diagnostic accuracy in pulsed Doppler Cerebrovascular studies. J Clin Ultrasound 10:227–232, 1982

16. Bharadvaj BK, Mabon RF, Giddens DP: Steady flow in a model of the human carotid bifurcation. Part I. Flow Visualization. J Biomechanics 15:5 349–362, 1982

17. Merode TV, Hick P, Hoeks APG, et al: Limitations of Doppler spectral broadening in the early detection of carotid artery disease due to the size of the sample volume. Ultrasound Med Biol 9(6):581–586, 1983

18. Spencer MP: Intracranial carotid artery diagnosis with transorbital pulsed wave (PW) and continuous wave (CW) Doppler ultrasound. J Ultrasound Med 2(10)(Suppl):61, 1983

19. Von Reutern GM, Budingen HJ, Freund HJ: The diagnosis of obstruction of the vertebral and subclavian arteries by means of directional Doppler sonography. Arch Psychiatr Nervenkr 222(2-3):209–222, 1976

SECTION II

CEREBROVASCULAR DIAGNOSIS

Ultrasound techniques for cerebrovascular diagnosis were conceived just 10 years ago and have been refined only within the past few years. Nevertheless, these procedures have attained widespread clinical application and now account for a large portion of the workload of many noninvasive vascular laboratories. In this section, the principles of ultrasound cerebrovascular diagnosis are presented in detail.

We begin with Chapters 4 and 5, by Dr. Dietrich, which describe the clinical relevance of noninvasive techniques and cerebrovascular anatomy. This basic material is followed by a discussion of Doppler cerebrovascular techniques (Chapter 6), contributed by the editor. Some of the techniques described in Chapter 6 have fallen into disuse with advancement in duplex scanning, but all currently used methods are included for the sake of completeness. The reader may wish to pick and choose among the contents of this chapter, but the editor suggests that the material on the posterior orbital examination and common carotid pulsatility be thoroughly studied. These procedures are an integral part of ultrasound cerebrovascular examination, even with advanced duplex instruments. Other material included in Chapter 6 may or may not be of importance to a given reader, depending on the instrumentation employed in a particular laboratory. State of the art duplex techniques for carotid examination are presented in Chapters 7 and 8. Chapter 9 deals with ultrasound vertebral examination, an area of controversy and clinical neglet. In this Chapter, Dr. White describes the currently available methods for vertebral examination and addresses the controversies surrounding this subject. In Chapter 10, Dr. Bernstein reviews non-ultrasound methods for noninvasive cerebrovascular diagnosis. In addition to describing these techniques, Dr. Bernstein outlines the advantages and limitations of each method and also indicates the potential for incorporation of these procedures with ultrasound studies. The reader is directed, in particular, to Dr. Bernstein's discussion of oculoplethys-mography and digital subtraction arteriography.

Edward B. Diethrich, M.D.

4

Clinical Applications of Noninvasive Cerebrovascular Screening

Diseases of the cerebrovascular system account for almost 200,000 deaths each year in the United States alone. The majority of these deaths is due to atherosclerosis, often aggravated by hypertension. In two-thirds of the people with symptoms of cerebrovascular insufficiency, the lesion lies in the extracranial carotid arterial system, primarily at the bifurcation of the common carotid artery into its internal and external branches. Other sites of potential atherosclerotic involvement include the aortic arch itself or any of its major branches: the innominate, left common carotid, left subclavian, and vertebral arteries.

Until this decade, detection of the atherosclerotic process in the cerebrovascular system had relied largely upon the demonstration of its resultant symptoms. Diagnostic techniques centered around palpation of arteries, auscultation of bruits, radionuclide cerebral blood flow measurements, and electroencephalography. Confirmation of the physician's presumptive diagnosis could be obtained only by aortic arch and cerebral angiography. The problem of accurately localizing atheromatous lesions was compounded by the reluctance to encourage an invasive study and a dearth of reliable noninvasive techniques. If the vascular impairment could not be adequately defined, it presented a major obstacle to prudent therapeutic intervention. Moreover, it was not feasible to consider screening the population for latent disease, which often accounts for sudden death from stroke.

Today, we have progressed impressively. We have at our disposal an array of noninvasive techniques we can employ safely to evaluate the extracranial cerebral vasculature: oculoplethysmography, carotid phonoangiography, ocular pneumoplethysmography, ophthalmosonometry, supraorbital Doppler ultrasonography, Doppler sonographic imaging, B-mode sonographic imaging, and most recently, digital subtraction angiography. These tests have been validated in numerous studies and their diagnostic criteria have been refined to enhance reliability and accuracy.

The use of ultrasound is especially valuable to vascular investigation. Other chapters in this text will review ultrasound techniques as they pertain to cerebrovascular examination. This chapter addresses the clinical applications of noninvasive screening in the detection of the stroke-prone patient.

THE MAGNITUDE OF THE PROBLEM

Death from stroke accounts for 18 percent of all cardiovascular-related fatalities, or about 10 percent of deaths from all causes. Cerebrovascular accidents occur almost equally in men and women, primarily in the elderly, but one-fifth of all strokes strikes persons under 65 years of age. Immediate mortality from stroke is almost 50 percent. Of the survivors, only 10 percent are left unimpaired and 30 percent are no longer capable of independent self-care. Long-term mortality in these people is 16 percent every year for men and 18 percent for women, with stroke being the terminal event in only 25 percent; myocardial infarction, cardiac failure, and other manifestations of the atherosclerotic process are the principal causes of death.[1-4]

Although the mortality for stroke is significant, stroke morbidity is particularly devastating. Cerebrovascular accidents leave many of their victims unable to pursue their normal occupations, and this, in combination with the number of stroke victims requiring chronic care, has a tremendous economic impact. In a single year it is estimated that cardiovascular diseases cost the nation well over $50 billion; certainly, stroke accounts for no small part of this fantastic sum.[2] However, we now have at our disposal diagnostic and therapeutic measures which, if used for screening and early detection in the high-risk population, can significantly reduce these figures.

Stroke Pathogenesis

Most strokes are due to either ischemia or hemorrhage. Cerebral ischemia is caused principally by embolism or thrombosis, while extravasation of blood is due to hypertensive intracerebral hemorrhage and rupture of saccular aneurysms or arteriovenous malformations. Cerebral hemorrhage is far more lethal than ischemic cerebral infarctions, accounting for almost 90 percent of the fatalities from stroke. It is far less common, however; atherothrombotic brain infarction is the most prevalent type of stroke, but it is fatal in only 20 percent of cases.[5]

Hemorrhage.   Intracerebral hemorrhages, the most serious complication of hypertension, may either be massive and fatal or small and compatible with some degree of recovery. Generally, hemorrhages arise from the penetrating branches of the middle cerebral, posterior cerebral, and basilar arteries. Sites of predilection are: putamen, 55 percent; cortex-subcortex, 15 percent; thalamus, 10 percent; pons, 10 percent; and cerebellar hemisphere, 10 percent.[4] As blood extravasates, it follows the path of least resistance, entering the ventricular system in more than 90 percent of cases. Intracerebral hypertensive hemorrhages almost never extends superficially through the cortex to the subarachnoid space. By contrast, ruptured saccular aneurysms, because they generally occur in the major vessels of the circle of Willis, often flood the subarachnoid space. Ischemic infarcts are also a frequent sequela of intracerebral hemorrhage due to aneurysmal rupture.

Embolism. There is conjecture as to the incidence of cerebral embolism as a cause of cerebral infarctions. Some clinicians contend that embolization may account for almost 80 percent of all cerebral infarctions while others maintain that only two to five percent of cerebral infarcts are embolic.[1,4,6] The former estimate seems plausible if one considers that fibrinoplatelet emboli may originate from sites of atherothrombosis and become lodged in vessels already compromised by atheroma, hence the assumption of a thrombosis at the point of occlusion. The heart is also the origin of many cerebral embolic events in cases of atrial fibrillation, valvular disease, and following myocardial infarction. Local emboli, particularly from ulcerative atherosclerotic lesions at the origin of the internal carotids, are common. Almost 90 percent of occlusions in the middle cerebral artery and 75 percent of those in the posterior cerebral artery are due to embolism. By contrast, occlusion of both the internal carotid arteries and the vertebral arteries is generally due to thromboses.

The major etiologic factor in stroke, through, is atherosclerosis. Atherothrombotic brain infarctions occur in men at half the rate of myocardial infarctions, while the incidence in women is the same for both types of infarction. Apparently the immunity to coronary atherosclerosis that women exhibit in the premenopausal years does not affect atherogenesis in the cerebrovascular system.

Atherosclerosis of the cerebral vasculature demonstrates the same proclivity for development in arterial bifurcations, branching and curves as it does elsewhere in the body. In decreasing order of occurrence, the most frequent sites for atheromatous formation in the cerebral circulation (Fig. 4–1) are the common carotid bifurcation in the neck, the lower basilar and upper vertebral arteries at or near their junction, the middle cerebral stem, the posterior cerebral artery as it winds around the cerebral peduncle, the anterior cerebral artery at the level of the corpus callosum, the supraclinoid portion of the internal carotid artery, and the origins of the subclavian, innominate, common carotid and vertebral arteries.[4,6]

Stroke is usually a condition of old age; nonetheless, the chances of a stroke before age 70 years are one in twenty.[3] The tendency for stroke to occur in the elderly is probably due to the relatively late onset and slow progression of atherosclerosis in the cerebrovascular system and the diminution of vascular integrity with advancing age.

Aside from age, the greatest contributor to stroke is hypertension. It plays a role in all major forms of stroke: it accelerates atherosclerosis, not only in the large vessels but also in small branches not usually involved with atherosclerosis in normotension (particularly the deep penetrating branches arising from the middle cerebral stem, posterior cerebral artery and basilar artery). Hypertension damages arterial walls leading to aneurysm formation and rupture, and atherosclerotic materials are more easily dislodged by increased turbulence and flow rates associated with hypertension. Diabetes also undermines vascular integrity, especially at the small-vessel level, and it hastens atherogenesis to the extent that diabetics, particularly those dependent on insulin, suffer an increased incidence of cerebrovascular accidents.

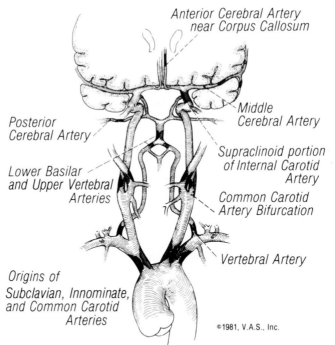

Anterior Cerebral Artery
near Corpus Callosum

Posterior
Cerebral Artery

Middle
Cerebral Artery

Lower Basilar
and Upper Vertebral
Arteries

Supraclinoid portion
of Internal Carotid
Artery

Common Carotid
Artery Bifurcation

Vertebral Artery

Origins of
Subclavian, Innominate,
and Common Carotid
Arteries

©1981, V.A.S., Inc.

Figure 4–1. The cerebrovascular anatomy showing the areas predisposed to atherosclerotic plaque formation.

The wide variation in clinical sequelae to cerebrovascular atherosclerotic occlusive lesions is due to the potential for development of collateral circulation. Of the collateral pathways explained in Chapter 5, the circle of Willis is undoubtedly the most important. There are at least nine congenital variations of this anastomotic ring (Fig. 4-2), but the ones most likely to contribute to a devastating outcome in a stroke are those in which there is no communication between the anterior and posterior circulation or there is vascular isolation of the left and right hemispheric carotid territories.[4,6]

Symptomatology

Two-thirds to three-fourths of the lesions responsible for premonitory signs of stroke are extracranial in location with the intracranial portion of the internal carotid artery, the middle cerebral artery and the vertebrobasilar system following closely thereafter.[5] Inasmuch as atherosclerotic lesions may be either occlusive or ulcerative, it is best to be cognizant of the pattern and location of lesions that give rise to certain symptoms.

Transient cerebral ischemic attacks (TIAs) are the main indicators of cerebrovascular insufficiency, and are significant as hallmarks of impending stroke. TIAs in the carotid and vertebrobasilar territories are different and must be judged independently. Carotid TIAs are more ominous. One-third of patients with carotid distribution TIAs develop completed infarctions within five years, 10 times the risk in the normal population.[3,6] Carotid TIAs have no uniform etiology,

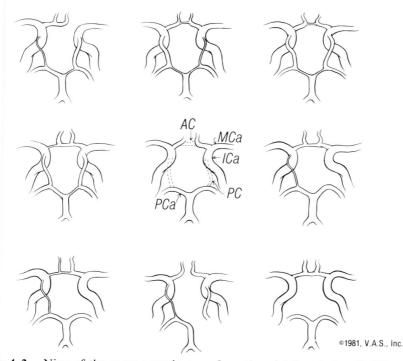

Figure 4–2. Nine of the more prevalent configurations of the circle of Willis, the most important collateral pathway. The center drawing depicts one configuration in which there is no communication between the anterior (AC) and posterior (PC) circulation. MCa = middle cerebral artery, ICa = internal carotid artery, PCa = posterior cerebral artery.

although the majority are associated with carotid atherosclerosis. They are manifested by well-defined hemiparesis, hemianesthesia, or dysphasia. Vertebrobasilar TIAs, on the other hand, are more nebulous; although more common, they are less likely to lead to stroke. They can also continue to recur indefinitely, whereas carotid TIAs either proceed to stroke, usually within two years, or diminish in frequency.[4] Vertebrobasilar TIAs are accompanied by feelings of rotation—vertigo and syncope—but paresthetic events are also common.

By ascertaining the level of brain involvement as reflected by the type of symptom, it is often possible to trace the probable origin. For instance, in the intracranial vasculature, certain vessels demonstrate a predilection for one type of occlusive mechanism over the other. The internal carotid and vertebral arteries are occluded primarily by thrombosis, while the middle and posterior cerebral arteries occlude 75–90 percent of the time by emboli.[6] Assessment of cerebrovascular insufficiency, however, is not an easy matter. Symptoms may be vague, masked by other pathologies or absent altogether. TIAs may arise for any number of reasons, even steal phenomena. In the case of vascular steal, an obstructing lesion induces a pressure gradient that steals blood from surrounding or communicating arteries and induces ischemia at a remote site. This is

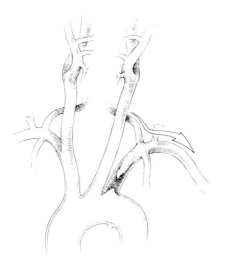

Figure 4–3. Occlusion in the proximal left subclavian artery may produce a steal of blood down the vertebral artery, leading to symptoms of vertebrobasilar insufficiency.

particularly true in lesions of the subclavian artery, in which blood can be stolen from the verebral artery, precipitating signs of vertebrobasilar insufficiency, with or without upper extremity claudication (Fig. 4-3). Moreover, neurologic disorders may elicit symptoms similar to cerebrovascular insufficiency, and this possibility must be entertained.

Collateral circulation, as well, may interfere with evaluation of cerebrovascular disease symptoms. Arterial occlusion may remain asymptomatic due to adequate perfusion by collaterals. In other cases, neurologic deficits due to a thrombosed cortical vessel may clear rapidly because of excellent collateral flow, suggesting an extracranial rather than intracranial occlusion.

A word must be said about the significance of carotid bruits in asymptomatic patients. Although there is controversy, current opinion tends to support the fact that these bruits may portend the development of cerebrovascular insufficiency and stroke and should be investigated noninvasively.[7–9] Unless corroborated by positive noninvasive tests, it is the consensus that asymptomatic carotid bruits are not in themselves an indication for an invasive study.

Clinical Cerebrovascular Evaluation

Evaluation of the cerebrovascular system should begin with a thorough history to define any symptoms and identify risk factors. Preliminary studies involve arterial palpation, auscultation, ophthalmoscopy and bilateral blood pressure recordings. Bilateral, simultaneous palpation of the branches of the external carotid artery (superficial temporal, facial and occipital arteries) is often helpful in identifying stenosis or occlusion of the ipsilateral internal carotid artery; palpation may cause increased collateral flow through the external branch and give rise to increased pulsation. Palpation of the common carotids at the angle of the jaw and low in the neck should be done next with the subclavian arteries and the radial arteries following thereafter. Diminished or absent pulses in the arteries or delayed pulses suggest proximal obstruction.

Auscultation of murmurs in the cervicocranial region should be carried out at the sites that have a propensity for the formation of atheroma, namely the carotid bifurcation, the subclavian-vertebral region, behind the orbits and beneath the mastoids. Murmurs are classified according to timing, duration, pitch, intensity and transmission characteristics, with the last two features and the point of origin being most important. Murmurs originating from the thorax are most often audible at the base of the neck over the common carotids or subclavian arteries. Murmurs in the brachiocephalic trunk transmit along the subclavian artery into the axilla, as well as up the carotid artery into the neck. Bruits in the carotid bifurcation are usually faintly transmitted to the cranial cavity.

The intensity of murmurs does not relate to the degree of stenosis. Intensity increases until the lumen is two-thirds stenosed; after that, the bruit softens, and completely disappears with occlusion. Once a lumen is two-thirds stenosed, the murmur will persist throughout systole: greater stenosis (approximately 90 percent) causes the murmur to fill the diastolic interval as well. Thus, a high-grade stenosis will give rise to a soft, high-pitched murmur that is accentuated during systole and continues into diastole. The following generalizations can also be made: (1) murmurs of high intensity, high pitch, and long duration suggest blood flow high in velocity through a small orifice; (2) low pitch murmurs of a high intensity or volume are generally associated with large orifices through which a large volume of blood is flowing under a high pressure gradient.

Ophthalmoscopy is of use in certain cases of cerebrovascular disease. Microemboli can appear in the retinal arterioles, and the three types are indicative of the level of embolization: (1) fibrinoplatelet emboli, white, cylindrical bodies, originate from mural thrombi in acute or imminent carotid occlusion; (2) cholesterol emboli are large, bright, refractile material usually cast off from ulcerating atheroma at the carotid bifurcation; and (3) calcific emboli, often observed in patients with aortic or mitral valve disease, are gray, ovoid, stationary bodies usually producing retinal infarction. Occlusion in the retinal venules suggests reduced arteriolar perfusion pressure perhaps caused by carotid artery disease. Hypertensive retinopathy and subhyaloid hemorrhages are also hallmarks of the presence of cerebrovascular disease.

Indications for Testing

With the advent of inexpensive, noninvasive testing procedures with established high reliability, it is within the scope of all physicians to provide stroke screening for those patients deemed at risk. To determine the risk, the following should be considered. (1) The majority of strokes are related to atherosclerotic disease, so a personal history of atherosclerotic heart disease or peripheral vascular occlusive disease places the patient immediately at high risk. The coincidence of coronary arterial disease and cerebrovascular disease is not uncommon.[1,3] Further, other cardiac impairments, such as left ventricular hypertrophy or enlargement with poor cardiac function, are precipitous of strokes. It is estimated that 75 percent of stroke patients have cardiac impairment.[3] (2) TIAs and other symptoms of cerebrovascular insufficiency should be investigated aggressively. Appropriate action at this point in the stroke process may well prevent a completed stroke. (3) Hypertension is a primary contributor to stroke. Not only does it aggravate atherosclerotic formations, but is is also the cause of cerebral hemorrhage, the most lethal form of stroke. The incidence of stroke rises dramatically in persons with elevated blood pressure, being proportional to the height of the pressure. (4) Diabetics suffer an increased number of strokes, particularly among those treated with insulin. (5) Other common risk factors for atherosclerotic disease, e.g., lipid levels, obesity, physical activity, smoking, etc., appear to have less relation to stroke occurrence than to coronary arterial disease. (6) The concept of the asymptomatic stroke-prone patient is gaining acceptance rapidly. Clues to the identification of this patient lie in a strong family history of stroke or heart disease, atherosclerotic disease elsewhere in the body, or the auscultation of a carotid bruit. Indeed, any candidate for cardiac, vascular or other major surgery should receive thorough cerebrovascular screening to help prevent the occurrence of a perioperative stroke.

STROKE SCREENING

There is now an array of noninvasive tests suitable for screening the stroke-prone or at-risk patient. Although palpation and auscultation give clues to cerebrovascular stenosis, they do not provide accurate definition of the existence of a lesion. Moreover, occlusions may not be appreciated at all by either method.

Noninvasive cerebrovascular screening tests today are designated as either indirect or direct.[10,11] In the former, the tests rely on hemodynamic alterations in the orbital and supraorbital circulation. Direct tests, as the name implies, examine the accessible portions of the extracranial carotid system, particularly the carotid artery bifurcation, the major site of atherosclerotic lesions in the cerebrovascular system.

The indirect tests include oculoplethysmography (OPG), periorbital Doppler ultrasonography, supraorbital photoplethysmography, opthalmodynamometry and forehead thermography. The first two of these are the most widely used. While these tests are reviewed in Chapter 10, there are several points that deserve comment.

All indirect tests, regardless of type, react to alterations in blood flow or pressure. To produce a detectable hemodynamic effect the diameter of a vessel in the carotid tree has to be reduced by as much as 50 percent,[12] leaving a significant gap in the evaluation of mild to moderate stenosis. At the other end of the spectrum, the tight stenosis cannot be distinguished from an occlusion because the hemodynamic effects of the two are similar. Because some indirect tests measure differentials and not absolute values in pressure or flow, equally severe bilateral disease may not be detected inasmuch as it produces no differential. Lastly, the indirect tests cannot detect nonstenotic ulcerative plaques, a considerable deficit in light of the embolic consequences of these lesions.

For these reasons, the major emphasis in the field of noninvasive cerebrovascular diagnostics has turned to the refinement of the direct investigation of the carotid artery. The original direct test, carotid phonoangiography, is joined by a burgeoning array of ultrasound techniques that are better able to detect the milder, non-flow-reducing changes in the artery.

The new direct tests are based on the use of the continuous or pulsed wave Doppler ultrasound subjected to various types of analyses: flow velocity waveform analysis, frequency spectral analysis, or flow velocity profiling. The introduction of real-time B-mode scanning has allowed visualization of the arterial wall as well, and in tandem with frequency spectral analysis, the resultant duplex scanning is a highly sensitive and specific test far superior to any indirect test.[5,11,13] More detailed information on these direct ultrasound tests appears in chapters 6–8.

In light of current technology, the best approach to stroke screening may lie in a cerebrovascular profile consisting of as many as three to four of the available procedures (mixing both indirect with direct, such as by using oculoplethysmography and carotid phonoangiography (OPG/CPA) supported by duplex scanning or other carotid imaging technique). Sensitivity and specificity are usually quite high with this combined testing system, but inconclusive or discordant results may impact even this highly reliable screening profile.

Aside from screening, noninvasive testing is also quite useful in following the progress of disease in mildly afflicted patients or in periodically reassessing the postoperative patency of endarterectomized vessels. Even in the operating room, B-mode scanning can be used to detect technical fault in the endarterectomy procedure.

DIAGNOSIS AND MANAGEMENT

The decision to proceed with more elaborate testing once the preliminary noninvasive screening procedures are completed is based on the correlation of test results with the patient's symptomatology and history. The construction of a prudent testing scheme is complicated by the variety of tests available, their costs and risks, and the ambiguities of certain cases (e.g., symptomatic patients with positive noninvasive tests, patients with atypical symptoms, patients with a history of atherosclerotic disease, and surgical candidates for vascular reconstruction).

Within the past few years, the development of two new testing procedures have helped immensely not only in clearing the confusion, but in lowering costs and reducing risks by obviating the need for invasive arteriography. As mentioned previously, real-time ultrasound duplex scanning is the best noninvasive test available today for providing anatomic images of accessible arteries (common, internal and external carotids). Adding the spectral analysis of blood flow at selected sites along the arteries overcomes the B-mode scan's deficiencies.

We routinely use duplex scanning to further investigate positive or borderline OPG/CPA findings in both symptomatic and asymptomatic patients. If a high-grade stenosis or occlusion is detected by duplex scanning, the indication for more definitive evaluation is clear. Until a few years ago, standard contrast arteriography was the ultimate in arterial definition. But with the advent of digital subtraction angiography (DSA), an alternative is now available.[11,13,14–17] Whether or not DSA is the technical equivalent of standard arteriography has been the subject of heated debate these last few years.[14–17] Though some investigators have not accepted DSA as a sole diagnostic test for dictating treatment,[14,17] we have found that a clear, high resolution DSA film low in artifacts offers more than sufficient documentation on which to base a surgical decision. We use the procedure routinely wherever possible to avoid invasive arteriography, although the latter is still applicable in patients whose symptoms indicate intracranial disease (cerebral hemispheric ischemia with reversible neurologic deficits or small, completed infarcts). DSA has also proven useful in avoiding an invasive procedure in ambiguous cases, particularly the asymptomatic patient with bruit and positive or inconclusive ultrasound findings of significant disease.

Should intravenous or intraarterial arteriography testify to the presence of a significant atherosclerotic lesion, surgical removal of the atheroma should be contemplated. A candidate for carotid endarterectomy must be thoroughly tested for coincident coronary arterial disease, inasmuch as the mortality associated with the operative procedure is due largely to myocardial infarction.[18] The timing and staging of the endarterectomy is also a consideration.

In the case of bilateral disease, endarterectomies are usually staged a few days apart, with the artery supplying the nondominant hemisphere or contributing less to the intracranial fill being done first. Carotid endarterectomy with contralateral internal carotid artery occlusion is a more hazardous procedure, but results are usually good. In the case of severe coronary arterial disease, the likelihood of a perioperative event in the carotid or coronary system should be determined, and it should be decided whether the carotid lesion should be addressed primarily, or if simultaneous operations should be performed.

It should be remembered that carotid endarterectomy is largely a prophylactic procedure, although it does provide symptomatic improvement of TIAs in 85 percent of patients.[1] There is a high morbidity and mortality connected to the procedure in patients with acute, progressive stroke. Moreover, less than desirable results have been obtained in patients with completed strokes. Hence, the endarterectomy is useful only as a preventive measure to circumvent a cerebrovascular accident in the stroke-prone patient.

However, surgery is not always possible. For inaccessible lesions that are producing TIAs, medical therapy may be of help. Today, platelet inhibitors are used to reduce the embolization of fibrinoplatelet aggregates from ulcerated plaques. Both aspirin and sulfinpyrazone have been studied in this regard, but the results are not encouraging.[18] While the occurrence of TIAs in patients thus treated is reduced, the drugs do not appear to offer protection against stroke. Anticoagulant therapy has been used in the past, but its risk of hemorrhagic complications makes antiplatelet therapy more attractive. Risk-factor reduction should also be undertaken, directed primarily to control of hypertension and reduction of cholesterol levels. Intervention in this fashion is showing great promise in reducing the incidence of strokes and myocardial infarctions.

SUMMARY

Death from disease in the cerebrovascular system is due primarily to atherosclerosis aggravated quite often by hypertension. Surgically accessible lesions in the extracranial vasculature are responsible for over two-thirds of the symptoms of cerebrovascular insufficiency. Yet, it was not until recently that we had at our disposal reliable, noninvasive diagnostic techniques that could localize these lesions, making possible more timely surgical intervention, more judicious use of arteriographic procedures, and routine screening for latent disease.

Strokes, which account for almost 200,000 deaths per year, are due to either ischemia or hemorrhage. The pathogenesis of stroke has been described, and a detailed discussion of symptomatology and its evaluation has been offered. The diagnosis of cerebrovascular disorders requires a thorough clinical evaluation and knowledge selection of appropriate noninvasive testing procedures. Criteria for selection of surgical candidates, a discussion of carotid endarterectomies, and alternative medical therapies have been reviewed in this chapter.

Edward B. Diethrich, M.D.
Medical Director
Arizona Heart Institute
P.O. Box 10,000
Phoenix, AZ 85064

REFERENCES

1. Callow AD: An overview of the stroke problem in the carotid territory. Am J Surg 140:181–190, 1980
2. Heart Facts, Dallas, American Heart Association, 1984
3. Kannel WB, Wolf PA: Risk factors in atherothrombotic cerebrovascular disease, in Meyer JS (ed): Modern Concepts of Cerebrovascular Disease. New York, Spectrum Publications, 1975. pp 113–134
4. Marshall J: The natural history of cerebrovascular disease, in Meyer JS (ed): Modern Concepts of Cerebrovascular Disease, New York, Spectrum Publications, 1975, pp 53–62
5. Jackson VP, Bendick, PJ, Becker GJ: Duplex carotid ultrasound. Indiana Med J 77:22–24, 1984
6. Fisher CM: Anatomy and pathology of the cerebral vasculature, in Meyer JS (ed): Modern Concepts of Cerebrovascular Disease. New York, Spectrum Publications, 1975, pp 1–43
7. Dorazio RA, Ezzet R, Newbitt NJ: Long-term follow up of asymptomatic carotid bruit. Am J Surg 140:212–213. 1980
8. Heyman A, Wilkinson WE, Heyden S, et al: Risk of stroke in asymptomatic persons with cervical arterial bruits. N Engl J Med 302:838–841, 1980
9. Wolf PA, Kannel WB, Sorlie P, et al: Asymptomatic carotid bruit and risk of stroke. JAMA 245:1442–1445, 1981
10. Abernathy M, Brandt MM, Robinson C: Noninvasive testing of the carotid system. AFP 29:157–171, 1984
11. Yao JST, Flinn WR, Bergan JJ: Noninvasive vascular diagnostic testing: Techniques and clinical applications. Prog Cardiovasc Dis 26:459–494, 1984
12. May AG, VandeBerg L, DeWeese JA, et al: Critical arterial stenosis. Surgery 54:250–256, 1963
13. Glover JL, Bendick PJ, Jackson VP, et al: Duplex ultrasonography, digital subtraction angiography, and conventional angiography in assessing carotid atherosclerosis. Arch Surg 119:664–669, 1984
14. Folcarelli D, Eikelboom BC, Riles JS, et al: Pitfalls of carotid artery surgery based on digital subtraction angiography. Bruit 7:13–17, 1983
15. Lusby RF, Ehrenfeld WK: Carotid artery surgery based on digital subtraction angiography. Am J Surg 144:211–214, 1982
16. Myerowitz PD: Digital subtraction angiography: Present and future uses in cerebrovascular diagnosis. Clin Cardiol 5:623–629, 1982
17. Russell JB, Watson JM, Modi JR, et al: Clinical use of digital subtraction angiography for evaluation of extracranial carotid occlusive disease. A comparison with standard arteriography. Surgery 94:604–611, 1983
18. Meyer JS: Medical and surgical treatment of cerebrovascular disease, in Meyer JS (ed): Modern Concepts of Cerebrovascular Disease. New York, Spectrum Publications, 1975, pp 159–178

Edward B. Diethrich, M.D.

5

Normal Cerebrovascular Anatomy and Collateral Pathways

The vascular system of the human brain differs significantly both anatomically and physiologically from other organs in the body. Although it accounts for only 2 percent of the body weight, the brain receives 15 percent of the cardiac output and consumes 20 percent of the body's oxygen supply in the basal state.[1] Cerebral arteries are little influenced by sympathetic nerves, unlike other arteries, but they are markedly affected by chemical changes in the blood.

Obstructive disease afflicting the cerebrovascular system can produce a wide array of sometimes ambiguous symptoms. Clinicians must attempt to identify the exact areas involved in the disease process; however, this is often made difficult by individual variability in the cerebral vasculature. Indeed, the extent of clinical symptomatology is entirely dependent on the ability of the collateral circulation to maintain adequate cerebral perfusion. Therefore, understanding the normal and collateral anatomy and the mechanisms of cerebral blood flow is essential to the diagnosis of obstructive disease in the cerebrovascular system.

This chapter addresses the anatomical and physiologic principles that influence the investigation of the vascular supply to the brain. It is important to stress the significance of appreciating the hemodynamics of the brain. Individuals vary considerably in their ability to compensate for alterations in cerebral blood flow, and the physician must be aware of the potential mechanisms for cerebrovascular collateralization in order to carry out a judicious evaluation protocol.

VASCULAR ANATOMY

The brain is supplied directly by four vessels: the two internal carotid arteries and the vertebral arteries. Any discussion of the cerebrovascular system must begin at the origins of these vessels, because obstructive disease, stenoses,

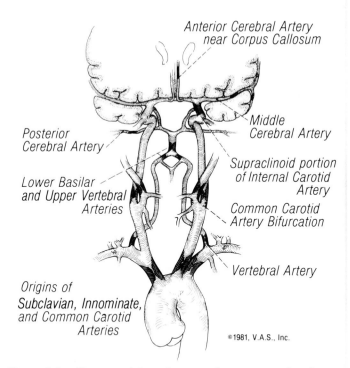

Anterior Cerebral Artery
near Corpus Callosum

Middle
Cerebral Artery

Posterior
Cerebral Artery

Supraclinoid portion
of Internal Carotid
Artery

Lower Basilar
and Upper Vertebral
Arteries

Common Carotid
Artery Bifurcation

Vertebral Artery

Origins of
Subclavian, Innominate,
and Common Carotid
Arteries

©1981, V.A.S., Inc.

Figure 5-1. Extracranial cerebrovascular anatomy showing the areas predisposed to atherosclerotic plaque formation.

ulcerative plaques or anomalies anywhere in the cerebrovascular tree may produce a stroke or symptoms of insufficiency.

The blood supply for the central nervous system[1-3] derives from the three great vessels arising from the aortic arch in the superior mediastinum: the innominate, the left common carotid and the left subclavian arteries (Fig. 5-1). The innominate artery travels upward, slightly posteriorly from the arch to the right of the neck for its 4–5-cm length, dividing into the right common carotid artery and the right subclavian artery at the upper border of the right sternoclavicular junction. The left common carotid artery ascends from the arch and passes beneath the left sternoclavicular joint. Neither common carotid has collateral branches, but each divides into the internal and external carotid arteries at the level of the upper border of the thyroid cartilage.

The internal carotids supply most of the anterior circulation to the cerebrum (Fig. 5-2). In their cervical portion, the internal carotid arteries may be relatively straight or may curve tortuously as they travel to the base of the skull. There are no branches of the internal carotid arteries in the neck. As they proceed intracranially, the internal carotid arteries give rise to the caroticotympanic branches in the petrous bone, the meningohypophyseal branches in the cavernous sinus region and the ophthalmic arteries immediately distal to the cavernous sinus. Eight millimeters beyond the clinoid process, within the dura mater, the internal carotid arteries give rise to the posterior communicating arteries, which joins with the posterior cerebral arteries. Further cephalad, the internal carotid

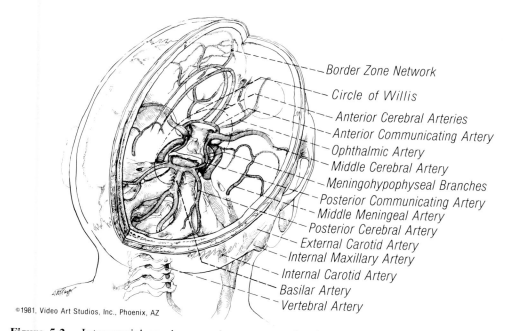

Border Zone Network
Circle of Willis
Anterior Cerebral Arteries
Anterior Communicating Artery
Ophthalmic Artery
Middle Cerebral Artery
Meningohypophyseal Branches
Posterior Communicating Artery
Middle Meningeal Artery
Posterior Cerebral Artery
External Carotid Artery
Internal Maxillary Artery
Internal Carotid Artery
Basilar Artery
Vertebral Artery

©1981, Video Art Studios, Inc., Phoenix, AZ

Figure 5-2. Intracranial cerebrovascular anatomy showing anastomotic connections of the circle of Willis. Note that the principal blood supply to intracranial structures is via the carotid arteries.

arteries divide into the middle and anterior cerebral arteries and give rise posteriorly to the anterior choroidal arteries.

The external carotid arteries normally supply no blood to the brain. However, several of their branches can become important collateral pathways should occlusion occur in the internal carotid or vertebral arteries. The branches of the external carotid artery are the ascending pharyngeal, the superior thyroid, the lingual, the external maxillary, and occipital, the facial, the posterior auricular, the internal maxillary, the transverse facial and the superficial temporal arteries. The external carotid branches most vital to collateral circulation are those in communication with the ophthalmic artery, and those that interconnect between the muscular branches of the occipital and vertebral arteries (Fig. 5-3).

The posterior circulation to the brain is supplied in large part by the vertebral arteries arising from the subclavian arteries. The vertebrals lie within the foramina transversaris of the upper cervical vertebrae and wind anteriorly into the subarachnoid space at the side of the medulla oblongata at the level of the atlanto-occipital interspace. They proceed cephalad and anteriorly until they reach the pontomedullary level, where they join to form the basilar artery. Four branches arise from the basilar artery as it courses upward before dividing into the posterior cerebral arteries. Branches of the basilar artery supply the entire pons and the superior and anterior aspects of the cerebellum. Branches of the vertebral arteries supply the medulla and the interior surface of the cerebellum.

The cerebral branches of the internal carotids and vertebral arteries are joined at the base of the brain by an arterial circle known as the *circle of Willis*.

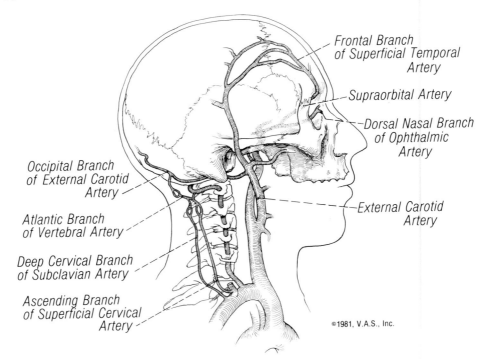

Frontal Branch
of Superficial Temporal
Artery

Supraorbital Artery

Dorsal Nasal Branch
of Ophthalmic
Artery

Occipital Branch
of External Carotid
Artery

Atlantic Branch
of Vertebral Artery

Deep Cervical Branch
of Subclavian Artery

Ascending Branch
of Superficial Cervical
Artery

External Carotid
Artery

©1981, V.A.S., Inc.

Figure 5-3. Extracranial cerebrovascular anatomy. Note the anastomotic connections between the external and internal carotid and between the occipital, cervical, and vertebral arteries.

This anatomosis is the most important element in intracranial collateral circulation and is also a common site of aneurysmal formation. It is a hexagonal arrangement of arteries composed of the anterior, middle and posterior cerebral arteries, which are joined together by the anterior and posterior communicating arteries (Fig. 5-2). Under normal circumstances, there is usually little mixing of blood via the communicating arteries. However, in instances of arterial occlusion in the carotid or vertebrobasilar vessels, this circle opens to function as a vital collateral pathway, as will be discussed later.

Component arteries of the circle of Willis can vary greatly in size, and there are at least nine congenital variations in the structure of the circle (Fig. 5-4). The most common anomalies involve absence or hypoplasia of one or both communicating arteries. Anomalous origin of the posterior cerebral artery from one or both internal carotid arteries has also been commonly encountered. Anomalies in the anterior portion of the circle are less commonly found, although among these, absence or hypoplasia of the proximal segment of the anterior cerebral artery between the internal carotid and anterior communicating arteries is more usual. Among the variations, the most significant in terms of decreasing collateral potential are those in which the anterior or posterior communicating arteries are absent or impervious. These conditions may isolate the anterior and posterior circulations or the left and right hemispheric carotid territories.

Anomalous formations can also occur in the extracranial circulation, most commonly involving the origins of the carotid and vertebral arteries. Most

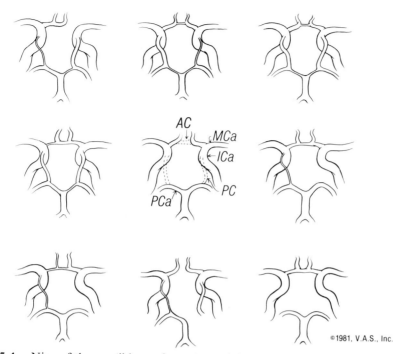

Figure 5-4. Nine of the possible configurations of the circle of Willis, the most important collateral pathway. The center drawing depicts one configuration in which there is no communication between the anterior (AC) and posterior (PC) circulation. MCa, middle cerebral artery; ICa, internal carotid artery; PCa, posterior cerebral artery;.

frequent is a close association between, or a sharing of the origin of, the innominate artery with the left common carotid artery. Less often, the left common carotid artery may arise from the innominate artery. Also seen is the anomalous origin of the left vertebral artery on the aortic arch between the left common carotid and subclavian arteries. Rarely, the right subclavian artery may have an aberrant origin on the aortic arch. Other abnormalities may occur in the cervical region, such as agenesis of the internal carotid arteries, but these are quite rare. Abnormalities in the vertebral arteries are usually limited to variations in size between the left and right, a common occurrence.

CEREBRAL HEMODYNAMICS

Before discussing the potential collateral pathways in the cerebrovascular system, it is best to explain the dynamics of cerebral blood flow[1,4] to help gain an appreciation of the importance of collateralization.

Despite the brain's large apportionment of the body's blood supply (15 percent of the cardiac output), there is little circulatory reserve, owing to the brain's high metabolic rate. Furthermore, the brain has no significant oxygen or glucose stores, making it entirely dependent upon the vascular system for maintenance.[1,2] This is the reason that even short episodes of interrupted cerebral flow can bring on symptoms of cerebral dysfunction, and cellular death can occur within 3 to 8 minutes of vascular failure.

Extrinsically, cerebral blood flow varies with the effective arterial perfusion pressure. Adequate perfusion relies upon systemic blood pressure, cardiac output and blood volume. Within the range of fluctuation possible for these extrinsic factors, blood flow can be modulated by a group of intrinsic factors that control cerebral vascular resistance. Among these factors are intracranial pressure, arterial oxygen tension, carbon dioxide tension, blood viscosity and vascular tone. Although the cerebral vessels are supplied with nerves, there has been little evidence that they play other than a minor role in controlling blood flow. Oxygen and carbon dioxide concentrations play the greatest roles in modulating cerebrovascular resistance, with carbon dioxide being the more significant factor.

Variations in cerebral blood-gas concentrations serve to provide constant blood flow within a wide range of systemic pressures and also provide local control to areas with varying demands.[1] For instance, if the brain requires more oxygen than is being supplied, it produces more carbon dioxide. This increase in carbon dioxide causes vasodilatation and increases blood flow until enough oxygen has been supplied to reduce the carbon dioxide concentration. This effect can happen either globally or locally.

Compensatory cerebral vasodilatation is also the mechanism that maintains cerebral blood flow when cerebral perfusion pressure drops as a person assumes an upright position. However, if the circulation is compromised by atherosclerotic disease, compensation may be insufficient, leading to symptoms of regional or diffuse hypoxia or anoxia.

COLLATERALIZATION

The vital role of collateral circulation in vascular occlusion has been appreciated for more than a century; however, its interplay in cerebrovascular occlusive disease has become an important diagnostic consideration only in the last two or three decades, helped largely by the advent of angiography and, later,[4-6] by noninvasive diagnostic techniques. Clinicians evaluating symptoms of cerebrovascular insufficiency and surgeons contemplating ligation of cervical arteries must be aware of the potential for collateral circulation and its influence on diagnostic tests and surgical procedures.

It was once believed that arteries in the brain were end arteries but it is now known that capillary and precapillary anastomoses are common. To better appreciate these collateral pathways, it should be noted that there are two types of arterial branches supplying the brain. The more important type in terms of neuronal function and nutrient supply for the central nervous system is the penetrating arteries. However, it is the diffuse circumferential or superficial arteries that spread over the entire surface of the cervical hemispheres, brain stem and spinal cord through which collateral circulation takes place. The circle of Willis and the major arterial trunks are included in this superficial system.

The routes for intracranial collateral circulation can be divided into three categories: large interarterial connections, intracranial-extracranial anastomoses and small interarterial communications (Figs. 5-2 through 5-5). The major pathway is the circle of Willis, providing communication between the two carotid arteries or between the basilar artery and either the right or left carotid artery. As described earlier, the anatomic variations possible within this arterial circle are normally of little importance unless occlusion in one of the cervical vessels occurs, demanding collateral blood flow.

Second only to the circle of Willis in importance is the complex intracranial-extracranial or pre-Willisian anastomoses. Perhaps the best known pre-Willisian anastomosis is that between the external and internal carotid arteries, via the orbital and ophthalmic arteries. Other external-to-internal carotid collaterals include the meningohypophyseal and caroticotympanic branches. Other important pre-Willisian anastomoses may be encountered clinically, including the following: (1) the occipital branch of the external carotid artery in communication with the atlantic branch of the vertebral artery; (2) the deep cervical and ascending cervical branches of the subclavian artery connecting with branches of the lower vertebral artery, the atlantic branch of the upper vertebral artery and the occipital branch of the internal carotid artery; and (3) the external carotid arteries communicating across the midline. Also included in the pre-Willisian group is the rete mirabile, or "wonderful net" of transdural anastomoses across the subdural space from the dural arteries to arteries on the surface of the brain.

Of lesser importance are the leptomeningeal collaterals forming the meningeal border-zone network. These connect the terminal cortical branches of the main cerebral arteries across the border zones along each vascular territory. Although these are not major collateral pathways, they may be sufficiently developed to interfere with the diagnosis of cerebrovascular insufficiency. Indeed, arterial occlusions may not become symptomatic because of adequate perfusion by the leptomeningeal anastomoses in the portion of the thrombosed artery's distribution. Likewise, excellent collateral flow around a thrombosed cortical vessel may induce rapid clearing of a neurologic deficit, leading the clinician to believe an extracranial occlusive process is involved.

It should be noted that there are no effective anastomotic pathways between neighboring cerebral artery branches, deep penetrating arteries, or the superficial and deep branches of the cerebral arteries.

The opening of collateral pathways is dependent largely upon the age of the individual and the time sequence of occlusion. In older individuals, collateral pathways are more likely to be hypoplastic or involved in the atherosclerotic process. Even collateral vessels of sufficient luminal size will not often be able to adapt rapidly enough to sudden occlusions, such as from embolism. Hence, collateral flow has a better chance of developing adequately in persons with slowly evolving atherosclerotic occlusions. When multiple atherosclerotic lesions are present, the adequacy of the collateral channels may be greatly lessened. Also affecting the adequacy of a collateral bed are the availability of multiple rather than single collateral sources and pathologic conditions of the vessels, reducing their capacity for dilation.

Extracranially, there are numerous cervicocranial collaterals. Occlusion of an internal carotid produces collateral circulation to the carotid siphon via the external carotid and ophthalmic artery (Fig. 5-5). The anterior and middle cerebral arteries in this case are also supplied from the opposite anterior cerebral artery and the posterior cerebral artery through the anterior and posterior communicating arteries. In the case of vertebral occlusion near its origin (Fig. 5-6), flow is shunted to the thyrocervical and costocervical axes with compensatory enlarge-

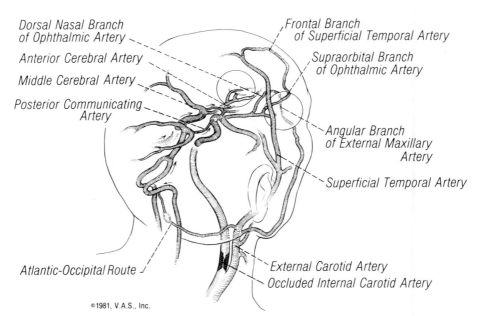

Figure 5-5. Major external carotid and vertebral collateral pathways associated with internal carotid occlusion.

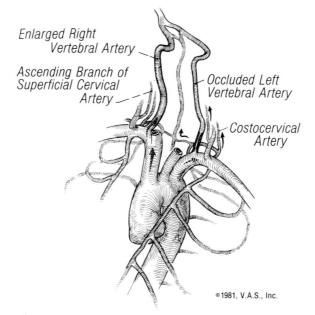

Figure 5-6. Major collateral pathways in vertebral occlusion.

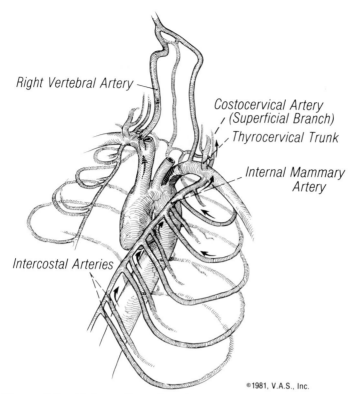

Right Vertebral Artery

Costocervical Artery
(Superficial Branch)

Thyrocervical Trunk

Internal Mammary
Artery

Intercostal Arteries

©1981, V.A.S., Inc.

Figure 5-7. Major collateral pathways in proximal subclavian occlusion.

ment of the opposite vertebral artery. Collateral circulation arising from occlusion of large branches of the aortic arch is through the intercostal and internal mammary arteries to the subclavian, and then through the branches of the thyrocervical and costocervical axes to the vertebral and carotid arteries (Fig. 5-7).

The simplest method of juding intracranial collateral potential is through a 5-minute common carotid compression test. If no changes are noted in consciousness, speech, extremity strength or fine finger control, then collateral flow can be judged sufficient. More specific information can be obtained by combining carotid compression with serial arteriography, electroencephalography, cerebral blood-flow measurement, ophthalmodynamometry or Doppler ultrasonography. Arteriography is a somewhat risky procedure and offers no hemodynamic data, but it does delineate the collateral flow pattern. Carotid compression with electroencephalographic (EEG) monitoring offers a more discrete endpoint, with the earliest signs of ischemia on the ipsilateral side indicating faulty collateralization. Isotopic measurement of cerebral blood flow, offering data on blood flow at the capillary level, can predict the tolerance of carotid ligation fairly well. If the cerebral blood flow is decreased by 25 percent or more during carotid ligation, then hemiparesis can be expected.

Carotid compression during ophthalmodynamometry or oculoplethys-mography can determine the collateral ophthalmic artery pressure, helpful in evaluating flow dynamics in the carotid and vertebral systems. Doppler ultrason-ography can be used to determine the direction of blood flow through the ophthalmic artery and also the lumen size of the internal and external carotid arteries. Collateral circulation, however, can interfere with sonographic results. For instance, ophthalmic flow can be in the normal anterior direction, even with an occluded internal carotid artery, owing either to stenosis of the ipsilateral external carotid artery or collateral circulation from the contralateral carotid artery through the circle of Willis or the internal maxillary artery. Variations in collateralization may also be responsible for differences in peak Doppler shift frequencies among individuals.

SUMMARY

The vascular system of the human brain can be afflicted by obstructive disease, which produces a variety of oftentimes nebulous symptoms. In attempt-ing to evaluate these symptoms and define the areas of disease involvement, the clinician must have a thorough knowledge of the vascular anatomy and an appreciation of the individual variability that may be encountered. The physician must also be cognizant of cerebral hemodynamics and the availability of collateral flow to interpret test results and characterize symptoms and arrive at an accurate diagnosis.

This chapter presents an in depth review of normal cerebrovascular anatomy and commonly encountered anomalies with a discussion of hemodynamics as it applies to the potential for collateralization. Commonly encountered extra- and intracranial collateral pathways have been defined along with methods of assess-ing the collateral flow.

Edward B. Diethrich, M.D.
Medical Director
Arizona Heart Institute
P.O. Box 10,000
Phoenix, AZ 85064

REFERENCES

1. Stephens RB, Stilwell DL: Arteries and Veins of the Human Brain, Springfield, IL, Charles C Thomas, 1969
2. Anson BJ, Maddock WG: Callander's Surgical Anatomy, Philadelphia, WB Saunders, 1958
3. Gray H: Anatomy of the Human Body, Phil-adelphia, Lea & Febiger, 1954
4. Meyer JS (ed): Modern Concepts of Cerebro-vascular Disease, New York, Spectrum Books, 1975
5. Fields WS, Breutman ME, Weibel J: Collat-eral Circulation to the Brain, Baltimore, Wil-liams & Wilkins, 1965
6. Strandness DE, Jr: Collateral Circulation in Clinical Surgery, Philadelphia, WB Saun-ders, 1969

William J. Zwiebel, M.D.

6

Doppler Cerebrovascular Techniques

Duplex sonography has become the predominant mode for ultrasound examination of the carotid arteries, and with good reason. The duplex technique combines physiological Doppler data with anatomical information supplied by the B-mode image in a way that is unique among ultrasound diagnostic techniques. The advantages of the duplex approach have made obsolete some Doppler techniques, but the reader should not be left with the idea that all "pure" Doppler methods have been superceded by duplex evaluation. The posterior orbital study and assessment of common carotid pulsatility, as described in this chapter are extremely valuable procedures that should be performed in the course of every duplex carotid examination. The periorbital examination, also described in this chapter, serves the same function as the posterior orbital study, namely, detection of external carotid collateral flow. Because the periorbital examination is difficult to perform, it has fallen into disuse and discussion of this test is included primarily for completeness.

The final technique described in this chapter is Doppler carotid imaging, which has proven to be quite accurate for detection of cervical carotid stenosis and occlusion. This technique has largely been supplanted by duplex imaging, but it remains in clinical use and is an effective diagnostic tool.

The reader may wish to pick and choose among the material contained in this chapter but the author strongly suggests that all readers become familiar with, and use routinely, the posterior orbital study and procedures for assessing common carotid pulsatility as described herein.

NONIMAGING DOPPLER TECHNIQUES

Nonimaging Doppler instruments (usually continuous-wave) may be used in the carotid circulation to detect external carotid collateral flow and to evaluate common carotid pulsatility. The Doppler component of a duplex instrument may be used to examine common carotid pulsatility, utilizing the same procedures as described herein for a nonimaging Doppler device. The duplex instrument cannot be used to assess external carotid collateral flow, however, unless a nonimaging Doppler transducer is included with the device.

Two procedures have been described for detecting external carotid collateral flow, the periorbital examination of Brokenbough[1] and the posterior orbital study of Spencer.[2] These are the only noninvasive tests, other than digital subtraction angiography, capable of detecting external carotid collateralization. As noted above, the posterior orbital examination is preferred for detecting external carotid collateral flow because it is more easily performed than the periorbital study. A second reason for favoring the posterior orbital technique is that it more directly

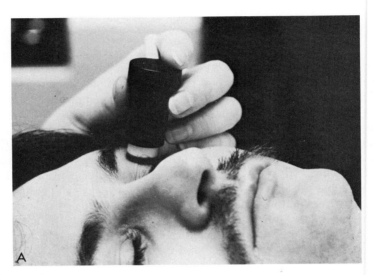

Normal

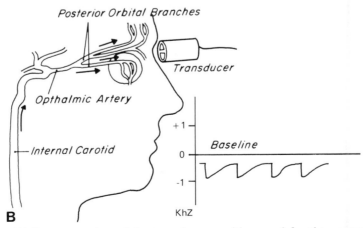

Figure 6-1. (A) Demonstration of the transducer position used for the posterior orbital examination. (B) Flow in the ophthalmic artery and its posterior orbital branches normally is directed out of the orbit, toward the transducer, producing downward deflections on the

interrogates ophthalmic artery flow than the periorbital examination. The latter principally examines the external carotid circulation. This distinction will become more clear upon reading the descriptions of these procedures.

Posterior Orbital Examination

The posterior orbital examination is based on detection and assessment of blood flow in the ophthalmic artery or its branches in the back of the orbit (Fig. 6-1). The examination requires a deeply focused, directional Doppler instrument with a relatively low frequency output (usually 4 or 5 MHz). The Doppler system must include a recording device capable of demonstrating flow velocity wave forms and flow direction, such as an analog, zero crossing recorder (see Chapter 1) or a digital frequency spectrum display.

Posterior Orbital Technique

A small amount of acoustic couplant is applied to the transducer, which is placed in contact with the closed eyelid. The ultrasound beam is directed into the orbit with medial angulation of approximately 15° to the body axis (Fig. 6-1A). Medial angulation of greater than 30° should be avoided, since excessive angulation renders directional information unreliable.[2] By carefully moving the transducer about in this general orientation, signals are detected from the ophthalmic artery or its branches in the posterior region of the orbit. As an aid for stabilization of the transducer, it is useful to rest the palm of the hand on the patient's forehead

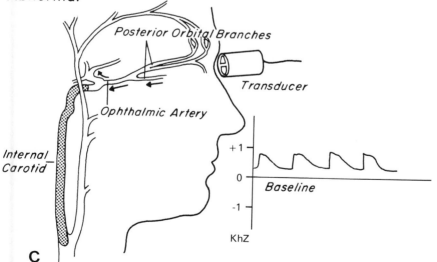

Doppler recording. (C) With internal carotid obstruction, posterior orbital flow is reversed and upward deflections are seen on the Doppler spectrum. Damped or biphasic signals may also occur with internal carotid obstruction.

as shown in Figure 6-1A. Also, the patient should be instructed to look toward the side opposite that being studied to avoid attenuation of the ultrasound beam by contact with the lens.

Interpretation of Posterior Orbital Signals

Flow in the ophthalmic and posterior orbital arteries is normally directed out of the orbit, toward the transducer and results in a downward deflection, with each heartbeat, on the recording device (Fig. 6-1B). (The convention is to display flow toward the transducer with downward deflections and flow away from the transducer with upward deflections.) Reversed posterior orbital flow (upward deflection) indicates external carotid collateral circulation (Fig. 6-1C), and the amplitude or frequency shift of the reversed signal roughly indicates the magnitude of collateral flow. Signal reversal should always be scrutinized carefully, however, since spurious flow reversal can occur when an abrupt curvature is present in the ophthalmic artery or when venous flow is mistaken for an arterial signal.[2] Whenever reversed signals are encounterd, one should search for another transducer position in which strong, normal-appearing, forward-flow signals are present. Such signals, if detected, should be regarded as the correct flow direction. Furthermore, arterial flow should be clearly pulsatile and should not vary in amplitude with respiration as venous flow does. Since orbital veins drain intracranially (into the cavernous sinus) a false impression of external carotid collateral flow may occur when venous signals are detected.

Bidirectional posterior orbital signals may occur in some cases of internal carotid occlusion. Spencer[2] believes that bidirectional signals result from simultaneous detection of forward flow in the posterior orbit and reversed flow in the anterior portions of the orbit. The downward component of the recorded signal is supplied by ophthalmic flow and the upward component by an external carotid branch. Damped posterior orbital signals indictate intracranial or ophthalmic artery flow reduction. The amplitude (strength) and frequency shift of a damped signal is abnormally low as compared with the contralateral posterior orbital signal, and the systolic waveform is broad with a sloping upstroke (Fig. 6-2). This type of signal, as well as very weak or absent posterior orbital flow, may occur when carotid siphon pressure is decreased due to carotid obstruction but collateralization has not developed. Alternatively, weak or absent signals may indicate ophthalmic artery occlusion.

Any deviation from a pattern of strong, forward posterior orbital flow with a sharp initial systolic component should be regarded with suspicion, and correlative abnormality in other segments of the ultrasound examination should be sought. Errors in detection of external carotid collateral flow can, in general, be avoided if both the posterior orbital and periorbital examinations (described below) are performed in every patient. However, to perform both studies is quite time consuming and we have used the periorbital examination only to confirm or refute questionable posterior orbital findings. The results of the peri- and posterior orbital examinations should coincide; if they do not, the sonographer should be immediately alerted to the possibility of error and should attempt to determine which examination is correct.

Posterior orbital flow will remain normally directed in the presence of

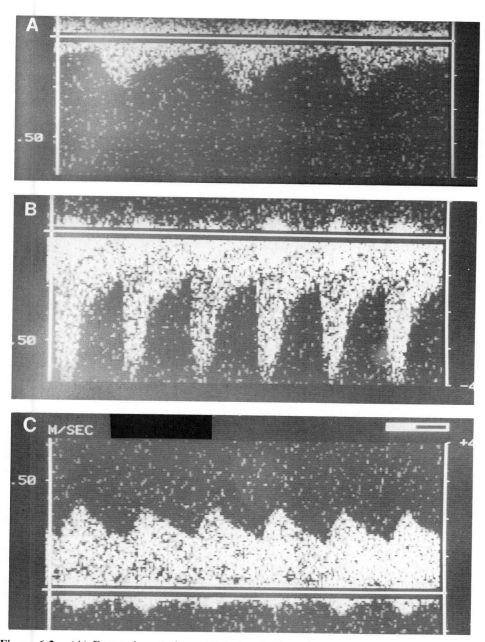

Figure 6-2. (A) Damped posterior orbital signal. Note the sloping initial component of the waveform (moving from left to right) and the relatively low frequency (height) of the waveform in comparison (B) to the contralateral normal posterior orbital signal. (C) Reversed, high volume posterior orbital flow.

hemodynamically significant internal carotid disease if satisfactory intracranial collateral circulation exists. In our experience, one-third of patients with occlusion of the internal carotid (a lesion of unquestionable hemodynamical significance) do not exhibit external carotid collateral flow.[3] Internal carotid obstruction may be predicated with the periorbital examination in the absence of external carotid collateral flow if common carotid compression maneuvers are used. The transducer is positioned to detect the posterior orbital signals and the ipsilateral common carotid is briefly (two or three heartbeats) occluded by digital compression. Normally, posterior orbital flow is significantly decreased, ceases, or, rarely, reverses direction with compression. If a severe internal carotid lesion exists but is compensated for by intracranial collateral flow, the posterior orbital signals will be unchanged by ipsilateral common carotid compression. In such cases, compression of the contralateral common carotid will severely diminish, terminate, or reverse the direction of the posterior orbital flow. If no change in the posterior orbital flow occurs with either ipsilateral or contralateral common carotid compression, intracranial collateral circulation has its origin in the vertebrobasilar system.

Both Barnes[4] and Brokenbough[1] have attested to the safety of carotid compression maneuvers. Only three transient neurologic deficits occurred in 5000 patients subjected to carotid compression in their experience. It is suggested, nonetheless, that compression be performed by a physician rather than a sonographer. Compression at the base of the neck is recommended, since the common carotid is accessible and relatively immobile at this point, and risk of dislodging atheromatous material is reduced. The safety of a common carotid compression can be enhanced greatly if B-mode imaging is used to detect plaque at the compression site. The compression maneuver should be excluded when major disease is evident.

In spite of the apparent safety of the common carotid compression maneuvers, we have not used this technique very often, because information from direct carotid examination (Doppler imaging or duplex) usually supplants that obtained through common carotid compression.

Periorbital Flow Assessment

The periorbital examination of Brokenbough is another method for detecting external carotid collateral flow and, thereby, for identifying hemodynamically significant internal carotid obstruction.[1,4] External carotid collateral flow is manifested with this technique through altered flow patterns in the distal (periorbital) branches of the ophthalmic artery. These branches arborize onto the forehead and anastomose there with external carotid branches. Normally, flow in the periorbital branches is directed out of the orbit and onto the forehead (Fig. 6-3A). If pressure in the carotid siphon and ophthalmic artery is reduced because of internal carotid blockage, two basic changes in periorbital flow may be observed. First, flow reversal may be detected in the periorbital branches, if external carotid collateral circulation is well established (Fig. 6-3B). Second, lowered ophthalmic-artery pressure may prevent periorbital flow from compensating for a sudden cessation of external carotid flow, induced by the examiner. This second change will be demonstrable even if external carotid collateral circulation is not strongly developed.

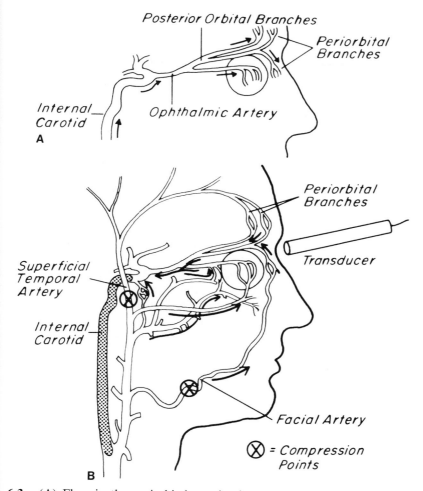

Figure 6-3. (A) Flow in the periorbital arteries is normally directed out of the orbit. Terminal periorbital branches anastomose with the external carotid branches on the face. (B) In the presence of a hemodynamically significant internal carotid obstruction, flow may reverse in the periorbital vessels. In other cases, flow out of the orbit may persist, but alterations in the periorbital signal will be detectable (see text). X's in panel B indicate points at which digital compression is applied to external carotid branches during the periorbital study.

Periorbital Technique and Instrumentation

The Doppler periorbital study is performed with a 10-MHz, superficially focused transducer. A directional instrument is preferred, since it allows direct detection of flow reversal, but a directional Doppler is not essential, since external carotid/ophthalmic artery flow dynamics can be adequately evaluated with a nondirectional device.

Flow signals must first be located through careful manipulation of the

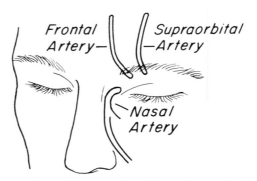

Figure 6-4.   Illustration of the location of the major periorbital vessels.

transducer over the periorbital vessels as they emerge from the orbital margin. Two branches, the frontal and supraorbital arteries (Fig. 6-4), are of particular interest and are routinely studied.

The frontal artery is located in the angle formed by orbital rim and the nose, and is found by placing the transducer near the inner canthus of the eye and gently moving it about until arterial signals are heard. The signals are then followed toward the orbital rim where the transducer is held in place over the artery (Fig. 6-5A). The supraorbital artery lies in the supraorbital notch, which can be readily palpated along the upper margins of the orbit (Fig. 6-5B). Once arterial signals are obtained in either the frontal or supraorbital artery, the transducer must be carefully held in place, because very slight movement will alter signal strength and character. Transducer stabilization is aided by gripping the probe between the tips of the fingers and thumb while resting the base of the hand on the forehead (Fig. 6-5), as described previously.

Periorbital Interpretation

The parameter first evaluated with a directional Doppler is periorbital flow direction, which can be recorded with a strip chart recorder or a directional frequency spectrum analyzer. For accurate determination of flow direction, care must be taken to point the transducer more or less into the orbit. Normally, flow should be out of the orbit (toward the transducer), and each arterial pulse should produce a downward deflection on the recording device. If strong, clearly reversed flow signals are obtained, external carotid collateral circulation may be tentatively diagnosed. Tortuosity of the periorbital arteries or improper direction of the transducer can cause spurious flow reversal, however.

The presence of flow reversal should always be confirmed by means of external carotid compression maneuvers. *These maneuvers constitute the entire periorbital examination if a nondirectional Doppler is used or if flow reversal is not detected initially.* With the Doppler transducer stabilized over one of the periorbital branches, digital pressure is applied sequentially with the free hand to the ipsilateral and contralateral facial and superficial temporal branches of the external carotid arteries. The facial artery is found by palpation along the lower border of the mandible (Fig. 6-6A), and the superficial temporal artery can be

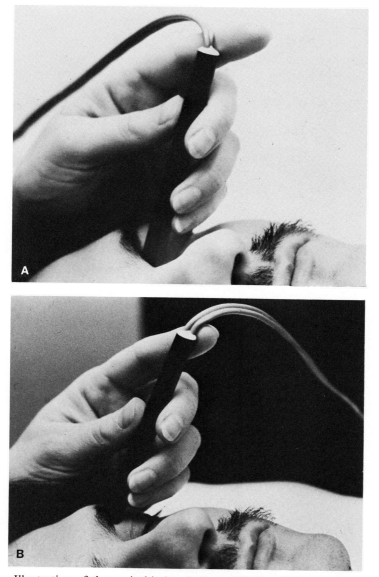

Figure 6-5. Illustration of the periorbital technique. (A) Transducer position for frontal artery examination. (B) Transducer position for supraorbital artery examination.

located in front of the ear and directly above the temporomandibular joint (Fig. 6-6B). It is important to locate these arteries at the beginning of the study, since it is very difficult to stabilize the Doppler transducer over the supraorbital vessel with one hand while searching for the facial and temporal pulses with the other. Normally, as each facial or temporal branch is compressed, the Doppler signal from the periorbital vessel should increase in amplitude (strength) and/or frequency, owing to enhanced flow out of the orbit (Fig. 6-7A), or should remain

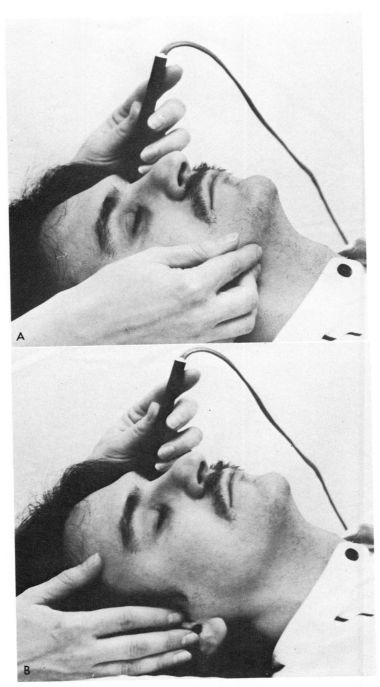

Figure 6-6. Periorbital compression maneuvers. (A) The facial artery is compressed as it courses around the mandible. (B) The superficial temporal branch is compressed immediately in front of the ear.

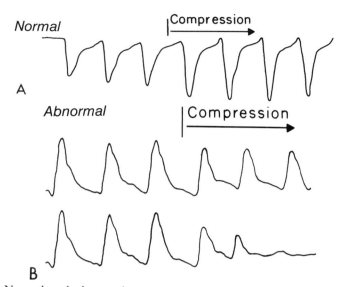

Figure 6-7. Normal and abnormal responses to compression maneuvers. (A) Normal periorbital flow is toward the transducer, producing downward deflections on the recording device with each pulse (inverted signals may occur in normal patients as discussed in the text). Facial or temporal artery compression either results in no change or increased strength of the signal (augmentation). (B) In the presence of severe internal carotid artery obstruction, compression maneuvers may cause diminution or cessation of flow, as shown.

unchanged. In the presence of external carotid collateral flow, the amplitude and/or frequency of the signal will be drastically reduced, or the signal will cease (Fig. 6-7B). If collateral flow is not well developed, or if pressure in the carotid siphon is only moderately reduced, the decrease in amplitude occurring with compression may be subtle. Normal and abnormal findings are summarized in Table 6-1.

To better understand the normal and abnormal responses to external carotid compression, imagine a patch of skin on the forehead supplied jointly by periorbital and external carotid branches. Compression of an external carotid branch reduces blood supply to the skin, but compensation for this reduction occurs normally via enhanced flow through the periorbital vessel. The strength of the periorbital Doppler signal increases, therefore, when the external carotid branch is compressed. If, however, carotid siphon and ophthalmic artery pressure is abnormally low, or blood is actually flowing retrograde through the periorbital branches to supply the brain, compensation for loss of external carotid supply will not be possible. Instead, a decrease in strength or cessation of periorbital Doppler signals will occur when the exernal carotid supply is terminated by digital occlusion. When an external carotid branch is compressed that does not supply blood to the area of skin in question, no change in the periorbital Doppler signal will occur. It may happen that only one of the four principal external carotid branches is the source of collateral flow. Therefore, abnormal periorbital findings

Examination Technique

Pulse velocity tracings used for evaluating carotid flow resistance may be obtained with a nonimaging Doppler transducer or a duplex instrument. The angle of incidence of the sound beam relative to the flow vector does not influence pulsatility findings since the ratio of systolic and diastolic flow velocities is important rather than absolute velocity measurements. Although qualitative assessment of pulsatility may be conducted with a simple zero-crossing flow meter the inherent inaccuracies of this device render it useless for quantitative pulsatility determination. In our experience, frequency spectrum analysis is essential for accurate assessment of carotid pulsatility. Furthermore, good quality flow tracings that reflect velocities along the diameter or in the center of the lumen are also essential for accurate pulsatility determinations. If signals are obtained off axis, near the vessel wall, inaccurate results are likely, since flow resistance near the vessel wall is greater than at mid stream. Furthermore, flow must be sampled in relatively disease-free segments of the common carotid, since luminal narrowing and turbulence will affect pulsatility patterns.

Examination Pitfalls

Caution should be exercised in interpreting pulsatility findings, since the overall status of cardiovascular physiology may profoundly effect the pulse-velocity tracing. Elevated peripheral resistance and pulse pressure in hypertensives may increase pulsatility in the absence of internal carotid obstruction. Spurious elevation of the pulsatility may, in addition, occur with tachycardia and diffuse peripheral vascular disease, and absence of diastolic flow may occur in low cardiac output states. Abnormal pulsatility should be symmetrical in these conditions, whereas, asymmetrical abnormality always suggests obstructive disease.

On several occasions, we have observed normal common carotid pulsatility in patients with severe internal carotid obstruction and very well developed external carotid collateral flow. It is possible, therefore, for external carotid collateral circulation to be of sufficiently low resistance to produce a normal common carotid pulsatility pattern. This should not pose a diagnostic problem, however, since the posterior orbital examination will easily detect external carotid collateral circulation in such patients.

DOPPLER IMAGING OF THE CAROTID BIFURCATION

The following discussion of Doppler imaging techniques will probably not be of interest to individuals who are using duplex instruments rather than Doppler imaging devices. The reader may wish, therefore, to skip ahead to Chapter 7, which is devoted to duplex carotid evaluation.

Examination of the cervical carotid vessels is possible with a hand-held Doppler transducer and is relatively simple in some patients. In other individuals, however, hand-held carotid Doppler examination is extremely difficult, primarily because of problems with sorting out the vascular anatomy at the carotid bifurcation. Pioneers in the field of carotid sonography used hand-held transducers to interrogate the carotid arteries, but the technical difficulties of this method quickly led to the development of Doppler imaging devices that produce maps of the carotid vessels.

Several continuous-wave and pulsed Doppler systems for imaging the cervical carotid vessels have been developed. All are similar in that they use a position-sensing device, coupled with a Doppler flowmeter, to create a two-dimensional picture of the carotid bifurcation (Fig. 6-11). The instruments differ to the extent that pulsed-Doppler is used in some systems and continuous-wave Doppler in others. Pulsed-Doppler systems offer the advantage of range gating that can be used to exclude unwanted signals from overlying veins. All Doppler imaging devices produce a relative crude image of the bifurcation (Fig. 6-12A), which is not diagnostic of and by itself, except in cases of vascular occlusion. All other diagnoses are based on abnormalities detected in the Doppler flow signal, and the image is used only for localization of flow abnormalities.

It is important at this point to distinguish between Doppler and duplex imaging. First, and most important, Doppler devices image flowing blood and thus reveal only the vessel lumen, which is crudely displayed. Duplex sonography, on the other hand, images the vessel wall with precise detail, including deposited plaque (Fig. 6-12B). Second, Doppler instruments in general provide physiological information about blood flow, while duplex devices supply both anatomical and physiological information. Finally, Doppler images are produced manually by repeated movement of the transducer across the vessel to "build up" an image on the display screen. With Duplex imaging, the sound beam is rapidly swept across the vessel by mechanical or electronic means to produce an instantaneous view of an entire segment of the vessel.

As noted earlier, duplex scanning is gradually replacing Doppler imaging techniques; nonetheless, Doppler imaging remains in use, and is an accurate and relatively inexpensive method for detecting carotid stenosis and occlusion.

Doppler Bifurcation Imaging Techniques

A typical Doppler carotid imaging device is schematically illustrated in Figure 6-11A. A deeply focused Doppler transducer (usually 4 or 5 MHz) is attached to a rigid arm, at a fixed angle of 60° from the body axis. The other end of the arm is attached to a set of potentiometers, which electronically link the position of transducer-arm assembly to the XY coordinates of a storage oscilloscope or TV monitor. This arrangement serves to orient the transducer in two dimensions. The location of arterial flow can accordingly be "mapped out" by moving the transducer up and down across the artery and gradually following the vessel along its course in the neck. The location of the carotid vessels may be ascertained by listening to the Doppler signals and simply following the arteries cephalad, but the mapping process is facilitated by an electronic gating system that activates the electron beam of the display screen only in areas where arterial flow is present. The operator establishes a threshold Doppler frequency shift corresponding to systolic flow velocity. With the threshold set, the electron gun of the display screen is switched on only during the systolic portion of the cardiac cycle and the image is written on the screen only in areas where arterial velocities are encountered. Areas of venous flow or other extraneous Doppler shifts are excluded from the image. With the threshold appropriately adjusted, a small

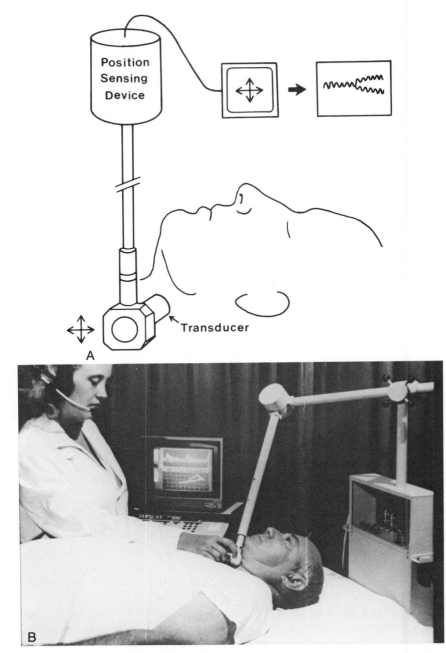

Figure 6-11. (A) Schematic diagram of the Doppler imaging system. The transducer is attached to a position sensing device. Horizontal or vertical movements produce proportionate deflections of the electron beam of the recording device. Bifurcation anatomy may be traced with this system as described in the text. (B) Photograph of a commonly used Doppler imaging system (DOPSCAN, courtesy of Carolina Medical Electronics, Inc., King NC).

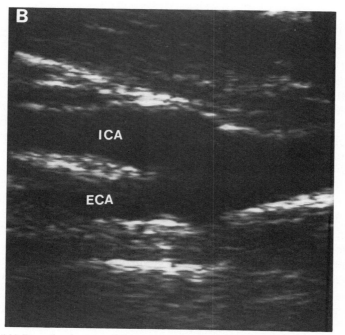

Figure 6-12. (A) Doppler image of the carotid bifurcation. The oblique line at the left of the image represents the border of the mandible. (B) B-mode carotid bifurcation image. ICA, internal carotid artery; ECA, external carotid artery.

portion of the vessel is imaged each time the transducer is moved up or down across the vessel lumen. Repeated adjustment of the threshold setting may be required with some devices in which the threshold is influenced both by the strength of the Doppler-shifted signals and by flow velocity.

The carotid mapping procedure is usually performed with the patient supine and the head gently extended (Fig. 6-11B). Having the patient lower the shoulder helps expose as much of the common carotid as possible. Mapping is begun with the common carotid at the clavicle and is continued cephalad to the common carotid bulb and from there into each of the bifurcation branches. It is important to search for a characteristic drop in Doppler frequencies and/or disturbed flow (Fig. 6-13; color plate 1) that identifies the bulbous portion of the common carotid artery. In many patients, the proximal internal and external carotid are superimposed on the image, and by knowing the position of the common carotid bulb, one may ascertain that an obstructive lesion is distal to the bifurcation rather than at it. Unfortunately, the decrease in frequency at the bulb will not occur when the lumen is narrowed by plaque, and this circumstance may result in improper localization of atheromatous lesions. Close attention should also be given to the pulsatility pattern in the bifurcation branch vessels. In all cases, the characteristic difference in flow resistance in the external and internal carotid described earlier in the chapter should be obvious in the audible signals or sonographic images. Observation of this difference in pulsatility ensures proper identification of the internal and external carotid as well as proper localization of diseased segments.

Imaging Pitfalls

Strongly attenuating atheromatous plaque can result in low-amplitude (weak) or absent Doppler signals over a portion of the carotid bifurcation and lead to considerable difficulty in mapping the carotid vessels. When this problem occurs, it is helpful to locate arterial signals farther distal in the external and internal carotid near the mandible and to follow the vessels back from that point to their junction with the common carotid. On other occasions, seemingly discontinuous segments of several vessels may be located, but assemblage of the bifurcation anatomy may be impossible. This difficulty usually occurs in the presence of: (1) major atheromatous disease of the bifurcation branches, (2) cervical collateral vessels, or (3) nearly occluded carotid segments with severely reduced flow. Apparent discontinuity of vascular anatomy may also occur in normal patients, however, because of vessel tortuosity and overlapping. In other normal or abnormal patients, portions of the arterial anatomy may be difficult to identify because the vessels lie deeply within the neck, out of the range of the transducer. This problem is especially likely to occur in obese individuals or those with short, "thick" necks. Since imaging difficulties may arise in both abnormal and normal individuals, one should not automatically conclude that a vessel is occluded when a flow signal cannot be heard. It is important to scrutinize common carotid pulsatility and periorbital/posterior orbital studies for evidence supporting or refuting the presence of occlusion.

A number of other pitfalls can occur with carotid bifurcation imaging.[3] Of principal importance, superimposition of the external and internal carotid arteries in the coronal plane can create a false impression of carotid occlusion—the internal carotid is usually assumed to be obstructed (Fig. 6-14). This error can be

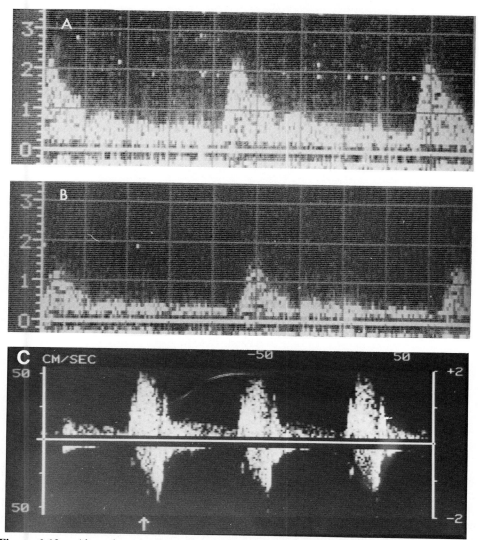

Figure 6-13. Alterations in flow observed in the bulbous portions of the common and internal carotid. (A) Waveform recorded from the "tubular" portion of the common carotid. (B) Waveform in the bulbous portion of the common carotid (same patient as in A. Note the reduced height of the signals corresponding to diminished velocities in the widened portion of the carotid vessel. (C) Biphasic flow observed at the junction of the common and internal carotid due to "swirling" of blood. Reversed flow or turbulence are common normal findings in this area.

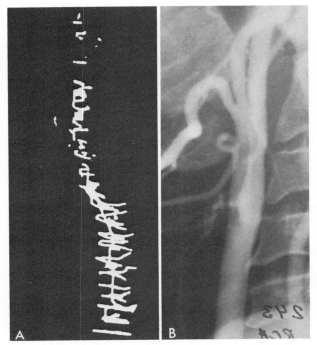

Figure 6-14. Superimposition causing false-positive diagnosis of internal carotid occlusion. (A) Only one vessel was detected through Doppler flow examination. (B) A lateral carotid arteriogram demonstrates superimposition of the external and internal carotid arteries. (From Zwiebel WJ, Crummy AB: Sources of error in Doppler diagnosis of carotid occlusive disease. AJR 137:231–242, 1981. With permission.)

easily eliminated if one finds a normal pulsatility profile in the ipsilateral common carotid and absence of external carotid collateral flow. The elusive vessel can usually be imaged by obliquing the patient's head to one side or another and rescanning the bifurcation to uncover the missing branch. A similar problem arises when the branch vessels lie immediately adjacent to one another, but this difficulty may be obviated by carefully imaging each branch based on high or low resistance characteristics evident in the Doppler shifted signals.

Significant error also may occur when the internal carotid is occluded and external carotid branches are mistaken for the normal bifurcations (Fig. 6-15). The principal means of preventing this mistake is to closely scrutinize the pulse-velocity characteristics of the Doppler signals heard in each of the bifurcation branch vessels. A distinct difference between the low- and high-resistance flow of the internal and external carotid should always be evident as mentioned previously. These characteristics may be detected aurally in the Doppler audio ouput or visually with frequency spectral analysis. To facilitate comparison of the signals in the branch vessels, the sonographer should routinely record short

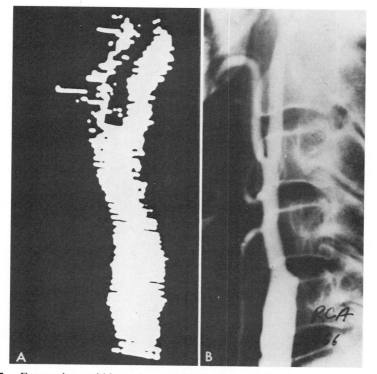

Figure 6-15. External carotid branches mimicking the carotid bifurcation. Comparison of the bifurcation image (A) and a lateral arteriogram (B) clearly indicates that external carotid branches were mistaken for the carotid bifurcation, resulting in false-negative diagnosis of internal carotid occlusion. (From Zwiebel WJ, Crummy AB: Sources of error in Doppler diagnosis of carotid occlusive disease. AJR 137:231–242, 1981. With permission.)

segments of Doppler signals, first in the external carotid, and then in the internal carotid. If external carotid characteristics are noted in both branch vessels, one should immediatly be suspicious that the internal carotid has not been imaged, and correlative findings should be sought in the common carotid pulsatility, as well as in the posterior or periorbital flow studies.

Another error of major significance that may occur with Doppler imaging is false-positive diagnosis of occlusion in the presence of very severe internal carotid stenosis with only a "trickle" of residual flow (Fig. 6-16). Flow velocity in a tiny internal carotid lumen may be too slow to be detected with the Doppler device and the vessel may be deemed occluded. The resulting error is particularly important because a potentially correctable stenosis is mistaken for an irremediable occlusion. The opportunity of surgically restoring flow in such cases might be denied if no further diagnostic evaluation is performed. This error is of clinical importance when either the common or internal carotid is mistakenly assumed to be occluded, but the latter situation is by far the more frequent. Detection of an abnormal resistivity index or of external carotid collateral flow does not help resolve this diagnostic dilemma, since these tests will be abnormal either in the presence of

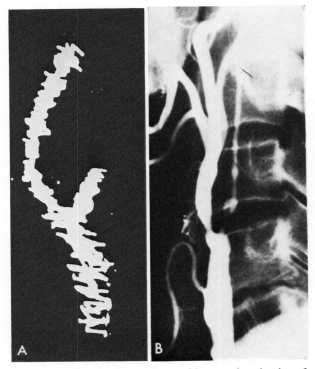

Figure 6-16. Severe internal carotid stenosis mistaken for occlusion. (A) Doppler examination indicated absence of flow in the area of the internal carotid. (B) Arteriography (performed 1 day later) demonstrates sluggish flow in a small caliber internal carotid lumen. (From Zwiebel WJ, Crummy AB: Sources of error in Doppler diagnosis of carotid occlusive disease. AJR 137:231–242, 1981. With permission.)

occlusion or severe internal carotid stenosis. B-mode imaging also is not helpful (see Chapter 7), since it is very likely that the tiny residual lumen will not be identified with currently available B-mode techniques. One must bear in mind, therefore, that the carotid Doppler study is a screening test and that all significantly abnormal studies including suspected occlusion, should be subjected to definitive diagnosis via arteriography, if the patient is thought to be a surgical candidate.

A final source of difficulty in carotid Doppler imaging is detection of more than two vessels at the carotid bifurcation. This problem is most commonly caused by imaging the internal carotid and two external carotid branches. In this circumstance, it is relatively simple to map the anatomy by noting which vessels exhibit high- or low-resistance flow characteristics. In other instances, the anatomic arrangement can be difficult or impossible to sort out, especially when seemingly discontinuous vessels are identified, when the Doppler signals are weak, or when one cannot be sure of differences in resistance patterns among the vessels. Careful scanning technique and correlation with common carotid pulsatility and periorbital or posterior orbital findings may document the patency and normality of vessels.

In some patients, the ultrasound results may remain uncertain despite the best effort of the sonographer, and such studies must be reported as nondiagnostic or equivocal.

Flow Signal Recording

The usual Doppler imaging technique is to first image the bifurcation and then carefully record the Doppler flow signals. The recording of flow signals is customarily begun at the clavicle and continued cephalad to the carotid bulb and sequentially into the bifurcation branches. Several methods for recording the Doppler signals are available. (1) Doppler frequency spectra may be recorded on film or on heat-sensitive paper at predetermined arterial sites as well as in areas where the sonographer detects abnormal flow, (2) flow-velocity information may be color-coded and displayed directly on the carotid bifurcation image. The color-coded image may be documented with still photography or continuously recorded on video tape in conjunction with the audible Doppler signals, (3) with more advanced systems, the bifurcation image, the audible Doppler signal, the frequency spectrum, and the sonographer's comments may be simultaneously recorded on videotape (Fig. 6-17; and Color plate 2).

Regardless of the recording method employed, abnormal flow signals must be localized as carefully as possible. The Doppler flow abnormalities of primary

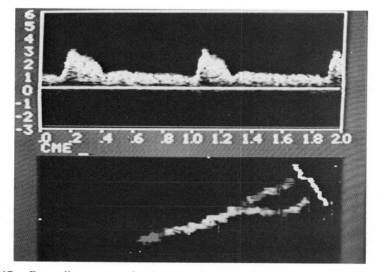

Figure 6-17. Recording system for Doppler imaging. The frequency waveform is illustrated in the upper panel and the bifurcation image at the bottom of the screen. A cursor (not visible) appears on the bifurcation image at the location from which the Doppler signals emanate. The combined frequency spectrum and bifurcation image may be recorded in real-time on videotape or may be "frozen" and recorded on hard copy images. (DOPSCAN, courtesy of Carolina Medical Electronics, Inc., King, North Carolina.)

Table 6-2
Reported Results, Doppler Imaging of the Carotid Arteries

Author	Barnes et al[9] 1976	Berry et al[10] 1980	O'Leary et al[11] 1981	Doorly et al[12] 1982	Wasserman et al[13] 1983
n vessels	82	226	216	190	132
n stenoses	25	83	107	53	56
% stenosis*	≥50	≥50	≥50	≥50	≥50
Sensitivity	92%	89%	96%	94%	89%
Specificity	70%	83%	91%	95%	91%
Accuracy	73%	85%	94%	95%	90%
Positive Predictive Value	47%	67%	91%	88%	89%
Negative Predictive Value	95%	95%	96%	98%	92%

* diameter reduction

importance are absence of flow, increased flow velocity, and turbulence. Through careful analysis of flow signals both aurally and with frequency spectral analysis, one can accurately diagnose occlusion and stenosis with Doppler imaging devices as indicated by the published results summarized in Table 6-2. A detailed description of Doppler flow signal analysis in normal and abnormal vessels is provided in Chapters 3 and 7. Those individuals using Doppler imaging devices should review all pertinent material in these chapters. It should also be noted that the Doppler imaging examination should always be accompanied by assessment of common carotid pulsatility and Doppler techniques for detection of external carotid collateral flow, as described in the preceding portions of this chapter.

CASE STUDIES

Case 6-1

A 71-year-old man was examined because of occasional episodes of light-headedness and a three-month history of persistent numbness on the right side of the face in a V1 and 2 distribution. Bruits were noted in the vicinity of both carotid bifurcations. The carotid Doppler findings are presented in Figure 6-18. What is your impression? Pay attention to the information on the data sheet (Fig. 6-18A).

Discussion. Posterior orbital flow is reversed on the left side and this finding is corroborated by abnormalities in the left periorbital study (see data sheet Fig. 6-18A). Common carotid pulsatility is abnormal bilaterally (Fig. 6-18D and E). Note that the common carotid spectra were obtained with a 10-MHz probe, accounting for the relatively high frequencies observed as compared with spectra

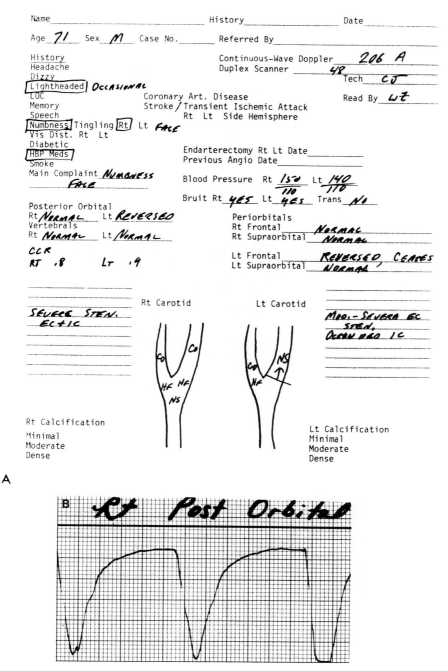

Name_____ History_____ Date_____

Age _71_ Sex _M_ Case No._____ Referred By_____

History   Continuous-Wave Doppler _206 A_
Headache   Duplex Scanner _____ _48_
Dizzy   Tech _CJ_
[Lightheaded] _Occasional_
LOC   Coronary Art. Disease   Read By _wt_
Memory   Stroke / Transient Ischemic Attack
Speech   Rt Lt Side Hemisphere
[Numbness] Tingling [Rt] Lt _Face_
Vis Dist. Rt Lt
Diabetic
[HBP Meds]   Endarterectomy Rt Lt Date_____
Smoke   Previous Angio Date_____
Main Complaint _Numbness_
Face   Blood Pressure Rt _150_ Lt _140_
                                            _110_   _110_
                           Bruit Rt _yes_ Lt _yes_ Trans _No_
Posterior Orbital
Rt _Normal_ Lt _Reversed_   Periorbitals
Vertebrals   Rt Frontal_____
Rt _Normal_ Lt _Normal_   Rt Supraorbital _Normal_
                                             Normal
CLR   Lt Frontal_____ _Reversed, Ceases_
RT _.8_   Lt _.9_   Lt Supraorbital _Normal_

_____   _____
Severe Sten. Rt Carotid   Lt Carotid   _Mod.-Severe EC_
_EC + IC_   _Sten._
_____   _Occlu Pro IC_
_____   _____
_____   _____
_____   _____

Rt Calcification   Lt Calcification
Minimal   Minimal
Moderate   Moderate
Dense   Dense

A

Figure 6-18. Case 6-1. (A) Data sheet. (B) right posterior orbital tracings.

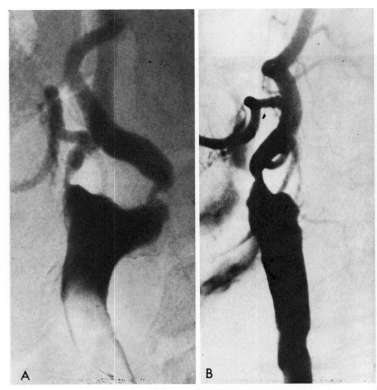

Figure 6-19. (A) Right and (B) left lateral carotid arteriograms.

shown in Figure 6-20D and E. On the right side, abnormal common carotid pulsatility (RI = 0.82) might be the result of systemic hypertension (see data sheet Fig. 6-18A), but on the left, diastolic flow is nearly zero and the tracing clearly is abnormal. The bifurcation images (Fig. 6-18F and G) show two branches on the right and only one branch on the left. Very high frequency signals are present at the right bifurcation. Since these exceed 12 KHz in systole, and diastolic flow is also very high, the findings indicate a stenosis of critical hemodynamic significance. Note on the data sheet (Fig. 6-18A) that the high-frequency signals (HF) on the right side are diffusely heard and that coarse sounds (Co) due to turbulence extend into both branch vessels. The latter finding suggests that the stenosis is at the common carotid bulb or involves both branches. Posterior orbital flow on the right side is not reversed, even though it appears that a hemodynamically significant lesion is present. One would not expect, however, to find external carotid collateral flow in the presence of a significant stenosis of either the common carotid or both the internal and external carotid. At the left bifurcation, one should conclude that the internal carotid is either very severely stenosed or occluded because only one branch is observed, external carotid collateral flow is present and common carotid pulsatility is abnormal. Moderate frequency elevation is observed in the remaining branch on the left side (see data sheet, Fig. 6-18A). Peak frequencies in this area were 8 KHz (no sonogram available), and this level of increased velocity is consistent with a moderate but not critical stenosis.

Arteriography (Fig. 6-19) confirms the Doppler findings. Note that on the right both the external and internal carotid are severely stenosed and that the left internal carotid is occluded. A minor stenosis is present in the left external carotid.

Case 6-2

A 56-year-old man presented with a two-month history of episodic blurred vision involving the left eye. A soft bruit was heard in the vicinity of the right carotid bifurcation. The Doppler findings are presented in Figure 6-20. Note information included on the data sheet (Fig. 6-20A). What is your diagnosis?

Discussion. First, note that left posterior orbital signals are weak and abnormal in appearance. (Fig. 6-20C). The sonographer questioned whether these signals were reversed or biphasic (see data sheet, Fig. 6-20A). Also, the left periorbtial examination is abnormal (see data sheet, Fig. 6-20A), with weak,

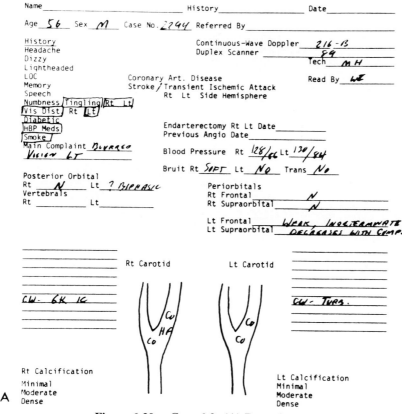

Figure 6-20. Case 6-2. (A) Data sheet.

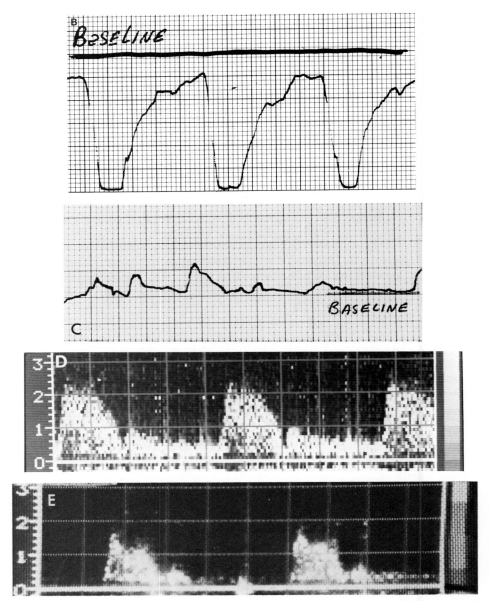

Figure 6-20. *(Continued)* (B) right and (C) left posterior orbital tracings. (D) right and (E) left common carotid sonograms.

indeterminate frontal artery signals and an abnormal response to compression during left supraorbital artery examination. Left common carotid pulsatility is also grossly abnormal (Fig. 6-20E). In spite of these findings, the left bifurcation image (Fig. 6-20G) is unremarkable and the sonographer noted only minor turbulence in the internal carotid orifice ("Co," data sheet, Fig. 6-20A). At the right carotid bifurcation, two distinct vessels are demonstrated with mild frequency elevation

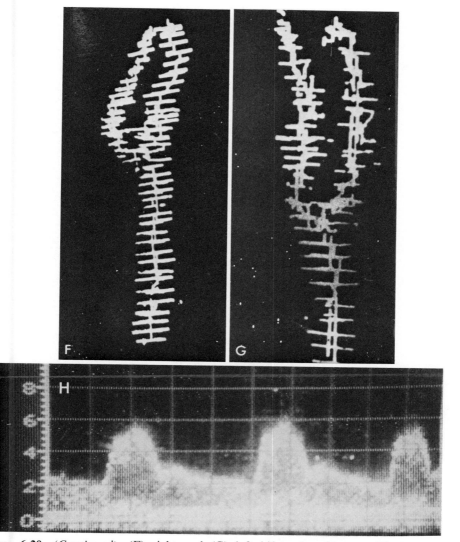

Figure 6-20. *(Continued)* (F) right and (G) left bifurcation images. (H) Frequency sonogram, proximal right internal carotid.

(6 kHz) in the internal carotid branch (Fig. 6-20H). This finding is consistent with a nonhemodynamically significant stenosis. Normal right common carotid pulsatility (Fig. 6-20D) and normal right posterior and periorbital studies support the impression of a nonhemodynamically significant lesion.

Arteriography (Fig. 6-21) demonstrates a minor stenosis of the right internal carotid as predicted. Note that the left carotid bifurcation contains fairly extensive plaque but only minor stenosis. Severe stenosis is present in the left carotid siphon and the left middle cerebral artery is occluded (Fig. 6-21C). This case illustrates the value of "indirect" Doppler examination of the carotid system.

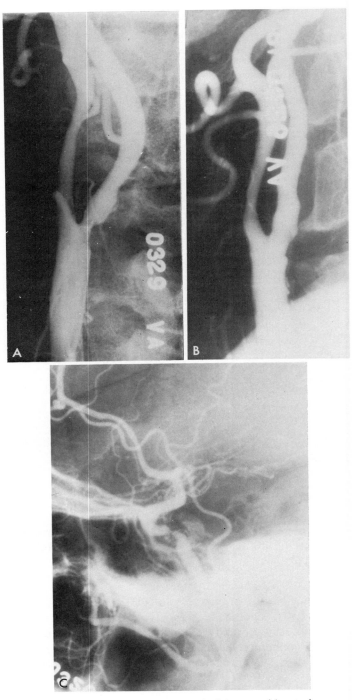

Figure 6-21. (A) anteroposterior and (B) lateral right carotid arteriograms. (C) Lateral ateriogram of the distal left internal carotid artery and cerebral branches.

Even though the intracranial abnormalities cannot be examined directly, their presence is revealed by extracranial flow abnormalities.

William J. Zwiebel, M.D.
Associate Professor of Radiology
University of Utah School of Medicine
and
Chief, Ultrasound and Body CT
Veterans Administration Medical Center
500 Foothill Drive
Salt Lake City, Utah 84148

REFERENCES

1. Brokenbough EC: Periorbital velocity evaluation of carotid obstruction. In Bernstein EF (ed): Noninvasive Diagnostic Techniques in Vascular Disease. St. Louis, C.V. Mosby, pp 212–220, 1978

2. Spencer MP: Technique of Doppler examination. In Spencer MP, Reid JM (eds): Cerebrovascular Evaluation with Doppler Ultrasound. The Hague, Martinus Nijoff Publishers, 1981, pp 77–80

3. Zwiebel WJ, Crummy AB. Sources of error in Doppler diagnosis of carotid occlusive disease. Am J Roentgenol 137:231–242, 1981

4. Barnes RW, Russel HE, Bone GE, et al: Doppler cerebrovascular examination: improved results with refinements in technique. Stroke (8)4:468–471, 1977

5. Machleder HI, Barker WF: Noninvasive methods for evaluation of extracranial cerebrovascular disease. Arch Surg 112:922–946, 1977

6. Moore WS, Bean B, Burton R, et al: The use of ophthalmosonometry in the diagnosis of carotid artery stenosis. Surgery 82:107–115, 1977

7. Planilo T, Pourcelot L, Pottier JM, et al: Étude de la circulation carotidienne par les methodes ultrasoniques et la thermographie. Rev Neurol (Paris) 126:127–141, 1972

8. Courbier R, Reggi M, Jausseran JM: Exploration of carotid arteries and vessels of the neck by Doppler techniques. In Dietrich ED (ed): Noninvasive Cardiovascular Diagnosis: Current Concepts. Baltimore, University Park Press, 1978, pp 61–73

9. Barnes RW, Bone GE, Reinertson J, et al. Noninvasive ultrasonic carotid angiography: prospective validation by contrast arteriography. Surgery 3:328–335, 1976.

10. Berry SM, O'Donnell JA, and Hobson RWII. Capabilities and limitations of pulsed Doppler sonography in carotid imaging. J Clin Ultrasound 7:405–412, 1980.

11. O'Leary DH, Persson AV, Clouse ME. Noninvasive testing for carotid artery sclerosis: I. prospective analysis of three methods. AJR 137:1189–1194, 1981.

12. Doorley TPG, Atkinson PI, Kingston V, Shanik DG. Carotid ultrasonic arteriography combined with real time spectral analysis: A comparison with angiography. J Cardiovasc Surg 23:243–245, 1982.

13. Wasserman DH, Hobson RWII, Lynch TG, Berry SM, Jamil Z. Ultrasonic imaging and oculoplethysmography in diagnosis of carotid occlusive disease. Arch Surg 117:1161–1163, 1983.

William J. Zwiebel, M.D.

7

Duplex Carotid Sonography

Before proceeding, the reader must understand the posterior orbital technique for detection of external carotid collateral flow and, in particular, must be familiar with normal and abnormal pulsatility patterns in the common, internal and external carotid. Knowledge of these subjects, covered in Chapters 3 and 6, is essential for thorough understanding of the material presented herein.

THE DUPLEX CONCEPT

The development of duplex ultrasound instrumentation combining high-resolution B-mode imaging with Doppler flow analysis represented a major advancement in ultrasound cerebrovascular diagnosis. Whereas, pure Doppler methods may only detect sizable atheromatous deposits that alter blood flow, plaque deposits of any size may be identified and examined with duplex instruments. The B-mode component of the carotid examination is extremely useful, because B-mode imaging frequently demonstrates plaque in patients with little or no Doppler abnormality. Patient managment may be significantly affected by identification of such plaque. Symptomatic patients with extensive carotid arteriosclerosis may be considered candidates for arteriography and subsequent surgery, even in the absence of major stenoses. In addition, B-mode imaging offers the potential for identification of surface irregularities and plaque hemorrhage that may cause embolization. Such abnormalities cannot be detected with Doppler methods alone.

The B-mode component of duplex imaging is not without limitations, however. This modality is useful only in areas where the carotid arteries are directly accessible to ultrasound examination, i.e., between the clavicle and mandible, and B-mode diagnostic capabilities are directly effected by image quality, which is often suboptimal in the distal internal and external carotid arteries. Furthermore, the severity of occlusive disease may, for reasons discussed below, be overestimated or underestimated with B-mode imaging. Published accuracy results with

B-mode imaging used independently from Doppler methods have been disappointing and work by the author and his associates[4] has documented the superior accuracy of duplex sonography over B-mode imaging. It is strongly recommended, therefore, that B-mode sonography should never be the sole method used in cerebrovascular ultrasound examination but always should be incorporated with Doppler in a duplex format.

RATIONALE FOR NONINVASIVE CEREBROVASCULAR EXAMINATION

The rationale for cerebrovascular ultrasonography was extensively discussed in Chapter 4, but the following objectives of duplex carotid sonography are worthy of emphasis. Sonographers should keep these goals in mind in the course of every carotid ultrasound examination. Duplex carotid sonography should (1) detect atheromatous disease in the carotid arteries and determine its extent and severity, (2) determine the magnitude of carotid obstruction, (3) detect external carotid collateral flow, and (4) detect severe carotid obstructive lesions outside of the cervical examination area (i.e., via abnormal common or internal carotid pulsatility, and detection of external carotid collateral flow).

The duplex examination must provide sufficient information for making a rational decision as to whether or not carotid atheromatous disease is present that may warrant surgery. If so, arteriography will be performed, in most cases, in anticipation of surgery. If not, arteriography will not be performed and a clinical judgment will be made concerning the need for medical therapy.

The clinical indications for ultrasound cerebrovascular study are outlined in Table 7-1. Assuming that vascular ultrasonography is an intermediary procedure between physical examination and arteriography, ultrasound should not be used when arteriography is mandatory. Furthermore, the diagnostic value of ultrasonography is limited for the most part to the carotid arteries. Ultrasound is not of

Table 7-1
Indications for Cerebrovascular Ultrasonography

Carotid	Asymptomatic Bruit, TIA, RIND, Completed Stroke with Minor Deficit—Use ultrasound to assess the extent and severity of carotid atherosclerosis and to detect major, surgically accessible obstructive lesions.
	Nonfocal Neurological Symptoms—Use ultrasound to detect major, surgically accessible occlusive lesions that might result in cerebral hypoperfusion.
Vertebrobasilar	Vertebral-Subclavian Steal—Use ultrasound to confirm clinically suspected steal syndromes.
	TIA or Poorly Localized Vertebral Basilar Symptoms—The use of ultrasound is confined primarily to searching for surgically remediable carotid obstructive lesions that might contribute to vertebrobasilar hypoperfusion.

great value in the vertebrobasilar system. Patients with clear cut vertebrobasilar symptoms are probably more effectively examined by intraarterial digital subtraction arteriography or standard selective arteriography, especially if vertebral or subclavian bypass surgery is a consideration. Symptoms of vertebrobasilar insufficiently may occasionally be an indication for ultrasound when the clinical objective is to rule out major carotid obstructive lesions that might contribute indirectly to reduced posterior fossa blood flow.

DUPLEX INSTRUMENTATION

B-mode ultrasound instruments designed for general purpose abdominal and obstetrical imaging are not effective for carotid examination because they do not have adequate spatial or gray-scale resolution. Highly sensitive instruments specifically designed for near-field work (high-resolution, superficial-structure scanners) are required for carotid study. The term high resolution has not been defined with respect to specific quantitative image characteristics; therefore, the editor is compelled to present his own unofficial definition. Axial and lateral resolution (in vivo) should be at least 1 mm since it is desirable to image plaque surface characteristics as small as 1 or 2 mm. Excellent sensitivity and wide dynamic range are also required, otherwise thrombus or plaque of low echogenicity simply is not visible. The author's definition, therefore, also includes adequate sensitivity for distinguishing low-echogenicity plaque from blood. A number of duplex devices are available commercially that meet these high-resolution spacial and sensitivity requirements.

Numerous transducer designs have been used in high-resolution duplex devices, including a mechanically oscillated transducer, a fixed transducer directed at an oscillating mirror and a rotating wheel containing several transducers. Transducer assemblies using a sector scan design produce a pie-shaped image, while other devices offer a rectangular image. The latter may be of advantage in scanning arteries lying close to the skin where the field of view of the sector image is quite narrow. Peak ultrasound frequencies employed in high-resolution instruments range between 7 and 10 MHz. Since ultrasound at such high frequencies is rapidly attenuated in tissue, the maximum effective depth of most of these devices is 4 cm. Real-time imaging, which is essential for detailed examination of the carotid arteries, is utilized in all of the available duplex systems. The Doppler components of the duplex instrument may be pulsed or continuous wave depending on the manufacturer's preference. Both types of Doppler technology have advantages and disadvantages as discussed in Chapter 2. In some cases, flow sampling and B-mode imaging may be conducted simultaneously, while with other systems the B-mode image must be "frozen" during Doppler applications. All pulsed Doppler devices are designed to allow the operator to select the precise location of Doppler sampling within the B-mode field of view. This is accomplished by varying both the Doppler line of site and the depth of the range gate from which the Doppler signals are accepted (Fig. 7-1). With most pulsed systems, the size of the range gate may also be varied to encompass more or less of the flow stream (Fig. 7-2).

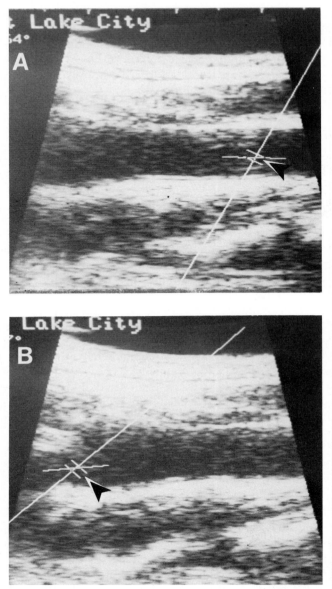

Figure 7-1. Illustration of changes in the position of the Doppler sample volume (arrowhead). (A) the sample volume is located at the right hand side of the image. (B) By changing the line of site of the Doppler transducer (the line extending through the image) and the position of the sample volume along that line, the Doppler sample volume can be placed at any location within the vessel.

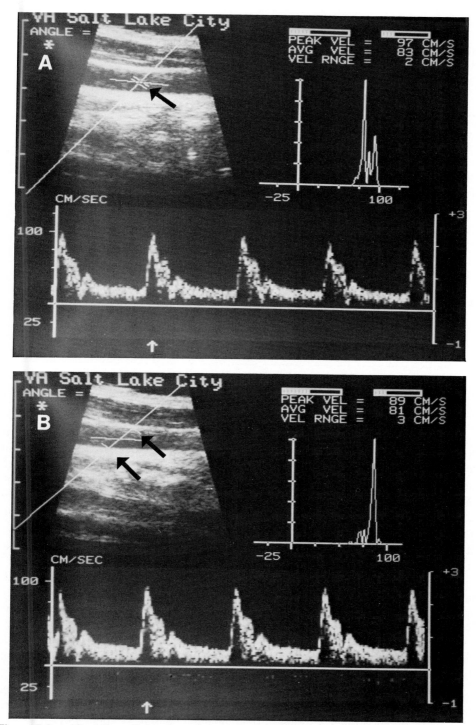

Figure 7-2. Alteration of the size of the sample volume. (A) A narrow sample volume (arrow, parallel lines) is demonstrated. (B) The sample volume (arrows) has been enlarged. Note that the spectrum at the base of the figure is somewhat broadened in comparison to that seen in (A) because all velocities in the flow stream are included in the wide sample volume.

Table 7-2
Reported Results, Duplex Carotid Sonography

Author	Clark & Hatten[12] 1981	Zwiebel et al[4] 1983	Bendick et al[13] 1983	Cardullo et al[10] 1983	Wetzner et al[14] 1984
n vessels	150	393	190	246	53
n stenoses	79	79	44	105	35
% stenosis	≥ 50	≥ 50	≥ 70	≥ 50	≥ 60
Sensitivity	94%	94%	91%	91%	94%
Specificity	90%	99%	97%	85%	89%
Accuracy	92%	95%	95%	87%	91%
Positive Predictive Value	95%	94%	89%	82%	94%
Negative Predictive Value	89%	89%	97%	92%	89%
Instrument Manufacturer	Advanced Technology Laboratory	Biodynamics + Carolina Medical Electronics	Diasonics	Diasonics	Diasonics

Through advancements in computer technology and transducer design, duplex instruments have been developed that superimpose a two-dimensional color-coded flow image on a two-dimensional B-mode image. Such devices are capable of imaging flow in real-time over the entire field of view of the transducer. This approach appears to represent a major technological advancement in ultrasound vascular imaging, but it is too early to assess the capabilities and limitations of this technique. A number of images produced by this type of instrument are included in this textbook (color plates 1,3,4), because these images are excellent for illustrating physiological and diagnostic principles.

Doppler signal processing capabilities vary widely among duplex instruments. All modern duplex devices utilize fast Fourier transform frequency spectrum analysis for processing Doppler shift information, but some systems also include sophisticated computing capabilities for measuring blood velocity ratios, spectral broadening and blood flow. These details will be considered further in the discussion of Doppler signal analysis in this chapter and in Chapter 8.

Although instruments of widely varying design are presently in clinical use, the methods and principles of examination described herein should, in general, be applicable to all duplex scanners. It is realized, however, that certain of the methods recommended may not be effective or possible with a specific duplex device. Excellent results for diagnosis of carotid occlusive disease have been reported with a variety of duplex instruments, as outlined in Table 7-2.

OVERVIEW OF THE DUPLEX EXAMINATION PROCEDURES

High-resolution carotid sonography is customarily performed with the patient in a supine position, the shoulders and head elevated on a pillow, and the head rotated toward the side opposite the carotid being studied. Examination of the entire carotid bifurcation may, at times, be accomplished with the patient's head and neck in a single position, but more often than not, the head and neck are moved to different positions to facilitate imaging various portions of the bifurcation branches. It is important not to extend the neck too severely. In addition to producing patient discomfort, overextension causes the sternomastoid muscle to contract, making it difficult to maneuver the transducer and to maintain skin contact. The patient may be examined in a sitting position if recumbency is not possible, but lack of stability generally makes the sitting position undesirable.

Recording

At the Salt Lake City Veterans Administration Medical Center, we routinely record the entire carotid examination on videotape, including verbal comments by the sonographer that indicate the location of abnormal findings. Hard copy images are also obtained to record specific flow measurements, such as common carotid pulsatility, and to document major B-mode or Doppler abnormalities such as large plaque deposits and flow abnormalities resulting from stenosis.

Image Orientation

With real-time imaging, the orientation of structures seen on the display screen is dependent on transducer position. In keeping with standardized ultrasound display formats, we routinely orient longitudinal images with the patient's head on the left side of the display screen. Transverse images are oriented as if viewed from the patients feet; hence, the patients right appears on the left side of the image. Some duplex instruments are not equipped with a switch to transpose the right and left sides of the image on the display screen, and this deficiency may limit the ability to standardize orientation. With such devices, we suggest that the images be displayed in whatever position allows best transducer access to the patients neck and that the sonographer verbally annotate the orientation during video tape recording.

The Common Carotid Artery

We routinely attempt to image the carotid bifurcation in three longitudinal transducer positions as illustrated in Figures 7-3A–C. It is best to begin the longitudinal examination with the transducer in an anterolateral position on the patient's neck (Fig. 7-3A), as near to the clavicle as possible. The proximal portion of the common carotid artery is usually the easiest area to examine, and beginning there enables the sonographer to get oriented. It is important to image as much of the proximal common carotid artery as possible and this is facilitated by having the patient lower the ipsilateral shoulder (Tell the patient, "reach down

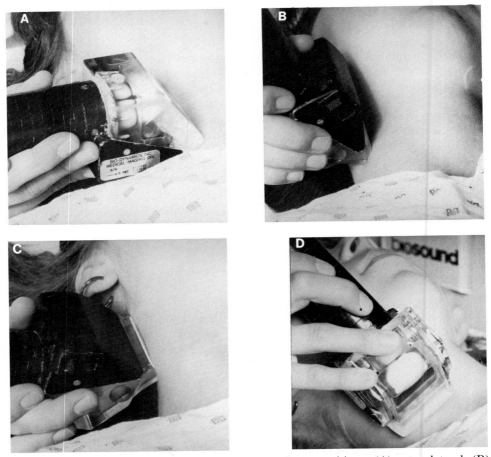

Figure 7-3. Illustration of standard B-mode transducer positions: (A) anterolateral; (B) lateral, 90° from (A); (C) posterolateral; and (D) transverse.

for your hip''). The common carotid artery can be identified by its pulsations and by prominent linear reflections adjacent to the vessel wall (Fig. 7-4). The internal jugular vein lies adjacent to the carotid artery, but the two vessels can easily be distinguished on B-mode images since the vein does not have a linear reflection along its wall, does not pulsate as sharply as the carotid artery and varies in size with respiration. Furthermore, Doppler signals in the jugular vein have a "windstorm" character that is distinctly different from arterial pulsation.

Once the common carotid artery is identified, it may be followed superiorly to the carotid bifurcation. The sonographer may then continue the examination into either the external or internal carotid arteries; however, it has become our practice to study the common, internal, and external carotid arteries sequentially. First, the common carotid artery is examined visually in two longitudinal planes at right angles to one another. When plaque is present in the common carotid artery, its position, extent and severity are studied and recorded on hard copy images. After the longitudinal examination is completed, the common carotid

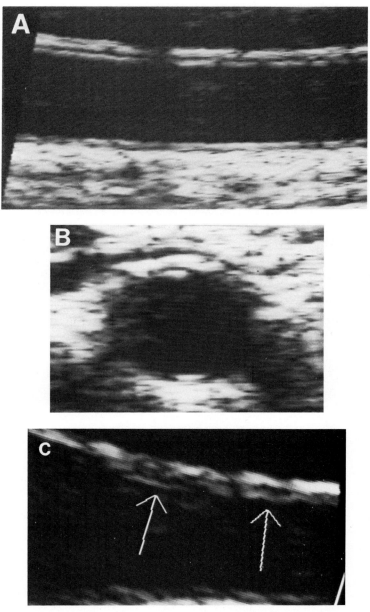

Figure 7-4. Demonstration of the normal intimal reflection. (A) Longitudinal and (B) transverse sections of the common carotid artery demonstrating a bright line along the inner margin of the artery wall. This line represents a strong, specular reflection from the intimal surface. (C) Minimal thickness plaque (arrows) is seen along the near wall of this vessel. Observe that the surface of this plaque does not parallel the prominent white line that represents the arterial adventitia. Also note the absence of the distinct lucent zone seen in A adjacent to the intimal line.

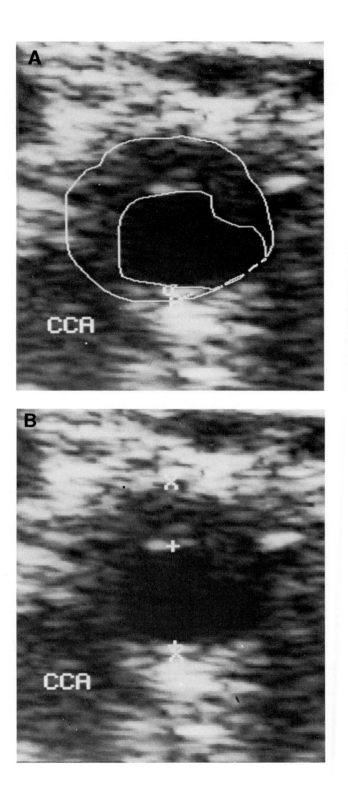

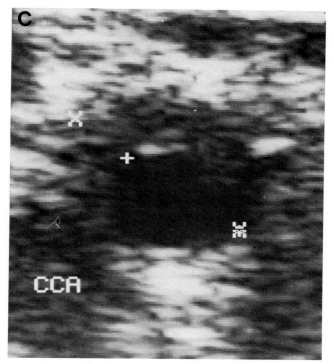

Figure 7-5. Measurement of plaque thickness in transverse sections. (A) In this transverse section of the common carotid artery (CCA), the outer circle represents the arterial wall and the inner circle the arterial lumen. The material between the circles is plaque. Note in B and C that measurements of plaque thickness and residual lumen diameter may vary greatly with the plane of measurement.

artery is examined in the transverse projection (Fig. 7-3D) beginning at the clavicle and continuing to the bifurcation. It is particularly important during transverse imaging to document the thickness of plaque deposits and the resultant severity of obstruction (Fig. 7-5).

Following visual inspection of the common carotid artery in longitudinal and transverse planes, we next evaluate common carotid flow signals. First, we measure the pulsatility, time averaged velocity and volume flow in a portion of the common carotid artery that is least affected by atherosclerosis. Next, flow characteristics in the stenotic and post-stenotic zones are scrutinized and recorded for common carotid obstructive lesions exceeding 40 percent decrease in diameter. Further discussion of these Doppler procedures is presented in Chapter 8.

The Internal and External Carotid Arteries

When common carotid artery evaluation is completed, the sonographer proceeds to the internal and external carotid arteries. Because the internal carotid artery is more important from a clinical perspective than the external carotid

Transducer Face

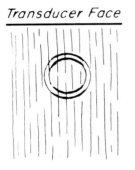

Figure 7-6. On transverse images, only those surfaces of the vessel that are relatively perpendicular to the sound beam are well visualized. Other portions of the vessel are poorly seen because of refraction and reflection.

artery, we tend to first concentrate our attention on the internal carotid (before fatigue takes its toll), but the sequence of examination is less important than unequivocal identification and careful study of both bifurcation branches.

It is useful to begin the examination of the external and internal carotid arteries in the transverse plane. Although good quality transverse scans may almost always be obtained in the common carotid artery, it is frequently impossible to obtain satisfactory transverse scans in the internal and external carotid branches. This difficulty is to be expected, considering physical limitations involved with scanning the curvilinear vessel wall in transverse planes (Fig. 7-6). Reflection and refraction from the curved wall surfaces deflect the sound beam and degrade the images. These problems are not encountered when the vessel is scanned longitudinally. Because good quality transverse images allow for accurate measurement of luminal narrowing, failure to obtain such images in the carotid branches represents a significant shortcoming of duplex imaging systems. In spite of these limitations, however, it is useful to attempt routine transverse imaging of the bifurcation branches. Images of reasonably good quality can sometimes be obtained beyond the bifurcation and may contribute significantly to identification of plaque, estimation of its severity and extent, and measurement of stenotic lesions. Moreover, even poor quality transverse images can be used to document the patency of the external and internal carotid arteries in cases where longitudinal imaging is difficult. Transverse images may also help to establish the relative position of the internal and external carotid arteries in the neck. This information, in difficult cases, can help a sonographer identify an appropriate plane for longitudinal imaging of the carotid branches.

The orientation of the branch vessels of the carotid bifurcation is extremely variable, with the result that it is not always an easy task to identify both the internal and external carotid arteries. When the internal carotid artery is occluded, one of the external carotid branches may be mistaken for the internal carotid artery; hence, correct identification of both vessels is imperative. Furthermore, if an obstructive lesion is present, it is critical that it be ascribed to the correct artery. Detection of a severe internal carotid stenosis may be an indication for angiography, but an isolated external carotid stenosis usually does not warrant further evaluation.

The external carotid artery can be recognized with certainty on longitudinal sections if one or more of its side branches is seen (Fig. 7-7), but these are not always found. Fortunately, there are other means of distinguishing between the

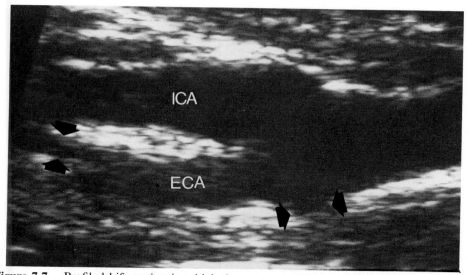

Figure 7-7. Profiled bifurcation in which the external (ECA) and internal carotid artery (ICA) may be clearly distinguished. The ICA is the larger of the two vessels and branches (arrowheads) are clearly seen to arise from the ECA.

external and internal carotid artery. (1) The external carotid artery is directed anteriorly toward the face, whereas the internal carotid artery is directed posteriorly and superiorly, roughly toward the mastoid process of the skull. (2) The external carotid artery is usually (but not always) smaller than the internal carotid artery. (3) Doppler signals in the external carotid artery have a high-resistance quality, in comparison to the internal carotid artery, which normally exhibits low resistance pulsatility features (Fig. 7-8). *We consider the pulsatility differences in the internal and external carotid arteries and the identification of external carotid branches to be the most important means for unequivocal identification of these vessels.* Further details concerning this important subject may be found in Chapters 3 and 6.

In spite of one's best efforts, it is sometimes not possible to be sure which vessel is the internal or external carotid artery, especially when the carotid bifurcation is severely diseased. When vessel identity is uncertain, one must be forthright and state that the location of abnormal findings cannot be determined. Diagnostic error severely detrimental to patient management could otherwise occur.

When the internal and external carotid arteries have been positively identified and transverse imaging is completed, the sonographer concentrates on longitudienal examination of each vessel. Generally, we are satisfied to image the external carotid artery in only one longitudinal plane, unless there is B-mode or Doppler evidence of major disease. We *always* prefer to obtain two longitudinal views of the internal carotid artery in planes approximately 90° from one another. The best planes for imaging the internal carotid artery are the anterolateral and posterior approaches (Fig. 7-3 A and C), but the other approach may work well in some

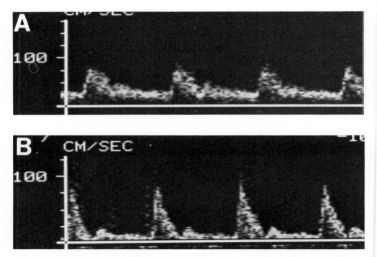

Figure 7-8. Comparison of pulsatility features of the internal and external carotid arteries. (A) The internal carotid pulse profile is characterized by broad systolic peaks and high volume diastolic flow. (B) In contrast, the external carotid pulse profile is characterized by sharp, narrow systolic peaks and relatively little diastolic flow.

individuals depending on the orientation of the carotid bifurcation. In the course of the B-mode examination, the sonographer should strive to accurately display the extent, severity, and surface characteristics of any plaque that is identified.

On longitudinal scans, problems can arise in determining whether atheromatous disease is located in the common carotid artery or in the orifice of one of the carotid branches. This important distinction can best be made if the carotid bifurcation is "profiled" with both the external and internal arteries seen simultaneously (Fig. 7-9). Profiling the bifurcation is frequently not possible, however. As an alternative, the sonographer should position the transducer at the bifurcation and shift back and forth between the branches several times to record the point at which the branches originate from the common carotid artery (Fig. 7-10), and to document the location of plaque deposits. This procedure is usually accomplished by gently sliding the transducer medially or laterally from one branch to the other. If the branches diverge quickly, a twisting motion may be helpful in shifting between the external and internal carotid.

If the carotid bifurcation is high in the neck (near the mandible), the field of view of the external and internal carotid artery may be restricted, and even an experienced sonographer may have difficulty obtaining adequate images of one or both bifurcation branches. The principal difficulties responsible for this problem are arterial tortousity or sharp medial angulation of the internal carotid artery relative to the skin line. With all ultrasound systems, it is possible to image only those surfaces of a vessel that are relatively perpendicular to the sound beam. In vessels that abruptly curve or "dive" away from the skin, it may be impossible to position the transducer such that the sound beam is perpendicular to the vessel wall (Fig. 7-11). In addition, vessels that are directed deeply into the neck may lie

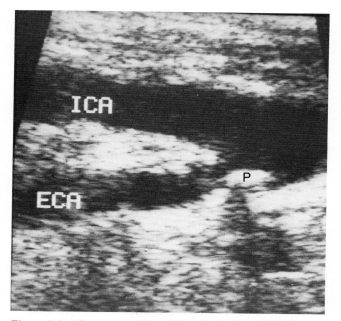

Figure 7-9.   Demonstration of the advantages of "profiling" the carotid bifurcation. The plaque (P) clearly is located in the orifice of the external carotid artery (ECA) rather than the internal carotid artery (ICA).

in the far field of the image where attenuation of the sound beam is greatest and resolution is poorest. Severe arteriosclerotic involvement may compound imaging problems, particularly when shadowing from plaque on the near wall of the vessel obscures large portions of the branch vessels or makes it difficult to follow the branches distally. We do not wish to cause unnecessary pessimism by pointing out these problems. With fairly diligent attention to detail and using a 10-MHz instrument, we were able to obtain satisfactory images of the common and internal carotid arteries in 89 percent of patients in at least one longitudinal plane, and we obtained satisfactory images in two planes in 67 percent of patients.[4]

Finally, sonographers should be aware of the existence of a "blind" area within the carotid arteries. This problem, as illustrated in Figure 7-10A, results from limitations of access of the sound beam to the carotid arteries. It is possible that small plaques located in the "blind" area may be overlooked on longitudinal imaging. Good quality transverse scans from different projections may obviate this problem.

Integration of the B-Mode and Doppler Components

In the course of longitudinal imaging of the internal and external carotid artery, we routinely evaluate Doppler flow signals. Doppler flow sampling is generally performed in only one plane (that which best displays the particular

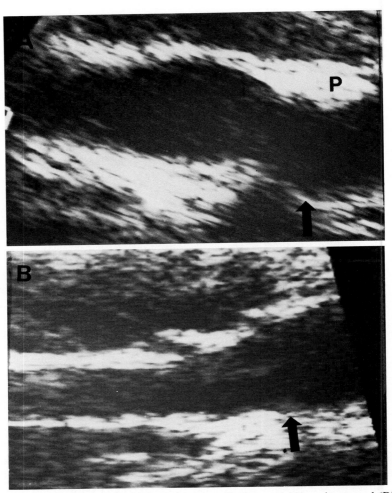

Figure 7-10. By shifting back and forth between the internal (A) and external (B) carotid arteries, the sonographer has determined that the orifice of each vessel lies approximately at the position of the arrows. The plaque (P) appears to span the junction of the common and internal carotid arteries.

branch vessel), but sampling in more than one plane may be needed to provide an adequate angle between the Doppler line of site and the flow stream. Doppler sampling should be performed throughout both branch vessels in as many locations as possible. With equipment having simultaneous B-mode and Doppler capabilities, Doppler sampling can be accomplished as a continuous sweep of the vessel. If the B-mode image must be frozen during Doppler operation, one should record frequency spectra in the proximal, mid- and distal internal carotid artery, and at one location in the external carotid artery. This minimal recording scheme applies to patients with little or no disease. When moderate or severe plaque is found, we carefully examine the flow characteristic of the prestenotic, stenotic,

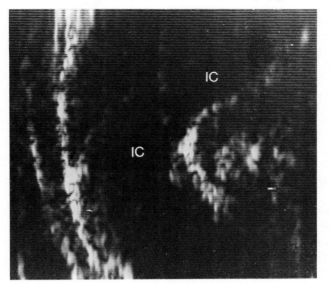

Figure 7-11. The internal carotid artery (IC) describes a very sharp curve. Its wall, as a result, is not perpendicular to the sound beam and is poorly-defined.

and poststenotic zones as described in Chapter 8. For internal carotid stenoses, we also compare peak stenotic zone velocities with common carotid systolic velocities. Hard copy recordings are made of significant Doppler and B-mode findings.

SUMMARY OF DUPLEX EXAMINATION PROTOCOL

1. Longitudinal B-mode imaging of the common carotid artery in two planes at right angles; document severity, extent, and characteristics of plaque.
2. Transverse B-mode imaging of the common carotid artery; document plaque thickness and degree of obstruction.
3. Common carotid artery Doppler examination. (1) Evaluate common carotid pulsatility; (b) measure time-averaged velocity and volume flow (these measurements are not possible with all instruments); (c) evaluate flow disturbances related to focal plaque deposits.
4. Transverse B-mode examination of the internal and external carotid arteries. (a) Determine visually whether both vessels are patent; (b) if image quality allows, evaluate plaque severity and degree of obstruction; (c) determine orientation of external and internal carotid arteries as an aid to longitudinal imaging.
5. Longitudinal B-mode examination of the internal carotid artery in two planes at right angles; evaluate severity, extent, and characteristics of plaque.
6. Doppler examination of the internal carotid artery. (a) Normal flow; document frequency spectra in proximal, mid- and distal locations; (b) evaluate

flow disturbances related to focal plaque deposits; prestenotic, stenotic, and poststenotic zones; (c) Document internal carotid/common carotid ratio.

7. Longitudinal B-mode imaging of the external carotid artery; evaluate severity, extent, and characteristics of plaque.

8. Doppler examination of the external carotid artery. (a) Normal flow; document frequency spectrum in one proximal location; (b) Evaluate flow disturbances related to focal plaque deposits; prestenotic, stenotic, and poststenotic zones.

NORMAL B-MODE APPEARANCE OF THE CAROTID ARTERIES

The normal common carotid artery has a uniform diameter to just below its bifurcation where a variable degree of widening occurs. The widened portion of the common carotid artery is oval in configuration as seen in transverse sections, while the remainder of the common carotid artery is round. A variable degree of localized widening also occurs in the proximal 1–2-cm of the internal carotid artery.

The arterial walls of the normal common, internal and external carotid arteries have an identical sonographic appearance, including uniform thickness and the presence of an echogenic line along the luminal surfaces (Fig. 7-4). This characteristic line probably arises from strong specular reflections at the intimal surface. In vitro correlative studies of ultrasound findings and arterial wall histology by Wolverson et al.[5] indicates that the intima and media produce a homogeneous band of medium echogenicity, and that the echogenic line does not specifically describe an anatomical structure other than the *surface* of the intima. The presence of the echogenic line along the inner arterial surface is not related to atherosclerosis and it should not be regarded as abnormal as long as it is smooth and projects no more than 1 mm from the remainder of the arterial wall. A thin, sonolucent line is typically seen beneath the echogenic intimal reflection (Fig. 7-4). Based on the Wolverson study,[5] this line also does not correspond to a specific histological structure, and its origin is unexplained. The author believes it represents the composite of intima and media sandwiched between the strong reflections from the intimal surface and the adventitial layer. The highly reflective outer border of normal arteries (Fig. 7-4) corresponds to the adventitial layer, according to Wolverson.[5]

The lumen of the carotid vessels should be echo free, however, artifactual intraluminal reflections are common, even with state of the art instruments. The sonographer, therefore, is faced with the challenge of differentiating between artifactual echoes and real ones from thrombus or plaque. One should be highly suspicious of echoes that can only be seen in one plane of section and cannot be documented from other perspectives (e.g., longitudinal and transverse planes). Echoes seen only in one plane are probably artifactual. It also is helpful to scrutinize the pulsation of the intraluminal echoes. Plaque will usually be seen to pulsate synchronously with the arterial wall; whereas artifactual echoes are stationary, except for those generated by the walls of the jugular vein.

One may occasionally detect reflections from blood cells in areas of sluggish flow, but this finding is only seen in the presence of significant obstruction.

ABNORMAL B-MODE APPEARANCE OF THE CAROTID ARTERIES

The histological composition of plaque and degenerative processes that occur within plaque are important factors in stroke pathogenesis; therefore, sonographic characteristics of plaque evident on B-mode examination may have important therapeutic and prognostic implications. Traditionally, duplex sonography has been used principally to identify and quantify obstructive lesions, but more recently, interest also has turned toward the important subject of characterizing the histological composition of plaque. The use of ultrasound for this purpose is in its infancy, and further development is likely within the next few years. The following summary represents the state of knowledge at the time of publication of this text.

Correlation of echo characteristics and plaque histology has been carried out by Wolverson et al.[5] These authors have confirmed that the relative proportion of lipid material, collagen, hemorrhage, and calcification within plaque determines its sonographic appearances.

Low Echogenicity Plaque

Fibrofatty plaque (Fig. 7-12A) containing a large amount of lipid material is the least echogenic type of plaque and may be so faintly echogenic as to be difficult to identify sonographically. This problem occurs because the acoustic properties of fibrofatty plaque are very similar to those of blood and because this type of plaque is acoustically homogeneous. Occasionally, we have had difficulty identifying fibrofatty plaque even when present in large amounts (Fig. 7-12B), but this problem generally has occurred when the image quality is poor. How frequently such difficulties arise with high-resolution imaging of fibrofatty plaque is unknown. To reduce the incidence of nonvisualization of plaque, it may be necessary to maintain receiver gain settings at relatively high levels. High gain levels may produce artifactual echoes within the vessel lumen with some instruments, but artifacts may be tolerable if plaque detection is assured.

Thrombus

The ability of high-resolution sonography to image thrombus within the vascular lumen has not been satisfactorily evaluated, and the limitations of high-resolution imaging in reference to vascular thrombus are unknown. Thrombus deposition on denuded or ulcerated plaque surfaces or in association with severe stenotic lesions, may generate considerable hazard of embolization. Failure to image thrombus may, therefore, result in significant error, and additional evaluation of the incidence of this problem is needed.

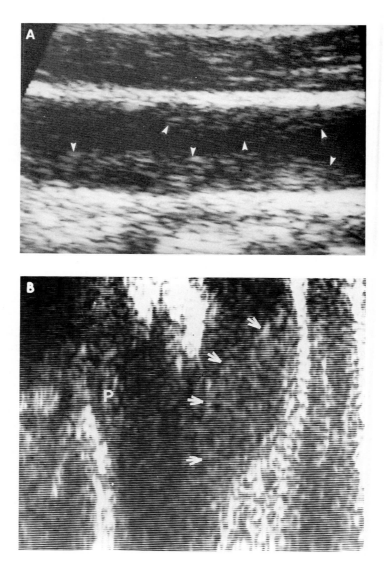

158

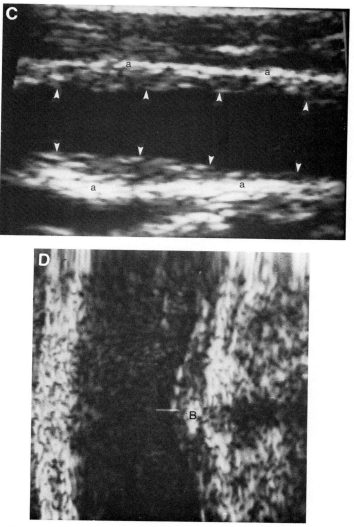

Figure 7-12. Plaque composition as indicated by B-mode sonography. (A) Fibrofatty plaque with a high lipid content (arrows) produces low level echoes. (B) Fibrofatty plaque may be difficult to image, even when present in large amounts. The large plaque deposit in the internal carotid artery (arrows) was overlooked with B-mode imaging until Doppler signals abnormalities indicated its presence. An additional small deposit (P) of fibrofatty plaque is present in the external carotid orifice. (C) Highly-fibrous plaque is more echogenic than fibrofatty plaque. Compare the echogenicity of this type of plaque with that shown in (A) and (B). (a, adventitial layer) (D) Calcification within a fibrous plaque produces a brightly echogenic focus (B) within the plaque, as well as shadowing distal to this focus.

Moderate-to-Strongly Echogenic Plaque, Without Shadowing

Wolverson et al.[5] found that predominantly fibrous plaque (Fig. 7-12C) was moderately or strongly echogenic and that the degree of echogenicity correlated with the amount of collagen within the plaque architecture. Uniformly fibrous plaque is homogeneous in echogenicity, but localized hypoechoic regions may be seen when large focal deposits of lipid material or thrombus are present within fibrous plaque.[6,7]

Brightly Echogenic Plaque With Shadowing

Bright reflections with acoustic shadowing are associated with "complicated plaque" containing dystrophic calcification (Fig. 7-12D). High-resolution imaging is extremely sensitive to calcification, and tiny areas on the order of 1 mm in diameter may be detected within plaque deposits.[5] Acoustic shadowing from large calcified deposits may be extremely troublesome. Such deposits obscure the remainder of the atheromatous deposit or the opposite wall of the vessel (Fig. 7-11), and may also prevent acquisition of Doppler flow information. In the presence of acoustic shadowing, it may be impossible to determine the severity and significance of arteriosclerotic involvement at a specific location.

Determining Plaque Severity and Extent

When plaque is identified, the sonographer should always evaluate its severity (thickness) and extent. Successful investigation for these features often requires a large dose of technical diligence, including the use of a variety of patient and transducer positions and repeated adjustment of gain level and other imaging parameters. Plaque develops asymmetrically in the arterial wall and spreads circumferentially and axially within the subintimal layer. As a result of this mode of development, plaque frequently has a crescentric configuration on cross section (Fig. 7-13A). Considering that the vessel and contained plaque represent a fairly complex three-dimensional structure and that a two-dimensional plane is used to image this structure, it is not surprising that the severity and the extent of plaque may readily be overestimated or underestimated, especially in longitudinal sections (Figs. 7-13A–C).

In completely normal vessels, false-positive diagnosis of plaque may result from scanning in oblique (off-diameter) planes of section. In such images, the poorly defined vessel margins are mistaken for arteriosclerotic deposits (Figs. 7-14D, and 7-14). Similarly, in diseased arteries, the severity of plaque may be overestimated or underestimated through malpositioning of the image plane. It is of great importance, therefore, to always scan along the vessel diameter when assessing plaque severity. Furthermore, carotid vessels should be studied in several planes of section whenever possible, and areas of arteriosclerotic involvement should be carefully scrutinized from different angles to establish the true severity and extent of disease. The appearance of plaque protruding into the vessel lumen can vary greatly as the image plane is moved.[3] This observation is nicely illustrated in Figures 7-13 and 7-15. Successful high-resolution carotid

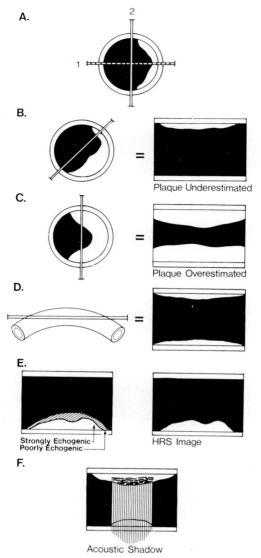

A.

B.

= Plaque Underestimated

C.

= Plaque Overestimated

D.

=

E.

Strongly Echogenic
Poorly Echogenic

HRS Image

F.

Acoustic Shadow

Figure 7-13. Sources of error in B-mode plaque diagnosis. (A) longitudinal images along line 1 will demonstrate the plaque deposit but longitudinal sections along line 2 will not. (B) A longitudinal section along the line shown will underestimate the severity of the plaque. (C) Longitudinal sections along this line will overestimate plaque severity. (D) Longitudinal sections through a curving vessel may suggest the presence of plaque when none is present, since portions of the vessel are not imaged directly along the vessel diameter. (E) Plaque severity may be underestimated when strongly echogenic plaque is visualized but overlying poorly echogenic plaque is not seen. (F) Acoustic shadowing may obscure plaque. (From Zwiebel WJ, Austin CW, Sackett JF, et al: Correlation of high-resolution, B-mode and continuous-wave Doppler sonography with arteriography in the diagnosis of carotid stenosis. Radiology 149(2):523–532, 1983. With permission.)

161

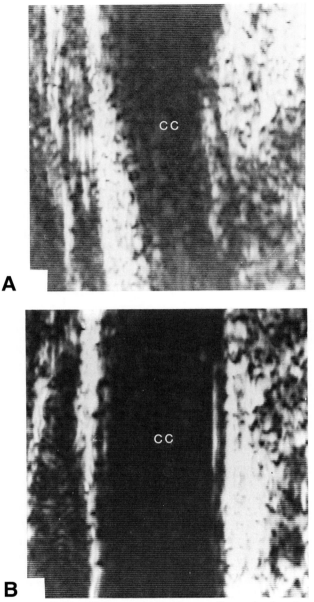

Figure 7-14. False positive plaque diagnosis due to off-diameter image planes. (A) In this off-diameter section of the common carotid artery (CC), it appears that plaque is present, resulting in stenosis. (B) The same artery is demonstrated to be normal by moving the transducer very slightly such that the plane of section is through the diameter of the vessel. Note the clearly seen intimal reflections.

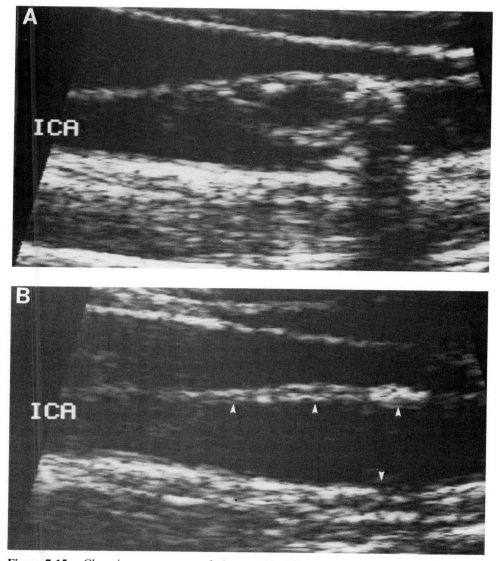

Figure 7-15. Changing appearance of plaque with different planes of section. (A) In this longitudinal view of the internal carotid artery (ICA), the lumen appears occluded by plaque. (B) In another section of the same vessel taken at right angles to A, the plaque is barely visible (arrowheads).

diagnosis clearly requires an ability to think three-dimensionally—a skill that both the sonographer and sonologist should foster.

The severity of plaque also may be underestimated if strongly reflective plaque components are imaged but overlying, less echogenic plaque is not seen (Fig. 7-13E). Since instruments with relatively poor gray-scale resolution and sensitivity can image only the strongly reflective components, they are prone to underestimate plaque thickness and extent.

Internal Plaque Characteristics

Relatively little research work has been done regarding correlation of plaque composition and internal characteristics with clinical manifestations of cerebrovascular disease, such as embolic phenomena and cerebral infarction. The most notable work in the field is that of Lusby et al.[6] who found that the presence of intraplaque hemorrhage correlated strongly with plaque surface denudation and platelet deposition. The implication of this finding is that intraplaque hemorrhage, with resultant thrombus accumulation, damages the overlying intimal surface and subsequently results in adherence of platelets or in frank intimal breakdown and ulceration. Other authors have inferred that intraplaque hemorrhage may cause sudden enlargement of plaque with resultant dramatic increase in carotid obstruction.[7] This process may account for rapid progression from minor carotid stenosis to critical levels of obstruction. Finally, complicated plaque containing hemorrhage, calcification, and lipid deposits is generally regarded as being more frequently symptomatic and dangerous than noncomplicated fibrofatty plaque. Hence, identification of such plaque may have important therapeutic implications.

Additional high-quality clinical research is needed to define the significance of sonographic findings of plaque composition; nonetheless, sonographers and sonologists would do well to scrutinize internal plaque characteristics both to develop skills in recognizing plaque composition and also to contribute to the general fund of knowledge in this field.

Surface Characteristics of Plaque

Evaluation of the surface characteristics of arteriosclerotic lesions is of considerable importance since irregularity is thought to be a common source of emboli that result in transient ischemic symptoms and cerebral infarction. Through careful scanning, one can frequently document a smooth, sharply defined surface (Fig. 7-10C), which probably indicates that the intimal layer over the plaque is intact (we have no histological proof of this). In other cases, gross surface irregularity or frank ulceration can be seen on B-mode images. The principal sonographic manifestation of surface irregularity is acute disruption of the contour of plaque as seen in longitudinal or transverse planes (Fig. 7-16). A large ulceration may also appear as an echogenic ring when the image plane is transverse to the mouth of the crater. Wolverson et al.[5], clearly confirmed that high-resolution sonography may detect plaque ulceration, but these authors also warn against overdiagnosis of plaque surface irregularity. From their experience, "ultrasound often showed minor surface irregularity of plaque simulating ulceration, when this was not present on gross inspection or histological examination".[5]

Even though it has been documented that B-mode sonography can detect plaque ulceration, the *accuracy* of ultrasound for in vivo ulcer diagnosis remains controversial. Two studies, based on surgical plaque correlation, have shown excellent results for ultrasound ulcer detection (Table 7-3); Johnson[8] found ultrasound 83 percent sensitive and 100 percent specific for ulcer detection and O'Donnel et al.[9] reported 100 percent sensitivity and specificity. Others, including the author have been unimpressed with sonographic ulcer detection, based on

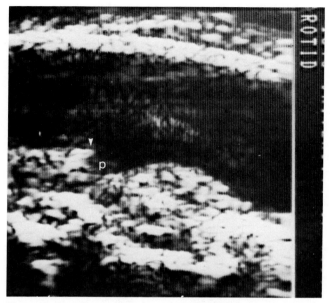

Figure 7-16. Demonstration of plaque ulceration. A sharply defined pit (p) is evident in the plaque surface with an overhanging lip (arrowhead). These findings are strongly suggestive of plaque ulceration.

Table 7-3
Reported Results, Carotid Ulcer Detection with
High Resolution B-Mode Sonography

Author	Cooperberg et al[1] 1979	James et al[2] 1982	Johnson[8] 1982	Cardullo[10] 1983	O'Donnell et al[9] 1983	Anderson et al[11] 1983
n vessels	52	158	32	246	79	100
n ulcers	18	34	6	51	27	21
Sensitivity	16%	0%	83%	51%	89%	24%
Specificity	97%	nd	100%	nd	87%	83%
Positive Predictive Value	75%	nd	100%	70%	28%	
Negative Predictive Value	44%	nd	96%	nd	80%	80%

nd = no data

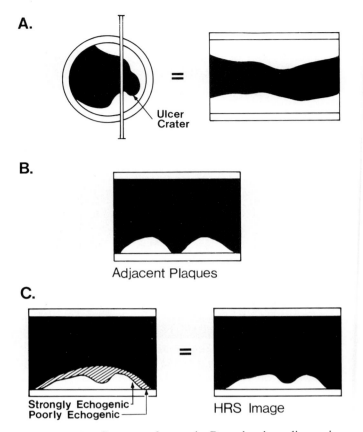

Figure 7-17. Sources of error in B-mode ulcer diagnosis. (A) The ulcer is excluded from view if the vessel is imaged along the longitudinal plane illustrated. (B) A gap between adjacent plaques is mistaken for an ulcer. (C) The poorly echogenic components of plaque deposit are not imaged while the strongly echogenic plaque is seen; false positive diagnosis of ulceration results. (From Zwiebel WJ, Austin CW, Sackett JF, et al: Correlation of high-resolution B-mode and continuous-wave Doppler sonography with arteriography in the diagnosis of carotid stenosis. Radiology 149(2):523–532, 1983. With permission.)

unfavorable results, including sensitivity levels from zero to 51 percent (Table 7-3).[1,2,4,10,11] Specificity for ulceration has been quite good in all reports, but this is a reflection of the small number of ulcers in each series. Studies demonstrating low sensitivity may be criticized since arteriography was used as the standard for comparison with ultrasound findings, and additional histological studies are clearly needed to resolve the issue. The author remains skeptical, however, about the performance of B-mode sonography for ulcer detection because of the following technical problems common to carotid B-mode examination: (1) Surface irregularity or ulceration may be readily overlooked if the vessel is not examined in multiple planes (Fig. 7-17A) or when image quality is poor. (2) A localized indentation between two adjacent plaques can be mistaken for an ulcer crater (Fig. 7-17B). (3) Brightly echogenic foci may be mistaken for surface irregularity if overlying, poorly echogenic plaque is not seen (Fig. 7-17C). In the latter instance, the space between the brightly echogenic areas is mistaken for a crater.

The author's philosophy concerning ultrasound diagnosis of plaque surface characteristics is: (1) if image quality is excellent and a clearly defined internal reflection is seen in several planes, the plaque may be deemed nonulcerated. (2) If normal image quality is excellent and a clearly defined crater or interruption of the plaque surface is seen, the plaque surface is described as irregular and potentially ulcerated. Visualization of a discrete crater in both longitudinal and transverse planes supports the impression of surface disruption. (3) If image quality is moderate or poor, surface characteristics usually cannot be commented upon. (4) The term "surface irregularity" is employed rather than "ulceration" since it is common knowledge that some irregular plaque surfaces seen at surgery are covered by an intact intimal layer, while other irregular areas are denuded of intima.

The detection of surface irregularity may be aided by the refinement of ultrasound devices that visually display color-coded flow information on the B-mode image. With such devices, it may be possible to document the movement of blood within ulcerations and thereby remove some of the uncertainty from plaque diagnosis.

B-Mode Diagnosis of Stenosis

Because arteriosclerotic plaque is deposited in the subintima and protrudes into the lumen, all plaque results in at least minimal reduction in lumen diameter. The point at which plaque is said to become stenotic is arbitrary, and B-mode diagnosis of carotid stenosis is based on visualization of plaque that appreciably reduces the lumen area. The severity of carotid stenosis can be evaluated with high resolution sonography through careful measurement of the diameter or area of the residual lumen. The usefulness of longitudinal sections for this purpose is limited since plaque asymmetry can lead to significant overestimation or under-estimation of narrowing, depending on the plane of section used (Fig. 7-14 and Fig. 7-16). Measurement of lumen narrowing is more accurate in transverse sections where asymmetry of plaque deposition is readily apparent, but it is frequently impossible, as noted previously, to obtain diagnostic-quality transverse images above the bifurcation. The examiner is forced, therefore, to rely on axial images for visual estimation of luminal narrowing in the external and internal carotid. The risk of errors in these cases may be reduced if two or more good-quality views are obtained in widely different planes of section, but Doppler assessment is clearly more accurate than B-mode imaging when the lumen is not well seen, especially in major obstructive lesions exceeding 50 percent diameter reduction. Furthermore, in the bulbous portions of the carotid bifurcation, Doppler evaluation of the hemodynamic effects of an obstructive lesions may be far more relevant than measurements of luminal narrowing. For example, a 50 percent stenosis in the bulbous portion of the internal carotid may have no flow limiting effects since the original diameter of the lumen far exceeded that of the distal, tubular portion of the internal carotid.

Improper B-mode scanning of regions of arterial-wall curvature may result in false-positive diagnosis of stenosis or occlusion in normal vessels, or in overestimation of the severity of obstruction in diseased arteries. The mechanism is the same as that mentioned in the preceding section on plaque. Close attention to image detail in the obliquely sectioned area will usually show that the vessel wall and plaque surfaces are not sharply defined, and that the intimal line is absent. The sonographer should then adjust the scan plane in an attempt to correctly display the vessel. Shadows from plaque pose another serious source of difficulty for B-mode diagnosis of stenosis or occlusion.

Duplex Diagnosis of Occlusion

Arterial occlusion is diagnosed with duplex sonography through these observations: (1) absence of arterial pulsations, (2) lumen filled with echogenic material, (3) sub-normal vessel size, and (4) absence of Doppler signals (Fig. 7-18). False-positive diagnosis of occlusion may occur when the lumen is obscured, either by acoustic shadowing or poor image quality. In such cases, diagnostic error is especially likely when portions of the vessel distal to the arteriosclerotic region cannot be seen, precluding the identification of distal pulsations or flow signals that might verify patency of the vessel. Duplex examination often cannot differentiate between occlusion and a severe stenosis with only a trickle of flow, because the flow velocity in the residual lumen is too sluggish to produce a detectable Doppler shift (see Fig. 6-16). Failure to detect pulsations or flow beyond the obstructing lesion in these instances is not diagnostic since absence of such findings may occur both in occluded vessels and in those that are severely stenosed. False-positive diagnosis of occlusion with duplex examination may be a very significant error, since a stenotic lesion is potentially remediable and occlusion is automatically assumed to be uncorrectable. We suggest, therefore, that arteriography be performed in all cases of severe occlusive disease even when the vessel is believed to be completely obstructed.

SUMMARY

Duplex vascular examination offers considerable advantage over independent use of B-mode or Doppler methods, since the duplex technique incorporates both anatomic and physiologic information. For carotid artery assessment, a standard examination protocol should be established that suits the needs of a given department. The examination protocol used at the author's institution has been outlined. Both Doppler and B-mode findings should be considered in formulating a diagnosis based on duplex examination.

The normal B-mode appearance of the carotid arteries has been described as well as sonographic findings associated with atherosclerotic plaque. When plaque is detected in the carotid arteries, the sonographer should determine (1) the thickness or severity of the deposit, (2) the extent of plaque deposition, (3) plaque surface characteristics, (4) the internal features of the plaque, and (5) the degree

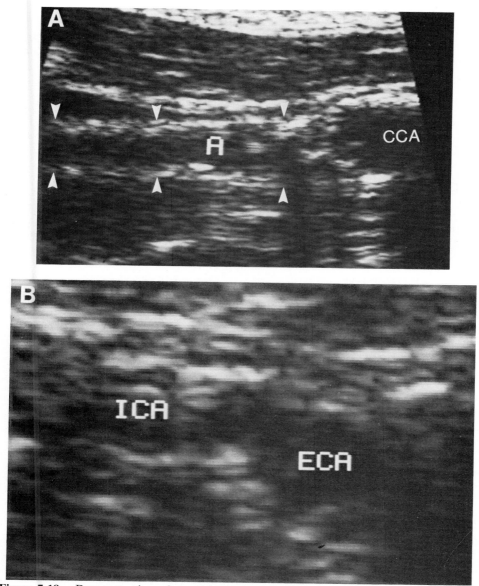

Figure 7-18. Demonstration of carotid artery occlusion. (A) The internal carotid artery (A, arrowheads) is considerably smaller than the adjacent common carotid artery (CCA), and the lumen of the internal carotid is filled with echogenic material. (B) On a transverse section, the internal carotid artery (ICA) is more echogenic and is much smaller than the external cartid artery (ECA). The internal carotid artery did not pulsate and flow signals were absent on Doppler examination.

of luminal obstruction. Doppler parameters employed in carotid diagnosis are discussed in detail in Chapter 8.

William J. Zwiebel, M.D.
Associate Professor of Radiology
University of Utah School of Medicine
and
Chief, Ultrasound and Body CT
Veterans Administration Medical Center
500 Foothill Drive
Salt Lake City, UT 84148

REFERENCES

1. Cooperberg PL, Robertson WD, Fry P, et al: High resolution real time ultrasound of the carotid bifurcation. J Clin Ultrasound 7:13–17, 1979

2. James EM, Earnest F, Forbes GS, et al: High-resolution dynamic ultrasound imaging of the carotid bifurcation: A prospective evaluation. Radiology 144:853–858, 1982

3. Comerata AJ, Cranley JJ, Cook SE: Real-time B-mode carotid imaging in diagnosis of cerebrovascular disease. Surgery 6:718–729, 1981

4. Zwiebel WJ, Austin CW, Sackett JF, et al: Correlation of high-resolution, B-mode and continuous-wave Doppler sonography with arteriography in the diagnosis of carotid stenosis. Radiology 149:523–532, 1983

5. Wolverson MK, Bashiti HM, Peterson GJ: Ultrasonic tissue characterization of atheromatous plaques using a high resolution real time scanner. Ultrasound Med Biol 6:669–609, 1983

6. Lusby RJ, Ferrell LD, Ehrenfeld WK, et al: Carotid plaque hemorrhage. Arch Surg 117:1479–87, 1982

7. Imparato AM, Riles TS, Gorstein F: The carotid bifurcation plaque: pathologic findings associated with cerebral ischemia. Stroke 3:283–245, 1979

8. Johnson JM: Angiography and ultrasound in diagnosis of carotid artery disease: A comparison. Contemporary Surgery 20:79–93, 1981

9. O'Donnell TF, Jr, Erodoes L, Mackey WC, et al: Correlation of B-mode ultrasound imaging and arteriography with pathologic findings at carotid endarterectomy. Arch Surg 120:443–449, 1985

10. Cardullo PA, Cutler BS, Wheeler HB, et al: Accuracy of duplex scanning in the detection of carotid artery disease. Bruit 8:181–186, 1984

11. Anderson DC, Loewenson R, Tock D, et al: B-mode, real-time carotid ultrasonic imaging. Arch Neurol 40:484–488, 1983

12. Clark WH, Hatten HP: Noninvasive screening of extracranial carotid disease: Duplex sonography with angiographic correlation. AJNR 2:443–447, 1981

13. Bendick PJ, Jackson WP, Becker GJ: Comparison of ultrasound scanning/Doppler with digital subtraction angiography in evaluating carotid arterial disease. Med Instrum 3:220–222, 1983

14. Wetzner SM, Tutunjian J, Marich KW: Focus on duplex scanning, a vascular diagnostic technology. Am Rev Diagnostics 1:31–36, 1983

William J. Zwiebel, M.D.

8

Analysis of Carotid Doppler Signals

The basic concepts of frequency spectrum analysis have been presented in Chapter 3. This chapter specifically concerns the application of frequency spectrum analysis to carotid diagnosis. As seen in the preceding chapter, B-mode imaging in its current form is an imprecise tool for measuring the severity of carotid obstruction, especially in the internal and external carotid. Furthermore, the physiological status of the circulation, as reflected by Doppler signals, frequently is more relevant than anatomic measurements of obstructive lesions. For these reasons, proper assessment of Doppler flow information is essential for accurate diagnosis of obstructive carotid lesions.

The simplest method for analysis of Doppler flow information is to convert the Doppler frequency shift into an audible signal that is analyzed aurally by the physician interpreting the study. Prior to the development of on-line, fast Fourier frequency spectrum analysis, the auditory technique was used exclusively and was quite accurate, assuming that the interpreter's ears were well attuned to the normal and abnormal qualities of carotid flow signals. Auditory analysis of Doppler signals remains a significant component of carotid flow assessment. Important Doppler characteristics including increased velocity, altered pulsatility, turbulence, and other flow disturbances are readily apparent in the audible Doppler output, and it is very important for the sonographer and sonologist to be cognizant of such abnormalities in the course of the duplex examination. Aural Doppler flow analysis has three major drawbacks, however, it is qualitative, completely subjective and considerable experience is required before accuracy can be assured.

Frequency Spectrum Analysis

The disadvantages of auditory Doppler evaluation led to the development of on-line, fast Fourier analysis devices for real time study of the Doppler shifted signal. Such frequency analysis devices have become increasingly more sophisticated with the development of each new generation of duplex scanners. State of

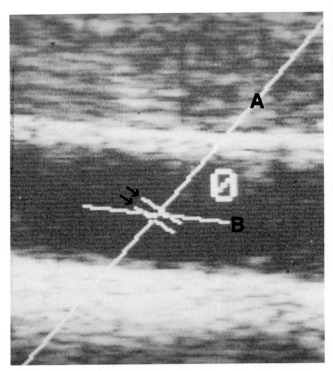

Figure 8-1. Illustration of the Doppler angle ⊕, which is formed by the Doppler line of sight (A) and the flow vector (B). The parallel lines (arrows) indicate the length of the Doppler sample volume.

the art frequency analysis instruments may be used not only to demonstrate the spectrum of *frequencies* within the Doppler output, but also to measure the spectrum of *velocities* within the blood stream. The process for converting the Doppler shift (in kilohertz) to flow velocity (in centimeters per second) requires knowledge of the "Doppler angle," which is the angle between the Doppler ultrasound beam and the flow vector or the vessel lumen (see Chapter 2). The operator of the duplex instrument informs the device of this angle by positioning an electronically generated line on the display screen, along the axis of flow (Fig. 8-1). When this angle is known, flow velocity becomes directly proportional to the Doppler shift and the instrument may digitally convert frequency shift values to velocity.

The standard format for displaying the Doppler shift frequency spectrum is shown in Figure 8-2. Time is represented on the X axis in divisions of a second. The Doppler frequency shift in kHz, or flow velocity in centimeters per second is represented on the Y axis. Blood flow away from the transducer is indicated above the display baseline and flow toward the transducer is registered below the baseline. The Z axis, or brightness of the image elements indicates the relative number of blood cells that are moving at a given velocity during a specific instant in time. The concept of the Z axis is somewhat difficult to understand, hence,

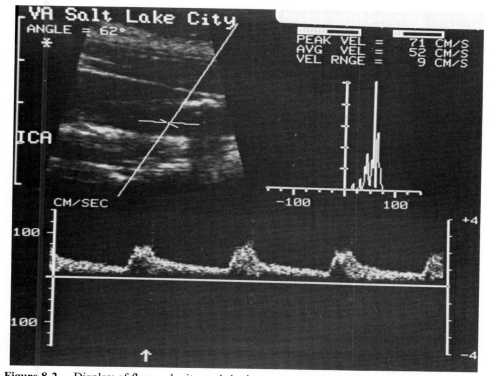

Figure 8-2. Display of flow velocity and the instantaneous Doppler spectrum. The image at the upper left demonstrates the position of the sample volume, the Doppler line of sight, and the flow vector. With knowledge of the Doppler angle (62°, in this case), the frequency spectrum at the base of the image may be represented both in centimeters per second (left hand margin) and in kilohertz (right hand margin). The graph in the upper right hand corner represents the distribution of velocities present at the moment in time indicated by the arrow at the bottom of the illustration. The peak velocity, average velocity, and the velocity range, at that moment, are automatically calculated (upper right).

further clarification may be helpful. The gray scale pattern in the image is directly related to the proportion of blood cells moving at specific velocities during specific moments of time. Imagine that the display screen is made up of a large number of tiny squares or "picture elements," each corresponding to a specific frequency shift, or velocity and a specific moment in time. Now let us examine just one picture element. If no blood cells are moving at the velocity (frequency shift) that corresponds to this particular element, it will be black. If a moderate percentage of the moving blood cells are at the velocity corresponding to this element, it will be gray. If a large percentage of the moving blood cells have a velocity corresponding to the picture element, it will be bright white.

Technically, the Doppler spectral display is called a "power spectrum" because it not only illustrates frequency shifts, but also demonstrates the relative power or flow energy concentrated at specific frequencies. For example, in laminar flow (Fig. 8-3; Color Plates 1, 2) the power or energy is concentrated in a narrow envelope near the maximum spectral frequencies. With turbulence, flow energy or power

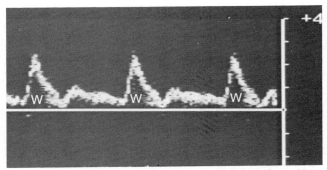

Figure 8-3. Spectral manifestations of laminar flow. Note that the frequency spectrum consists of a discrete white line that encloses a well defined window (W). This appearance indicates laminar flow, in which the majority of blood cells are moving at similar velocities.

becomes more uniformly distributed across a wide range of frequencies (spectral broadening), and in severe turbulence flow energy may be concentrated at lower frequencies.

With some duplex instruments, it is possible to dissect a moment in time from the spectrum display and illustrate the spectrum of frequencies or velocities present at that particular instant (Fig. 8-2). This capability is useful for evaluating spectral broadening, as discussed below. With sophisticated spectrum analysis devices, it also is possible to determine the average velocity of flowing blood over a period of time (the time averaged velocity). If the time averaged velocity across the flow stream is known and the diameter or area of the vessel is also known, blood flow may be calculated in cubic centimeters per second, and sophisticated spectrum analysis instruments are equipped to perform these flow calculations (Fig. 8-4). Other functions of sophisticated spectrum analysis devices include the calculation of velocity or frequency ratios that are useful for quantifying luminal obstruction (e.g., the systolic/diastolic ratio and the internal carotid/common carotid ratio). Diagnostic application of these Doppler signal analysis features are discussed below.

SPECTRAL FEATURES OF CONTINUOUS WAVE AND PULSED DOPPLER INSTRUMENTATION

Comparison of continuous wave and pulse wave (pulsed) Doppler instrumentation has been covered in Chapters 2 and 3, but a brief review and a few comments are in order before proceeding with carotid frequency spectrum analysis.

A continuous wave Doppler records frequency shifts from all moving objects within the ultrasound beam. In contrast, pulsed Dopplers may be range gated such that Doppler shifts will be recorded only from a specified location (range) along

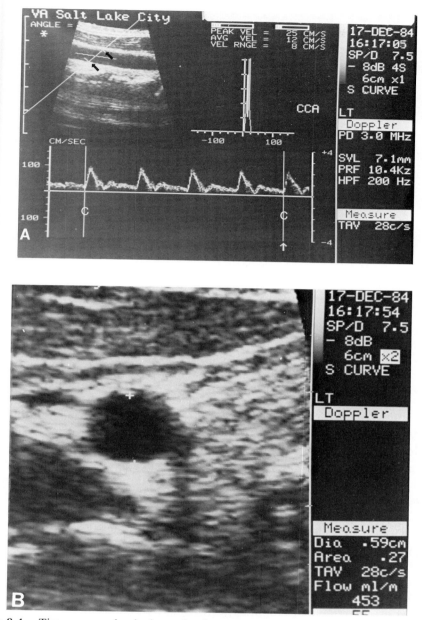

Figure 8-4. Time averaged velocity and volume flow determinations. (A) For measuring the time averaged velocity, the sample volume (arrows, upper right) is positioned to include the entire lumen. Electronic cursors (C, bottom) are then placed on the frequency spectrum to encompass as many cardiac cycles as possible. The instrument then computes the time averaged velocity (TAV, lower right), which in this case is 28 cm/sec. (B) Volume flow is then determined by measuring the diameter of the lumen (cursors) and converting the diameter to an area measurement (lower right). With knowledge of the time averaged velocity and the vessel area, the instrument calculates flow in ml/min. In this case, flow is 453 ml/min (lower right).

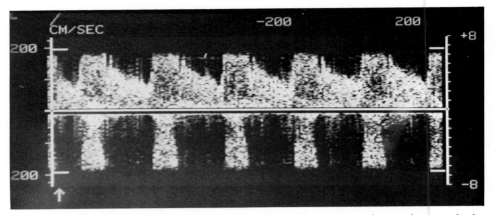

Figure 8-5. Demonstration of aliasing. In this frequency spectrum, the maximum velocity that can be measured is approximately 180 cm/sec. Components of the flow profile that exceed that velocity are projected below the baseline.

the Doppler sound beam (Fig. 8-1 and Fig. 8-2; see also Fig. 7-1 and Fig. 7-2). The region from which Doppler signals are accepted is termed the sample volume, and the use of a small sample volume has distinct advantages for identifying the source of the signal and for determining whether or not turbulence exists within an artery.[1,2] In normal arterial flow, a range of velocities exists across the arterial lumen. With a large sample volume or with a continuous wave Doppler, the entire spectrum of velocities will be demonstrated. The advantage of pulsed, range gated Doppler lies in ability to sample flow in highly specific locations; thus flow signals from one vessel may be clearly distinguished from signals arising in another vessel (e.g., internal versus external carotid artery). Furthermore, a small sample volume positioned directly in the center of the vessel will more accurately confirm the existence of a narrow range of central velocities corresponding to laminar flow. The principal disadvantage of a pulsed Doppler signal is limitation of the maximum frequency shift that may be accurately recorded. As a rough rule of thumb, pulsed Doppler signals cannot detect frequency shifts greater than one-half of the Doppler pulse repetition frequency (see Chapter 2). When the maximum frequency shift is exceeded, a condition termed "aliasing" occurs, in which a portion of the forward flow spectrum is cut off and either is demonstrated below the display base line (Fig. 8-5) or is mixed with other parts of the spectrum (depending on equipment design). The maximum frequency shift detectable with a given pulsed Doppler depends on the instrument design and specific operating circumstances, but it is not uncommon for aliasing to occur in severe carotid stenoses using commercially available duplex instruments. The practical implications of aliasing may be relatively unimportant for diagnosis of carotid stenosis, however, since stenoses with flow velocities that exceed the aliasing cutoff of most instruments are clearly of hemodynamic significance. Aliasing may represent a more serious problem during Doppler examination of deep-lying abdominal vessels.

INTERPRETATION OF DOPPLER FLOW SIGNALS
ASSOCIATED WITH CAROTID STENOSIS

Frequency Spectral Findings at Different Points in the Stenotic Lumen

Sonographers must be aware of and search carefully for the typical flow abnormalities that exist at various locations in the vicinity of an arterial stenosis.[3,4] These flow patterns are beautifully illustrated in superimposed B-mode and color coded Doppler images. Proximal to the stenosis, a laminar flow pattern will be detected, assuming that this part of the vessel is normal (see color plate 1). With very severe stenosis, pulsatility may be increased proximal to the lesion, as discussed in Chapter 3.

Within the stenotic zone, velocities are increased, but flow generally remains laminar (Fig. 8-6A; Color Plates 2,3). Some spectral broadening may occur in the stenotic zone, however, when there is a markedly parabolic distribution of velocities across the lumen (see Chapter 3), when the lumen is irregular, or when the Doppler sample volume includes a portion of the poststenotic turbulent flow. The audible Doppler signals in the stenotic zone typically have a high pitched, smooth sound and the pitch rises in proportion to the increase in velocity. In some stenoses, the area of highest velocities may be confined to a very small region; hence, *it is imperative that the examiner search carefully in the vicinity of any stenotic lesion to ensure that the region of maximal velocity has been detected.*

As the stenotic jet rushes into the poststenotic lumen, the flow stream spreads out rapidly producing disturbed flow patterns or frank turbulence in proportion to the severity of stenosis (Fig. 8-6B; color plate 4). Maximal turbulence occurs within 1 cm beyond the stenosis,[4] and in very severe lesions, turbulence in this region may cause the arterial wall to vibrate, producing (1) high amplitude, low frequency signals in the Doppler spectrum, (2) loss of definition of the upper border of the spectrum, (3) simultaneous bidirectional flow (above and below the baseline), and (4) a gruff, bruitlike sound in the audible Doppler output.

About 1 or 2 cm beyond the stenosis, frankly turbulent (swirling) flow subsides and the high amplitude, low frequency spectral pattern gives way to a more uniform degree of spectral broadening indicative of moderately disturbed flow (Fig. 8-6C). The audible signal in this zone has a bubbling or fluttering quality.

Laminar flow usually is re-established within 3 cm beyond the stenosis,[3,4] but the distance over which flow disturbances may extend varies in proportion to the severity of the lesion.

Systolic Velocity Measurements

The principal Doppler parameters used in determining the severity of arterial stenoses are the peak systolic and diastolic Doppler shifts observed in the stenotic zone. Increases in the stenotic zone Doppler shifts bear a well defined relationship to the magnitude of luminal narrowing. Stated simply, as the lumen area is reduced, flow velocity must increase in order for the same volume of blood to transverse the narrowed segment. Stenotic velocity increases do not continue

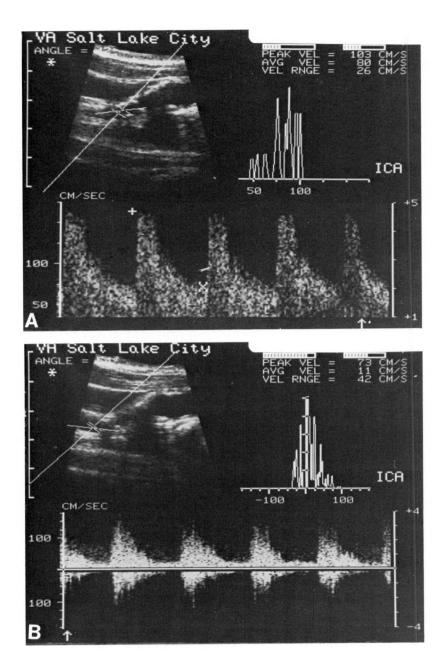

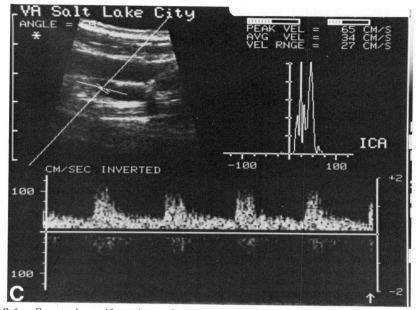

Figure 8-6. Spectral manifestations of stenosis. (A) In the stenotic zone, systolic (†) and diastolic (x) velocities are increased in proportion to the severity of the stenosis. In this case, flow is somewhat turbulent in the stenotic zone. (B) In the immediate post stenotic region, severe turbulence is manifested by "filling in" of the spectrum with high intensity, low velocity signals and by flow reversal due to swirling motions. (C) Farther down stream in the post stenotic zone, less severe turbulence is indicated by low intensity filling-in of the frequency spectrum and relatively little flow reversal.

uninterrupted to the point of occlusion, however, because of the effects of increased resistence to flow. In the carotid system, peak systolic velocities occur with a lumen of 1–1.5-mm diameter, and as a stenosis progress beyond that point, velocity falls off rapidly.[5] The 1–1.5-mm measurement for peak velocity occurrence assumes that the stenotic segment is very short. If the length of the stenotic segment is relatively long (greater than the original vessel diameter), then peak velocities will be lower than expected and will occur at residual diameters larger than 1.5 mm.

The relationships among velocity, Doppler frequency shift, luminal narrowing and flow are described in Figure 8-7, which is adapted from Spencer.[5] In this figure, note first the relationship between diameter and area reduction (horizontal axis). In a cylindrical vessel, a diameter reduction of 50 percent corresponds to an area reduction of approximately 75 percent, and a diameter reduction of 70 percent decreases the luminal area by 90 percent! Second, note that blood flow (cubic centimeters per minute) remains stable in the carotid system until diameter reduction approaches 60 percent. Beyond this level of obstruction, flow decreases precipitously. Third, observe that as lumen diameter decreases, flow velocity and Doppler shifted frequency rise in inverse proportion to the luminal size. Finally, note that peak velocities occur at about the same point in which flow begins to fall off (70 percent decrease in diameter). Beyond this point, velocity and Doppler

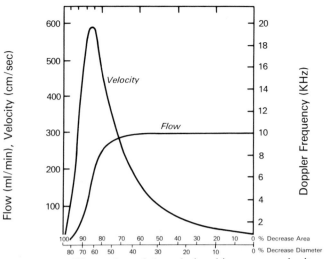

Figure 8-7. Illustration of the relationship among velocity, flow and lumen size in carotid stenosis. As the diameter decreases (from right to left) the velocity increases in a reversed parabolic fashion. Peak velocities occur at approximately 60–70% decrease in diameter. Thereafter, the velocity falls off rapidly to zero. In contrast, blood flow remains stable until the diameter is reduced by 50–60%. Flow falls off very rapidly to zero thereafter. Note also the relationship of percent decrease in diameter and percent decrease in area as shown at the base of the figure. Adapted from Spencer MP: Full capability Doppler diagnosis, in Spencer MP, Reed JM (ed): Cerebrovascular Evaluation with Doppler Ultrasound. The Hague, Martinus Nijhoff Publishers, 1981, p 213. With permission.

shift frequency abruptly decline to normal or subnormal levels, and it is possible for stenoses in this range to be underestimated based on measurement of peak systolic velocity.

Garth et al.[6] confirmed that peak systolic velocities greater than 100 cm/sec in the internal carotid are highly predictive of greater than 50 percent stenosis. In a study conducted by the author,[7] it was determined that peak systolic frequency shifts in the stenotic zone could be used clinically to classify patients within four categories of luminal narrowing, but peak systolic frequencies did not precisely relate to luminal obstruction, particularly in moderately severe stenoses from 40 to 60 percent in diameter. Stenotic zone velocities may be influenced by blood pressure, cardiac output, peripheral resistence, arterial compliance and the presence of contralateral carotid obstruction. Therefore, the examiner must always bear in mind that stenotic zone velocities may be considerably below or above the theoretical value for a given degree of obstruction, and it is possible to under- or overestimate the severity of such stenoses if other Doppler and B-mode findings are not considered.

Systolic Velocity Ratios

Because peak stenotic velocity shifts may be influenced by a variety of physiological factors, some investigators suggest that accuracy may be improved by comparison of peak stenotic zone frequency (or velocity) with the peak systolic frequency/velocity in a normal portion of the carotid system. Spencer and Reid[5] proposed comparison of the peak systolic frequency in the internal carotid stenotic zone with peak frequency in the normal, distal portion of the internal carotid. The validity of this approach was verified by Ritgers et al.[8] who found such ratios to be the most accurate of a large number of spectral parameters tested. The problem with the internal-to-internal carotid ratio is that it may be difficult to obtain Doppler signals far enough distally to ensure that normal flow is recorded.

Blackshear et al.[9] suggested the use of an internal carotid stenotic zone/common carotid ratio (Fig. 8-8). These investigators determined that a normal internal/common carotid systolic ratio is less than 0.8, and they found ratios exceeding 1.5 in all internal carotid stenoses with diameter reduction of 55 percent or more. Garth et al.[6], using velocity measurements rather than frequency, confirmed the validity of the 1.5 internal-to-common carotid ratio as an indicator of ≥ 50 percent stenosis and also found this ratio to be superior in accuracy to absolute stenotic zone velocities. Although peak velocity ratios have been worked out for internal carotid stenoses, the applicability of these ratios for common or external carotid lesions has not been clearly determined.

Diastolic Velocity Measurements

As arterial stenosis increases in severity, flow velocity rises initially only in systole. As luminal narrowing progresses beyond 50 percent, diastolic velocities also increases[10] and the ratio of systolic to diastolic velocities falls. With severe stenoses that exceed 70 percent decrease in diameter, very high velocities are present throughout the entire cardiac cycle and the ratio of systolic to diastolic velocity is drastically reduced. It is possible to grade stenotic lesions based on this changing velocity or frequency relationship (Fig. 8-8), and it has been tentatively established that a systolic/diastolic ratio of less than three in the stenotic zone is highly indicative of 70 or 80 percent diameter luminal narrowing.[11]

Spectral Broadening

Poststenotic flow disturbance (spectral broadening) is worthy of attention during duplex examination for two reasons. First, the presence of severe turbulence may be the only indication that a major stenosis is present in a severely diseased artery; e.g., when Doppler signals in the stenotic zone are blocked by calcification. Second, the severity of poststenotic disturbed flow is a rough indicator of the severity of carotid obstruction. Spectral broadening due to disturbed flow is first noticed along the down slope of systole and extending into diastole (Fig. 8-9A). Broadening progresses from this appearance to eventual fill-in of the entire spectral window as the stenosis becomes increasingly severe

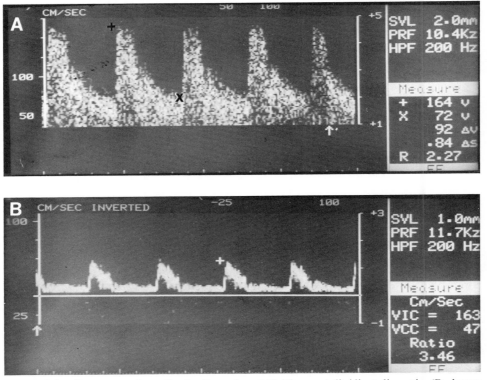

Figure 8-8. Demonstration of velocity ratios. (A) The systolic/diastolic ratio (R, lower right corner) is 2.27, a finding that suggests a stenosis in the range of 60 to 80% decrease in diameter. (B) Shown is the common carotid spectrum in the same patient as A. The internal carotid-to-common carotid velocity ratio is 3.46, as shown at the lower right.

(Fig. 8-9B). Severe turbulence is manifested as an exaggerated form of spectral broadening in which high amplitude, low frequency signals predominate, the upper border of the spectrum becomes indistinct and local flow reversal is seen below the spectrum baseline, assumedly due to swirling motion (Fig. 8-9C).

A variety of qualitative and quantitative schemes has been proposed for relating spectral broadening to lumen narrowing[1–4,6,10,12–16] and the medical literature on this subject is quite confusing. The best *qualitative* measure of spectral broadening appears to be complete fill-in of the spectral window, which is an easily recognized end point. Unfortunately, this degree of spectral broadening may be associated with various levels of carotid obstruction.

The significance of spectral broadening in the diagnosis of carotid stenosis may be summarized as follows: (1) Observation of spectral broadening is useful for evaluation of stenotic lesions but the specificity of this finding is poor. (2) Spectral broadening increases in severity in proportion to the magnitude of stenosis, but the proportionality of this relationship is difficult to define. (3) Filling in of the spectral window suggests a stenosis in the range of 50 percent or greater diameter reduction, but less severe lesions may also cause this degree of spectral broadening. (4) Severe, frankly turbulent postenotic flow is probably the most definitive form of spectral broadening and is highly suggestive of a very severe stenosis exceeding 70 percent decrease in diameter.

DOPPLER DIAGNOSIS OF OCCLUSION

As discussed previously, absence of a detectable Doppler shift signal is an indication of arterial occlusion. The pitfalls of this finding bear restatement. A Doppler shift signal cannot be detected in very severe stenoses with only a trickle of residual flow as illustrated in Figure 6-16, and such stenoses probably will be misdiagnosed as occlusion.

DOPPLER DIAGNOSIS OF NON-STENOTIC PLAQUE

Plaque that does not appreciably narrow the arterial lumen may cause flow disturbances that result in spectral broadening (Fig. 8-10), but the correlation of spectral broadening with nonstenotic plaque is relatively poor. Moderately severe but smooth plaque may produce little or no spectral broadening. Conversely, spectral broadening may be found in normal or minimally diseased vessels, especially in the presence of abnormal flow states such as systemic hypertension. Doppler techniques clearly are not useful for detecting nonstenotic carotid disease.[17] Fortunately, the introduction of duplex imaging has made the accurate diagnosis of nonstenotic plaque possible, regardless of its flow effects.

PUTTING THE DUPLEX EXAMINATION TOGETHER

We have discussed in Chapters 7 and 8 a variety of B-mode and Doppler parameters that indicate the severity of carotid atheromatous disease, and we have seen that the accuracy of each parameter is subject to certain limitations. It is the craft of the diagnostician to weigh and assemble all of the available ultrasound findings in determining the severity of carotid lesions. If one parameter does not fit with the rest, the diagnostician must assess the significance of this observation in relation to other findings and perhaps re-examine the patient in reference to the discrepant results. The diagnostician must also judge Doppler findings in light of the overall condition of the cardiovascular system. Blood pressure, cardiac output, aortic valvular disease, collateral flow and a host of other physiological factors may affect both normal and abnormal Doppler findings. Figure 8-11 summarizes the various Doppler parameters that must be integrated in the diagnostic process.

ILLUSTRATIVE CASES

As an additional aid to the reader, the following case examples are presented to illustrate the complex process of formulating a diagnosis based on duplex ultrasound data.

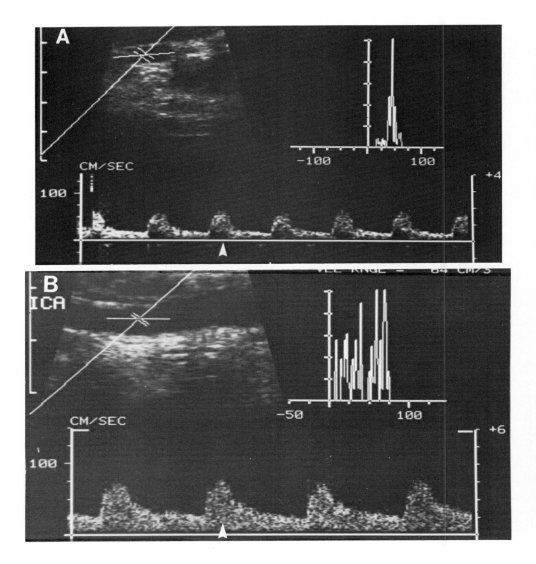

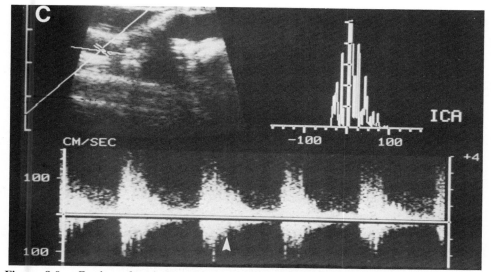

Figure 8-9. Grades of turbulent flow. (A) Minor turbulence is indicated by spectral broadening at peak systole, late systole and into diastole. Note that approximately 50% of the window persists beneath the spectral envelope. The velocity range (upper right) is approximately 50 cm/sec. at the moment in time indicated by the arrowhead. (B) Moderate turbulence is indicated by fill-in or the spectral window. The velocity range is approximately 75 cm/sec. at the moment in time indicated by the arrowhead. (C) Severe turbulence is characterized by spectral fill-in, poor definition of the spectral borders, and forward and reversed flow. The velocity range is approximately 125 cm/sec at the point in time indicated by the arrowhead.

Case 1

This 75-year-old male was studied because of bilateral asymptomatic cervical carotid bruits noted incidentally at physical examination. The duplex carotid examination is shown in Figure 8-12. What is your diagnosis?

Discussion. Posterior orbital signals are normal bilaterally (Fig. 8-12A and B). Extensive, moderately thick plaque is demonstrated in the common carotid (Fig. 8-12C and 8-12D). Although the lumen diameter is reduced by up to 50 percent in a single plane, area reduction is not sufficient to result in appreciable increase in flow velocities (Fig. 8-12E). Note that right common carotid pulsatility is normal. Moderately severe plaque is present in the right internal carotid orifice and adjacent portion of the common carotid bulb (Fig. 8-12F). Even though this plaque reduces the lumen diameter by approximately 50 percent, velocities were not increased in the right internal carotid (Fig. 8-12G). More severe plaque deposition is evident in the right external carotid orifice (Fig. 8-12H). This plaque results in visible narrowing of approximately 60 percent; however, the Doppler signals (Figs. 8-12, I and J) suggest that the stenosis is of greater severity. Normal velocities in the external carotid are 100 cm/sec or less at peak systole. Note that right external carotid systolic velocities exceed 200 cm/sec (Fig. 8-12I), and there

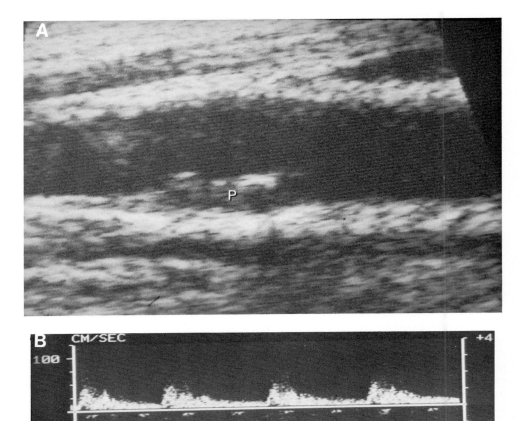

Figure 8-10. Disturbed flow resulting from nonstenotic plaque. (A) Plaque (P) in the bulbous portion of the common carotid produces mild narrowing of the arterial lumen. (B) Broadening is evident in this Doppler recording adjacent to the plaque.

is considerable turbulence in the poststenotic zone (Fig. 8-12J). Systolic velocity measurements for external carotid stenoses are not as well defined in relation to degree of luminal narrowing as for internal carotid stenoses; nontheless, this stenosis clearly is a severe lesion of at least 70 percent decrease in luminal diameter. Note in comparison with the arteriogram (Fig. 8-13) that the orifice of the right external carotid is appreciably narrowed in comparison with more distal portions of the vessels. Now compare the diameter of the proximal right internal carotid to its distal portions. Because plaque was deposited in the bulbous portion of the internal carotid, very little narrowing is present relative to more distal portions of the vessel, and no increase in velocity is observed.

At the left bifurcation, moderately thick plaque is noted in the common carotid (Figs. 8-12, K and L), without increase in flow velocity (Fig. 8-12M). Common carotid pulsatility is normal. The internal carotid is relatively poorly visualized (Fig. 8-12N). Some plaque is seen, but it does not appear that the lumen is severely narrowed. The absence of severe narrowing is indicated by normal

DIAMETER STENOSIS	GRAY-SCALE WAVEFORM (cm/sec)	PEAK SYSTOLIC VELOCITY	PEAK SYSTOLIC FREQUENCY (4.5MHz, 50°)	PEAK SYSTOLIC FREQUENCY (3.0MHz, 50°)	VELOCITY HISTOGRAM (cm/sec)	VELOCITY RANGE (50% amplitude)	FREQUENCY BANDWIDTH (50% amplitude)	VELOCITY RATIO[1]	SYSTOLE/DIASTOLE RATIO[2]
0-40%	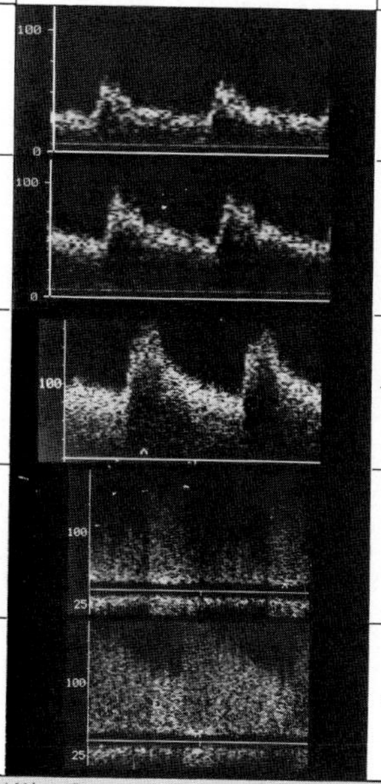	<80cm/sec	<3kHz	<2kHz	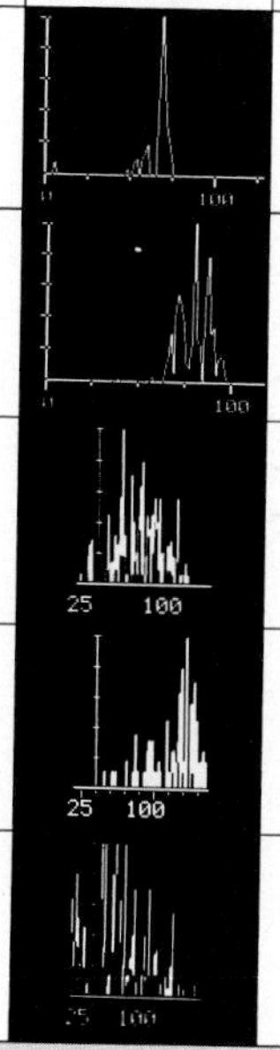	<30cm/sec	<1kHz	<1	>3
40-60%		80-120cm/sec	3-4.5kHz	2-3kHz		<40cm/sec	<1.5kHz	<1	>3
60-80%		120-175cm/sec	4.5-6.5kHz	3-4.4kHz		>40cm/sec	>1.5kHz	>1.5	>3
80-99% Grade I[3]		>175cm/sec	>6.5kHz	>4.4kHz		>50cm/sec	>2kHz	>1.8	<2
80-99% Grade II[4]		>175cm/sec	>6.5kHz	>4.4kHz		>50cm/sec	>2kHz	>1.8	<2

[1] Velocity Ratio = peak systolic velocity (at stenosis) ÷ peak systolic velocity (normal CCA)
[2] Systole/Diastole Ratio = peak systolic velocity ÷ end diastolic velocity
[3] Grade I (Highly turbulent, pulsatile flow, may obscure)
[4] Grade II (High turbulence, loss of pulsatility indicates >95% stenosis)

Figure 8-11. Summary of spectral findings associated with carotid stenosis. Moving from left to right, the following parameters are listed: (1) Diameter stenosis indicates the decrease in luminal diameter. (2) Peak systolic velocity refers to the velocity in the stenotic zone of an internal carotid stenosis. (3) End diastolic velocity refers to the lowest velocity observed in the internal carotid stenotic zone during diastole. (4) Systolic velocity ratio is the ratio of the internal carotid stenotic zone peak velocity to the peak velocity in a normal portion of the common carotid artery. (5) Diastolic velocity ratio is the ratio of the internal carotid stenotic zone end diastolic velocity to the end diastolic velocity in a normal portion of the common carotid artery. (6) Spectral broadening is the velocity range at peak systole as measured in centimeters per second. This measurement is not available on most duplex instruments. (From work by Baker et al., 1986.)

187

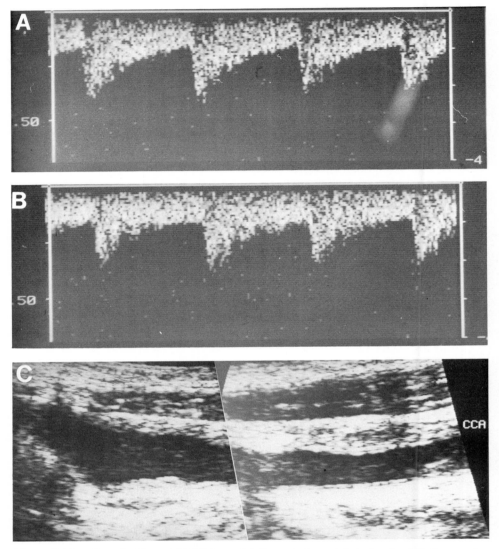

Figure 8-12. Case 1. (A and B) Right and left posterior orbital signals. (C) Composite, longitudinal view of the right common carotid artery (head toward left).

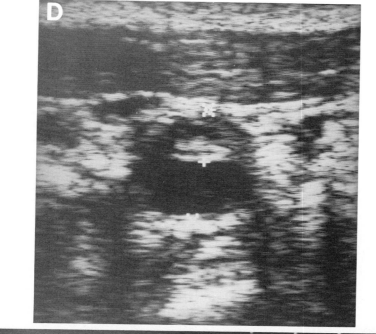

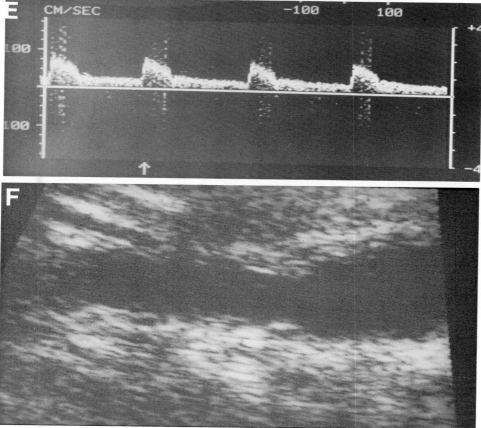

Figure 8-12. *(Continued)* (D) Transverse section, right common carotid artery at point of maximal narrowing. (E) Frequency spectrum, right common carotid artery in the area of narrowing. (F) Longitudinal view, right internal carotid orifice.

189

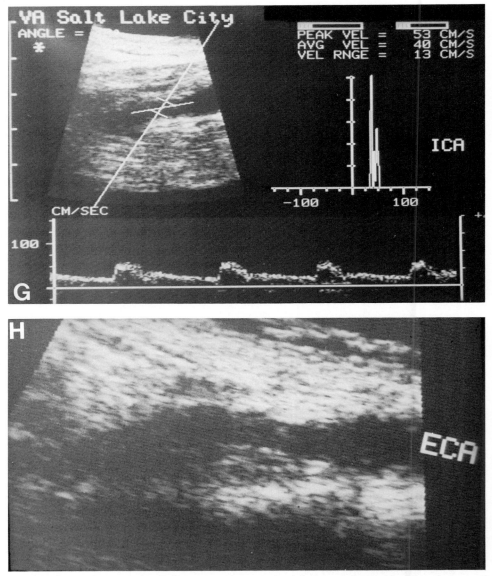

Figure 8-12. *(Continued)* (G) Frequency spectrum, right internal carotid orifice, in area of plaque. (H) Longitudinal view, right external carotid (ECA) orifice.

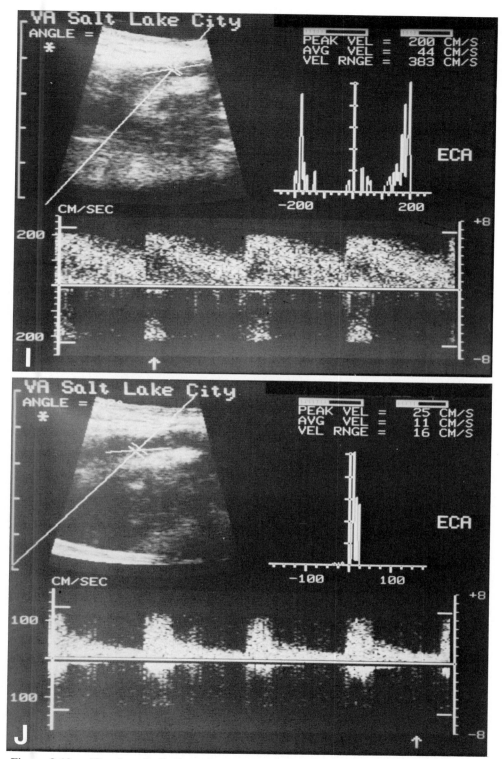

Figure 8-12. *(Continued)* (I) Stenotic and (J) poststenotic spectra of the right external carotid artery.

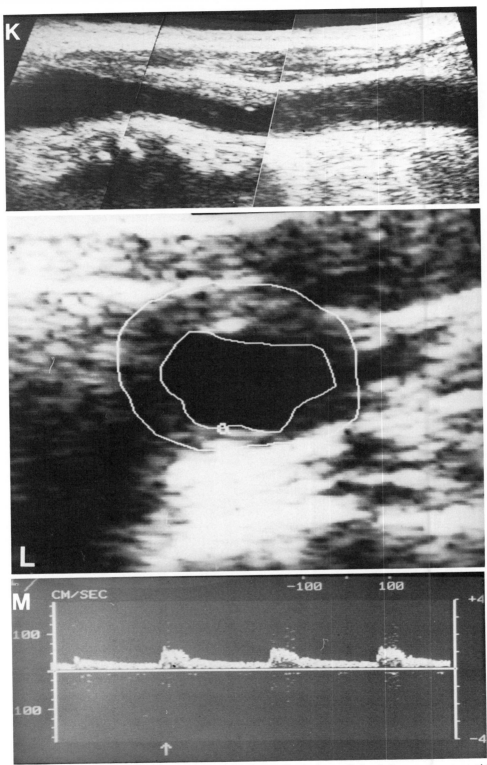

Figure 8-12. *(Continued)* (K) Composite longitudinal view of the left common carotid artery. (L) Transverse scan, left common carotid artery at point of maximal narrowing. (M) Frequency spectrum, left common carotid artery at narrowest point.

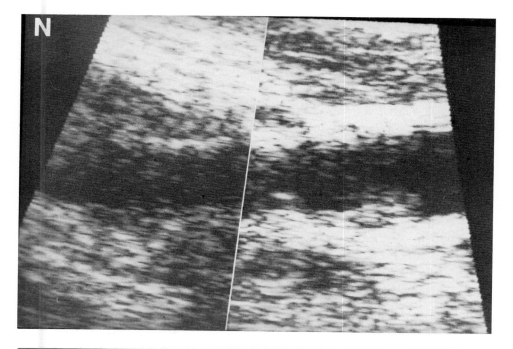

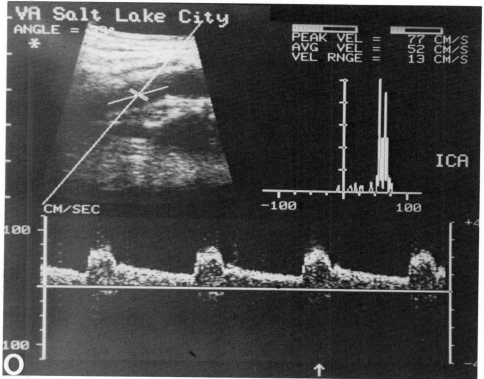

Figure 8-12. *(Continued)* (N) Composit longitudinal view of the left internal carotid orifice. (O) Representative frequency spectrum, left internal carotid artery in area of plaque.

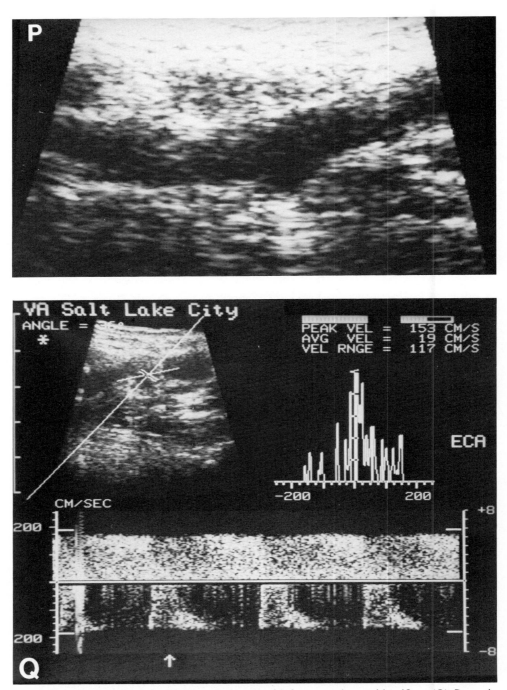

Figure 8-12. *(Continued)* (P) B-mode image of left external carotid orifice. (Q) Stenotic and

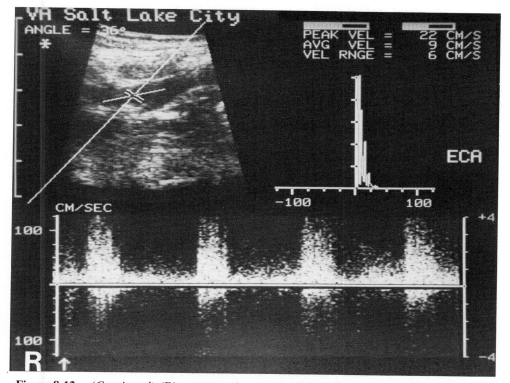

Figure 8-12. *(Continued)* (R) poststenotic spectra of the left external carotid artery near its orifice.

flow velocities in the internal carotid (Fig. 8-12O). The left external carotid is difficult to image (Fig. 8-12P) but clearly is abnormal as indicated by very high stenotic zone flow velocities (Fig. 8-12Q) and severe poststenotic turbulence (Fig. 8-12R). The arteriogram (Fig. 8-13) confirms the ultrasound findings of a relatively minor internal carotid stenosis and a severe external carotid stenosis on the left side. Common carotid narrowing is not fully appreciated in this single plane view.

This case is significant in that the principal stenoses are in the external carotid arteries. The presence of extensive plaque, particularly at the right bifurcation, led to arteriography and subsequently to right carotid endarterectomy.

Case 2

This 64-year-old woman presented with a history of dizziness. She was found to be hypertensive (BP 190/90) and a harsh right cervical bruit was noted. The duplex carotid examination is presented in Figure 8-14. What is your impression?

Discussion. The posterior orbital findings (Figs. 8-14, A and B) are an immediate tip-off that severe internal carotid obstruction is present bilaterally. On the right side, the frequency of the signal is quite low indicating that posterior orbital flow is fairly sluggish. Also note that the right waveform has a somewhat damped appearance. The frequency of the left posterior orbital waveform is

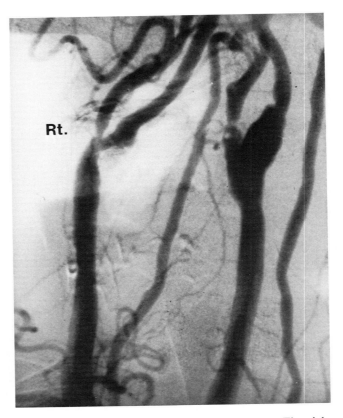

Figure 8-13. Arteriographic findings for case 1. The right (Rt.) and left carotid bifurcations are seen on an arch arteriogram.

considerably greater, suggesting that this is a more important collateral circuit. Nonetheless, the waveform does have a somewhat damped appearance probably because of resistance in the collateral bed. (There is no evidence of major external carotid obstruction on this side [Figs. 8-14, M and N].) The common carotid waveforms (Figs. 8-14, C and D also provide evidence of bilateral internal carotid obstruction. On the right side, pulsatility is somewhat greater than normal, while the left common carotid waveform is grossly abnormal and is clearly indicative of major internal carotid obstruction. Note that diastolic flow on the left returns to zero. Relatively minor plaque deposition is present in the right common carotid, but in the right internal carotid there is evidence of major plaque that almost occludes the lumen (Fig. 8-14F). Flow signals in this region are grossly abnormal. Systolic velocities approaching 400 cm/second are detected in the stenotic zone (Fig. 8-14G) with resultant aliasing on the pulsed Doppler spectrum. The systolic/diastolic ratio in the stenotic zone is grossly abnormal, measuring 1.51 from the continuous wave spectrum (Fig. 8-14H). The internal carotid/common carotid ratio in this case is 10 to 1. Severe poststenotic turbulence is demonstrated in Figure 8-14I. There is no question that the right internal carotid is severely

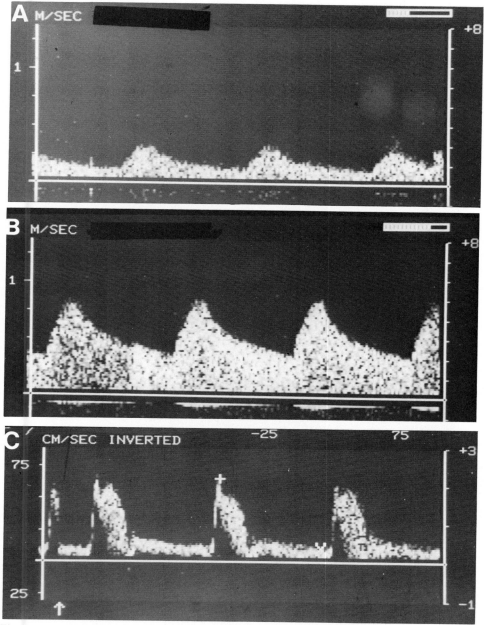

Figure 8-14. Case 2. (A and B) Right and left posterior orbital flow. (C) Right common carotid frequency spectrum.

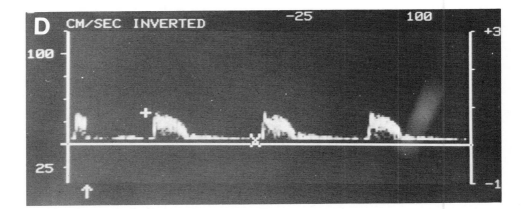

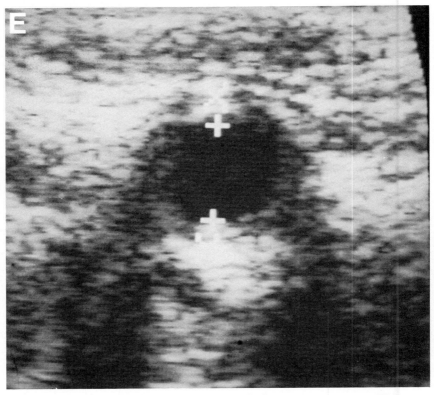

Figure 8-14. *(Continued)* (D) Left common carotid frequency spectrum. (E) Representative transverse section of the right common carotid at the point of maximal plaque deposition. (x, arterial wall. +, lumen.)

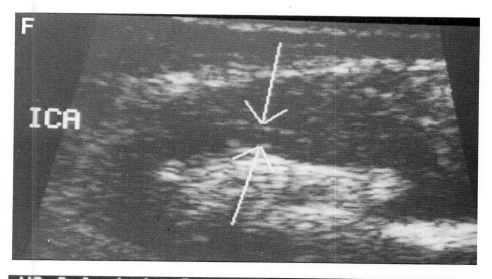

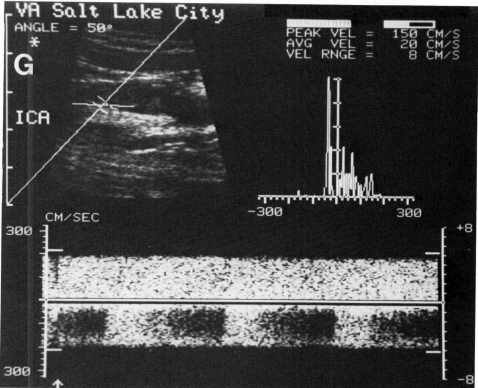

Figure 8-14. *(Continued)* (F) Longitudinal view of the right internal carotid artery. Arrows indicate the apparent residual lumen. (G) Pulsed Doppler spectrum of the right internal carotid artery at the same point as the arrows shown in F.

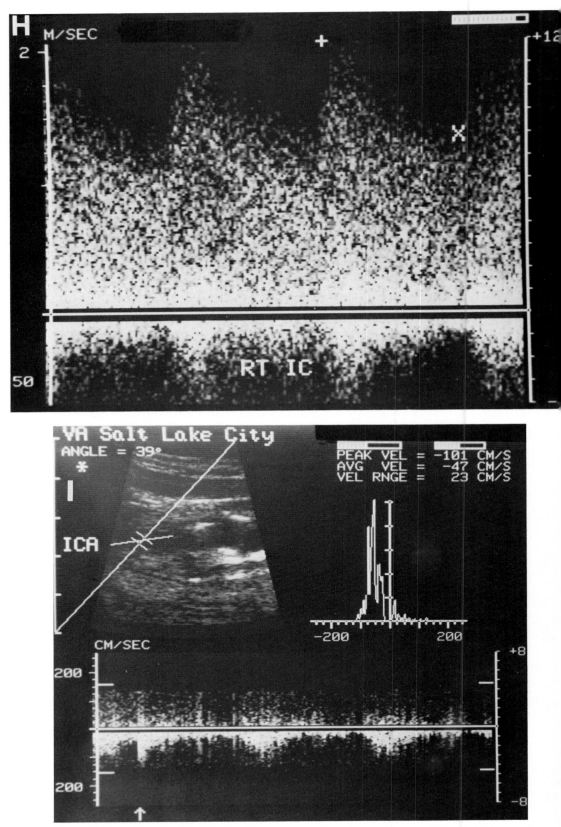

Figure 8-14. *(Continued)* (H) Continuous wave Doppler spectrum of the right internal carotid artery at approximately the same point as the arrows in F. (I) Pulsed Doppler spectrum of the right internal carotid artery, slightly downstream from the arrows in F.

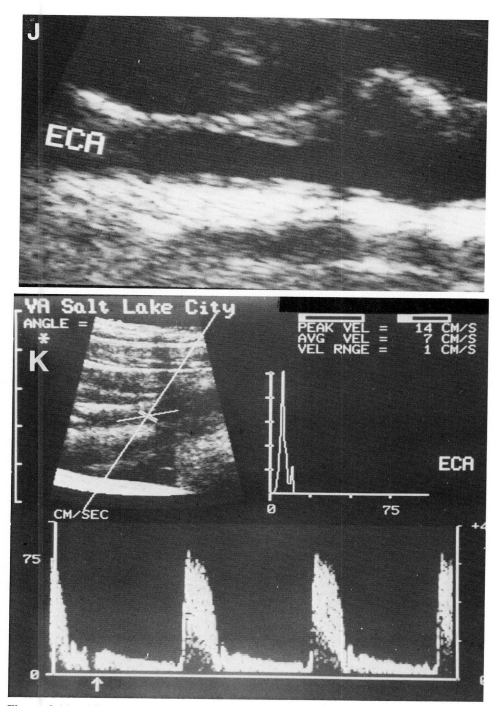

Figure 8-14. *(Continued)* (J) Longitudinal image of the right external carotid artery (ECA). (K) Frequency spectrum representative of the narrowed portion of the right external carotid artery.

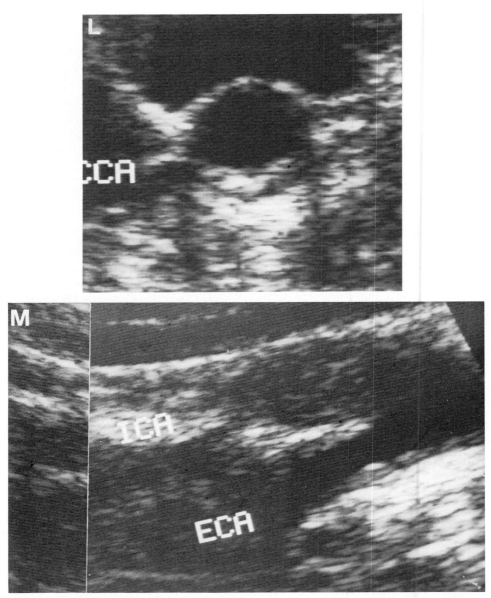

Figure 8-14. *(Continued)* (L) Transverse view of left common carotid artery (CCA) at the point of greatest plaque thickness. (M) Composite view of the left external (ECA) and internal (ICA) carotid arteries. Flow could not be detected in the internal carotid artery.

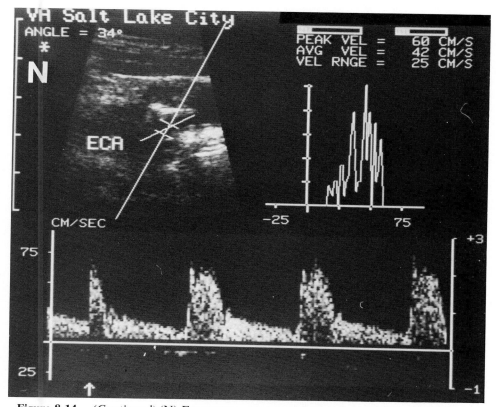

Figure 8-14. *(Continued)* (N) Frequency spectrum of the left external carotid artery.

stenosed. A moderate amount of plaque is present in the right external carotid orifice (Fig. 8-14J), but velocities in the external carotid (Fig. 8-14K) are not elevated, even in the presence of external carotid collateral flow. One would expect higher velocities through the narrowed portion of this lumen if external carotid flow were very well developed, which does not appear to be the case. Considering both the B-mode and spectral findings, the obstruction of the right external carotid probably does not exceed 40, or at most 50 percent.

At the left bifurcation, fairly minor plaque deposition is evident in the common carotid as illustrated in Figure 8-14L. The internal carotid artery is filled with echogenic material, no pulsations were observed and Doppler signals could not be obtained. It was assumed, therefore, that this vessel was occluded. Note the difference in appearance of the internal and external carotid lumens (Fig. 8-14M). External carotid flow (Fig. 8-14N) is normal with the exception of some turbulence related to the plaque at its orifice. Luminal narrowing here is minimal (20–30 percent).

The arteriographic findings (Fig. 8-15) confirm the ultrasound results, except that the large ulceration in the right internal carotid was not seen on the B-mode study. Failure to identify this ulceration emphasizes the problems associated with ultrasound diagnosis of plaque surface abnormality.

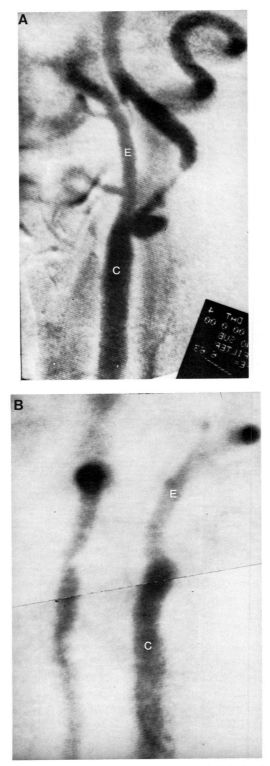

Figure 8-15. Arteriographic findings for case 2. Lateral digital subtraction arteriograms of the right (A) and left (B) carotid bifurcations are shown. C, common carotid artery; E, external carotid artery.

Case 3

This 74-year-old male had a right hemispheric cerebral infarction three years before examination. Carotid ultrasonography was requested because of an incidentally noted, low intensity right cervical carotid bruit. What is your impression?

Discussion. Right posterior orbital flow is reversed (Fig. 8-16A) indicating severe stenosis or occlusion of the right internal carotid artery. The right common carotid is severely narrowed by a large amount of low echogenicity plaque (Figs. 8-16, C and D). Visually, the degree of narrowing appears to be about 70 percent of the original diameter, and this degree of narrowing is confirmed by increased velocity in the stenotic zone (Fig. 8-16E) exceeding 200 cm/sec. Only one branch vessel could be identified on the right side and a spectrum from that vessel is shown in Figure 8-16F. Note that there is quite a lot of diastolic flow consistent with a low resistance type of circulation. This vessel, in fact, is the external carotid, but the low resistance appearance results from external carotid collateral flow to the brain. The flow pattern is also somewhat turbulent since the recording is made downstream from the severe right common carotid stenosis.

On the left side, moderate thickness plaque is present throughout much of the common carotid (Fig. 8-16G) with maximal narrowing of approximately 60 percent (Fig. 8-16H). The frequency spectrum in the area of maximal common carotid narrowing (Fig. 8-16I) supports the visual finding of approximately 60 percent stenosis. Note that peak frequencies reach approximately 180 to 200 cm/sec, but that the diastolic flow velocities are quite low. Peak systolic velocities in this lesion are higher perhaps than one would expect because the right internal carotid occlusion results in increased left common carotid flow. Images of the bifurcation branches (Fig. 8-16, J and L) demonstrate minimal to moderate thickness plaqueing that is more severe in the internal carotid than in the external carotid. The degree of narrowing, nonetheless, does not appear to be very great. The internal carotid is not seen very well, but normal flow velocities (Fig. 8-16K) exclude the possibility of major stenosis. Flow velocities also are normal in the external carotid (Fig. 8-16M). Flow in both the external and internal carotid is somewhat turbulent due to the presence of plaque. The possibility of surface irregularity is raised on the basis of the internal carotid image (Fig. 8-16J), but the findings are equivocal due to poor image quality.

Arteriographic findings. A lateral arteriogram of the right carotid bifurcation is shown in Figure 8-17A. The severe stenosis of the common carotid is confirmed as is occlusion of the internal carotid. Note the prominence of the external carotid artery resulting from its function as a collateral vessel. The left carotid bifurcation is seen in Figure 8-17B and C. It is difficult to judge the maximal degree of common carotid narrowing since the vessel is diffusely enlarged and the original diameter cannot be determined; however, the findings seem to be consistent with a 50–60 percent stenosis. The results in the left internal and external carotid also are quite consistent with the ultrasound diagnosis of moderate plaque deposition without major stenosis. Note that there is no evidence of surface irregularity in the internal carotid, even though the B-mode image (Fig. 8-16J) suggested irregularity.

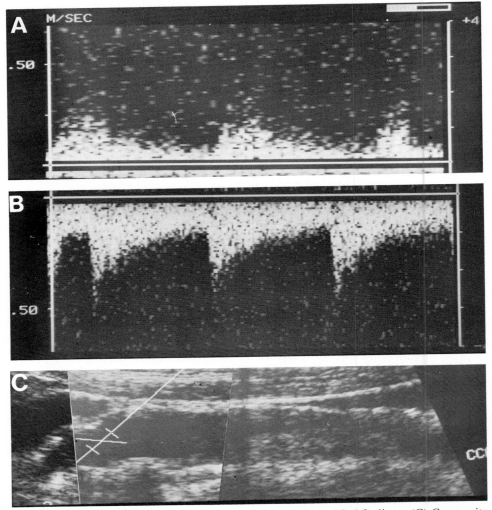

Figure 8-16. Case 3. (A) and (B), right and left posterior orbital findings. (C) Composite view of the right common carotid artery, including the orifice of the only branch vessel identified on the right side.

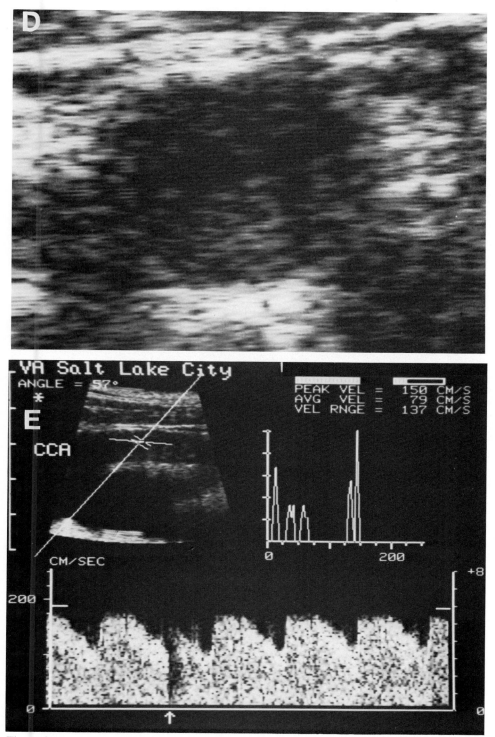

Figure 8-16. *(Continued)* (D) Transverse section of the right common carotid artery at its narrowest point. (E) Frequency spectrum in the stenotic portion of the right common carotid artery.

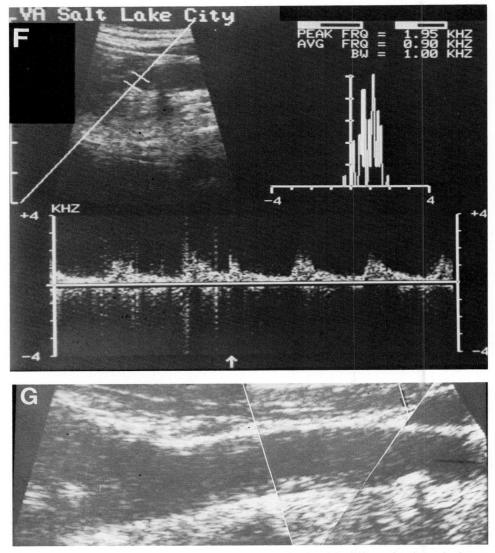

Figure 8-16. *(Continued)* (F) Frequency spectrum in the right bifurcation branch shown in C. (G) Composite longitudinal view of the left common carotid artery showing the origins of the branch vessels.

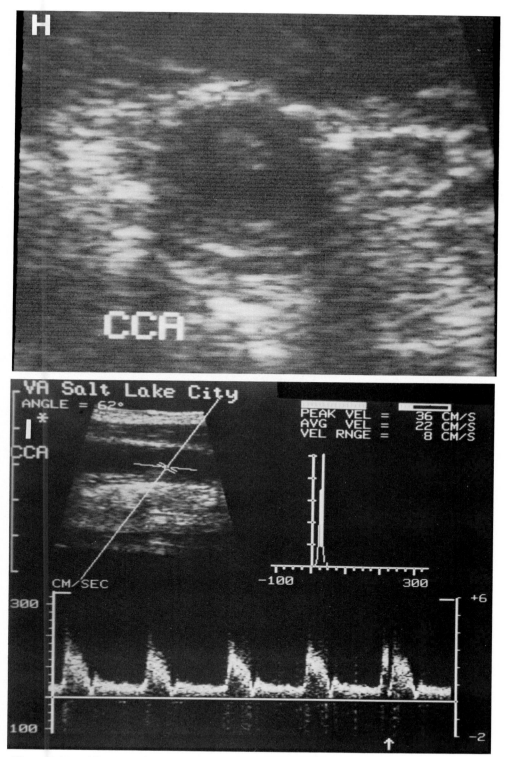

Figure 8-16. *(Continued)* (H) Transverse view of the left common carotid artery (CCA) at the point of maximal plaque thickness. (I) Frequency spectrum of the left common carotid artery at the point of maximal plaque deposition.

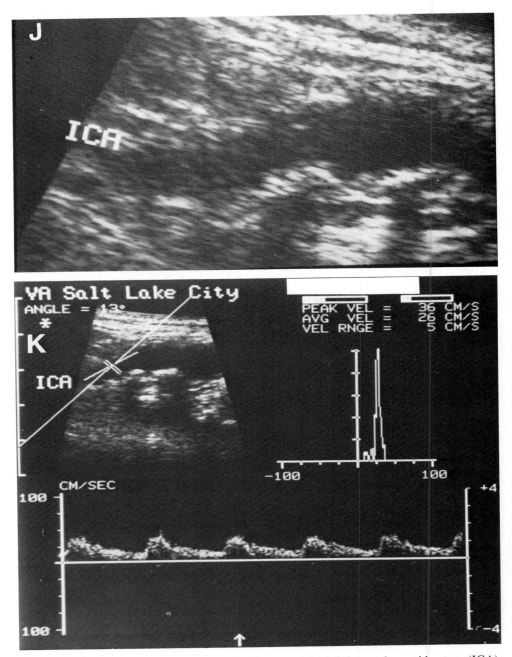

Figure 8-16. *(Continued)* (J) Longitudinal image of the left internal carotid artery (ICA). (K) Representative frequency spectrum adjacent to the plaque in the left internal carotid artery.

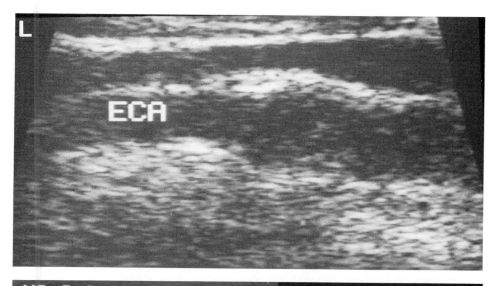

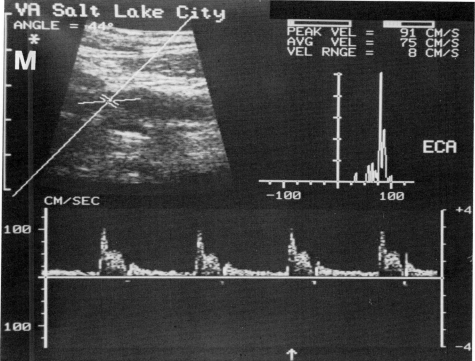

Figure 8-16. *(Continued)* (L) Longitudinal image of the left external carotid artery (ECA). (M) Representative frequency spectrum from the left external carotid artery.

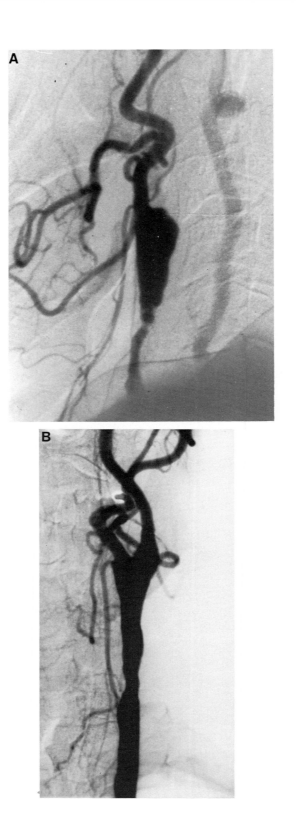

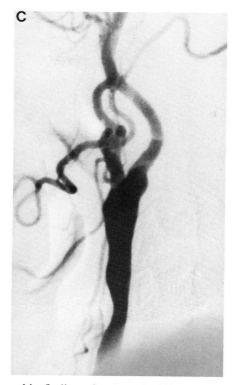

Figure 8-17. Arteriographic findings for case 3. (A) Lateral view of the right carotid bifurcation. (B) Anteroposterior and (C) lateral views of the left carotid bifurcation.

Case 4

This 78-year-old male was admitted for evaluation of iliofemoral occlusive disease. Five years previously, he had suffered a relatively minor left hemiparesis from which he had recovered with only minimal residual left arm weakness. Doppler results are shown in Figure 8-18. What are your conclusions based solely on these Doppler findings?

Discussion. Posterior orbital signals are strong and normally directed bilaterally (Figs. 8-18, A and B). However, common carotid pulsatility is markedly abnormal on the right (Fig. 8-18C). Note the difference in pulsatility and level of diastolic flow on the right side as compared with the left (Fig. 8-18D). The abnormal pulsatility pattern in the right common carotid artery clearly indicates a hemodynamically significant obstruction either of the internal carotid or of the common carotid distal to the point of examination. Common carotid flow measurements (Figs. 8-18, E and F) are indicative of reduced flow in the right carotid system. Note that the diameter and area on the right side are smaller than on the left. The difference in the time averaged velocity on the right and left is quite dramatic (7 cm/sec, right; 20 cm/sec, left) as is the difference in blood flow (184 ml/min, right; 672 ml/min, left).

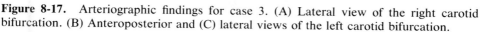

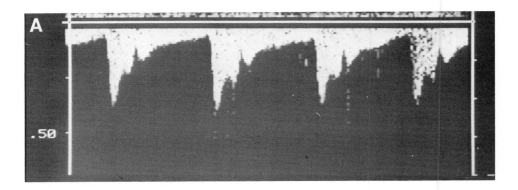

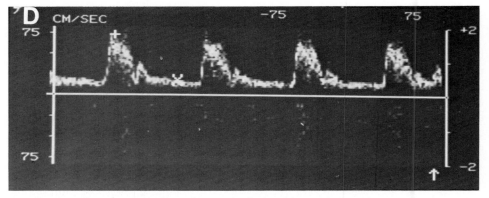

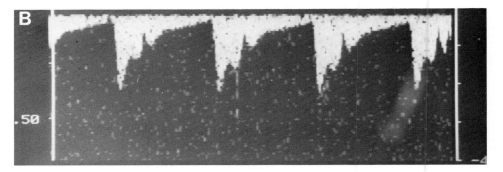

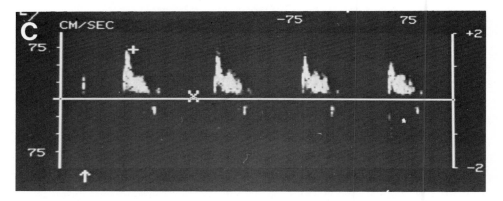

Figure 8-18. Case 4. (A) and (B) right and left posterior orbital tracings. (C) and (D) right and left common carotid pulsatility findings (center stream).

214

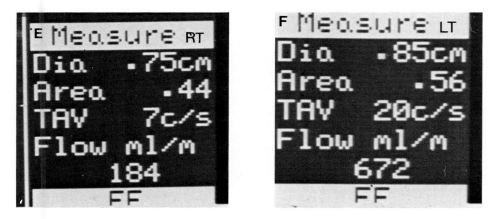

Figure 8-18. *(Continued)* (E) and (F) right and left common carotid flow statistics. Dia, diameter; TAV, time-averaged velocity in cm/sec.

If only these data were available one could correctly diagnose a hemodynamically significant obstructive lesion on the right side. The fact that posterior orbital flow is normally directed and symmetrical, indicates that intracranial collateral circulation is well established.

Arteriography (not shown) demonstrated occlusion of the right internal carotid.

William J. Zwiebel, M.D.
Associate Professor of Radiology
University of Utah School of Medicine
and
Chief, Ultrasound and Body CT
Veterans Administration Medical Center
500 Foothill Drive
Salt Lake City, Utah 84148

REFERENCES

1. Knox RA, Phillips DJ, Breslau PJ, et al: Empirical findings relating sample volume size to diagnostic accuracy in pulsed Doppler cerebrovascular studies. J Clin Ultrasound 10:227–232, 1982

2. van Merode T, Hick P, Hoeks APG, et al: Limitations of Doppler spectral broadening in the early detection of carotid artery disease due to the size of the sample volume. Ultrasound Med Biol 6:581–586, 1983

3. Reneman RS, Spencer MP: Local Doppler audio spectra in normal and stenosed carotid arteries in man. Ultrasound Med Biol 1:1–11, 1979

4. Douville Y, Johnston KW, Kassam M, et al: An in vitro model and its application for the study of carotid Doppler spectral broadening. Ultrasound Med Biol 4:347–356, 1983

5. Spencer MP, Reid JM: Quantitation of carotid stenosis with continuous-wave (C-W) Doppler ultrasound. Stroke 3:326–330, 1979

6. Garth KE, Carroll BA, Summer EG, et al: Duplex ultrasound scanning of the carotid arteries with velocity spectrum analysis. Radiology 147:823–827, 1983

7. Zwiebel WJ, Zagzebski JA, Crummy AB, et al: Correlation of peak Doppler frequency with lumen narrowing in carotid stenosis. Stroke 3:386–391, 1982

8. Rittgers SE, Thornhill BM, Barnes RW:

Quantitative analysis of carotid artery Doppler spectral waveforms: Diagnostic value of parameters. Ultrasound Med Biol 3:225–264, 1983

9. Blackshear WM, Phillips DJ, Chikos PM, et al. Carotid artery velocity patterns in normal and stenotic vessels. Stroke 1:67–71, 1980

10. Langlois Y, Roederer GO, Chan A, et al: Evaluating carotid artery disease. The concordance between pulsed Doppler/spectrum analysis and angiography. Ultrasound Med Biol 1:51–63, 1983

11. KW Marich: Personal communication. Diasonics Inc., Sunnyvale, CA.

12. Sheldon CD, Murie JA, Quin RO: Ultrasonic Doppler spectral broadening in the diagnosis of internal carotid artery stenosis. Ultrasound Med Biol 6:575–580, 1983

13. Johnston WJ, deMorias D, Kassam M, et al:

Cerebrovascular assessment using Doppler carotid scanning and real-time frequency analysis. J Clin Ultrasound 9:443–449, 1981

14. Barnes RW, Rittgers SE, Putney WW: Real-time Doppler spectrum analysis. Arc Surg 117:52–57, 1982

15. Keagy BA, Pharr WF, Thomas D, et al: A quantitative method for the evaluation of spectral analysis patterns in carotid artery stenosis. Ultrasound Med Biol 6:625–630, 1982

16. Brown PM, Johnston KW, Kassam M, et al: A critical study of ultrasound Doppler spectral analysis for detecting carotid disease. Ultrasound Med Biol 5:515–523, 1982

17. Zwiebel WJ, Austin CW, Sackett JF, et al: Correlation of high-resolution B-mode and continuous wave Doppler sonography with arteriography in the diagnosis of carotid stenosis. Radiology 149:523–532, 1983

Denis N. White, M.D., F.R.C.P.

9

Vertebral Ultrasonography

The brain is the most important organ in the body, since the quality of life enjoyed by an individual depends more upon its health than that of any other organ. The prevention and treatment of disease of the brain is, therefore, of the utmost importance to public health. By far the commonest cause of brain disease are occlusive vascular disorders. The reason for this predominance lies in the formidable metabolic requirements of the brain. This organ, which constitutes only 2 percent of the total body weight, needs a blood supply of 900–1100 ml/min, which is approximately 12–15 percent of the resting cardiac output; furthermore, it utilizes between 20–25 percent of the resting total body oxygen consumption and approximately 70 percent of the total resting fasting glucose output of the body.[1] Even relatively minor flow reduction in such a high-demand organ results in serious dysfunction.

Statistics referable to the mortality and morbidity of stroke are covered in detail in Chapter 4 and will not be repeated here. It is interesting to note, however, that in China, stroke is an even more serious problem than in Western countries. Out of a population of nearly 1 billion, almost 2 million Chinese die yearly from stroke. In the two decades before 1979, the mortality in a district near Shanghai from cerebrovascular disease rose to 1.94 per 1000 population, exceeding that from all other causes including malignancy and heart disease.[2]

Since the intracranial vasculature is largely inaccessible to radical treatment for arteriosclerotic occlusive disease, physicians have concentrated on the diagnosis and radical treatment of occlusive disease in the cervical arteries that feed the circle of Willis from which the cerebral blood supply arises. Such investigations have become increasingly used in the last three decades as angiography became safer and more widely adopted. The risks and difficulty of angiography, however, have stimulated the desire to develop safer and nonintrusive techniques for the diagnosis of such arteriosclerotic lesions in the cervical arteries. It is somewhat anomalous to reflect that the development of nonintrusive techniques aimed at replacing angiography depends for its success upon the prior development of accurate techniques such as angiography. Only under these circumstances is it possible to evaluate the accuracy of the noninvasive methods when the results of both techniques are compared in the same patient.

Peculiarities of the Vertebral Artery

Noninvasive techniques have enjoyed considerable success in the investigation of carotid occlusive disease, but so far, this has not been the case with vertebrobasilar disease, and it is important to consider the reasons for this difficulty. Some of the problems are technical and instrumental and will be considered in the body of this chapter. Other difficulties result from the vertebral artery itself and these can be classified into anatomical, pathogical, or surgical.

Anatomical Peculiarities

The common carotid artery and the origins of the internal and external carotid arteries are relatively superficial in the anterolateral portion of the neck, making them readily accessible for direct examination by nonintrusive techniques. This is not the case with the vertebral arteries, which are more deeply placed in the neck and, during their midcervical course, are largely obscured by bone as they pass through the transverse processes of C6 to C2 (see Fig. 5-3). For this reason, Doppler vertebral examination is subject to difficulty and limitations not encountered in carotid studies. Details of the anatomy of the vertebral artery have been described in Chapter 5. There are, however, a few points of considerable importance to the ultrasonographer that need re-emphasis.

Usually both vertebral arteries arise from the subclavian arteries, but in about 8 percent of normal persons, the left vertebral artery arises directly from the aorta. In such people, visualizations of that vertebral artery may be difficult angiographically. Moreover, in such patients, it is obvious that left subclavian artery occlusive disease will never result in a steal syndrome via that vertebral artery. Less commonly, on the right side both the common carotid and vertebral arteries may arise at the termination of the innominate artery; in such cases, subclavian occlusive disease will again cause neither vertebral nor carotid steal syndromes but innominate occlusive disease may do so. Anomalous origin of both the left and right vertebral artery is very difficult to visualize directly by any ultrasonic imaging technique, because the vessel origin lies within the chest rather than the neck. Ultrasonographers therefore have to examine the vertebral arteries ignorant of the possible existence of an anomalous origin, which may seriously affect the interpretation of their findings.

Moreover, unlike the common carotid arteries, which are usually of nearly equal size, the verebral arteries are usually unequal in size with a significant difference in 73 percent of normal persons and a two-to-one difference in diameters in 20 percent.[3,4] Although the flow velocity in such asymmetrical vertebral arteries remains equal, as do the frequencies of the Doppler shifted energy backscattered by the blood within them, the amplitude of the signals backscattered by the smaller artery is reduced, and this may make its detection by ultrasonic techniques difficult.

Low in the neck the vertebral artery, near its origin, lies in close proximity to a number of other arteries of similar size, making its identification difficult without the aid of spatial imaging techniques. These arteries include the inferior thyroid, ascending cervical, superficial cervical and suprascapular arteries all originating from the thyrocervical trunk of the subclavian artery (See Figs. 5-6, and 5-7). The thyrocervical trunk lies just lateral to the vertebral artery, and overlies it when scanned from the usual supraclavicular, anterolateral scanning plane. The internal thoracic artery runs inferiorly from the same region and the costocervical trunk arises more laterally from the subclavian artery, but their branches do not overlie the vertebral artery when viewed from the usual scanning plane, hence are not so easily confused with the vertebral artery.

High up in the neck, the occipital artery and its numerous muscular and meningeal branches also run in close proximity to the vertebral artery and may overlie and be confused with it. This is especially likely to occur because of the 90-degree, 180-degree, and 90-degree turns that the vertebral artery takes as it encircles the lateral mass of the atlas and then turns upward and forward through the foramen magnum. Moreover, in the presence of distal obstructive disease of the vertebral artery, its own spinal and meningeal branches may enlarge to form a collateral circulation and add further to the number of arteries of significant size present in this region.

The vertebral arteries are unique in that while they, like many other arteries, are paired, both arteries join to form the basilar artery from which the arteries to the brain stem, cerebellum, and posterior cerebrum arise. In the presence of occlusive disease of one vertebral artery, the blood flow to the basilar artery can be maintained by the other vertebral artery, which, by means of only a small increase in its overall diameter, can completely compensate for the flow that would have occurred through the obstructed vessel. This is obviously a much more efficient method of developing a collateral circulation than occurs in, for example, the internal carotid artery, where multiple, small, indirect anastomotic channels between the external carotid artery and the intracranial circulation must be enlarged in an attempt to compensate for reduced flow. The ease with which the second vertebral artery may compensate for occlusive disease of the first is one reason for the reluctance of surgeons to operate directly upon the vertebral arteries for obstructive disease.

Normally, the blood from the two vertebral arteries remains separate in its course through the basilar artery so that each vertebral artery supplies blood to the ipsilateral cerebellum, brain stem, and posterior cerebral artery. The anterior and posterior communicating arteries in the anastomotic circle of Willis normally do not mix blood from the left and right carotid and vertebral arteries. In the presence of occlusive disease of any of these four main arteries, however, the anastomotic circle may become functional and of importance in compensating for reduction in flow or pressure in one or more of the branches. Unfortunately, variants in the anatomy of the circle of Willis are the rule; Fields[5] found such anomalies to be present in 59 percent of 2727 brains. This is one reason that the same occlusive lesion, whether it be in the vertebral or carotid system, may result in very different symptoms and signs of neurological disease in different persons. In bilateral occlusive vertebral disease, the presence and size of the posterior communicating arteries will determine the degree to which the carotid system can compensate for any deficiencies in blood flow.

Pathological Peculiarities

Although atherosclerosis is a generalized disease, there are important differences in the type of atheroma that may develop in the vertebral arteries as compared with that in the carotid arteries. It has long been conventional to divide the atheromatous lesion into fibrous and fatty plaques. The former may be an earlier stage of the fatty lesion and capable of healing[6] but most authorities believe that the big, fibrous lesion is a late stage of the fatty plaque that has been covered with organized mural thrombi. It is the fatty plaque that breaks down, ulcerates, and forms a source for the emboli that cause transient ischemic attacks (TIA). Such fatty plaques progress causing increasing stenosis and eventually occlusion of the artery. In the carotid arteries, atheroma is usually of the lipid type and develops in the region of branches such as the origin of the common carotid artery, its bifurcation and siphon, and the origin of the cerebral arteries. In the vertebral system, lipid atheromatous deposits only tend to occur in the basilar artery. At the origin and termination of the vertebral arteries, the much less progressive multiple fibrous type of atheromatous lesion is more usual. This type of lesion causes medial atrophy with dilatation and elongation of the vessel but not ulceration at these sites,[7] though occlusions may occur at the termination of the artery in the region of the foramen magnum. Figure 9-1 shows the sites of atherosclerosis in the carotid and vertebral systems for three different age groups. The "step-ladder" lesions in the vertebral arteries in the oldest group should be noted; they are associated with osteophytes from degenerative disease of the cervical vertebrae that presumably damage and compress the vertebral arteries as a result of movements of the neck. Since stenoses have to be severe before they reduce the blood flow, atherosclerosis in the vertebral arteries tends to be a less malignant condition than in the carotid artery.

Since ulcerated fatty atheromatous plaques most often occur in the basilar rather than the vertebral arteries, TIA symptoms are relatively uncommon manifestations of vertebral atheromatous disease. Classical vertebral TIA symptoms include visual-field defects, diplopia, dysarthria, dysphagia and hemifacial sensory symptoms possibly associated with contralateral long-tract motor and sensory symptoms. With vertebrobasilar insufficiency due to occlusive atheromatous lesions, dizziness is by far the most common symptom and is the cause of much diagnostic difficulty, since it does not have the distinctive vertiginous features of labyrinthine dysfunction. Vertebral insufficiency symptoms are, therefore, difficult to distinguish from the common episodes of dizziness or unsteadiness that occur in many circulatory, neurological, epileptic and emotional disturbances. Such patients constitute a significant fraction of any medical and especially neurological practice. In every such patient, the possibility that the dizziness may result from vertebral-basilar ischemia must be considered, therefore, it is understandable that physicians eagerly seek a nonintrusive test for vertebrobasilar insufficiency that does not involve the rigors of vertebral angiography.

Surgical Peculiarities

Finally, the radical treatment of vertebrobasilar occlusive disease is severely limited. The vertebral arteries are accessible only in the lower neck, but even at the origins of the vertebral arteries, few surgeons are willing to attempt recon-

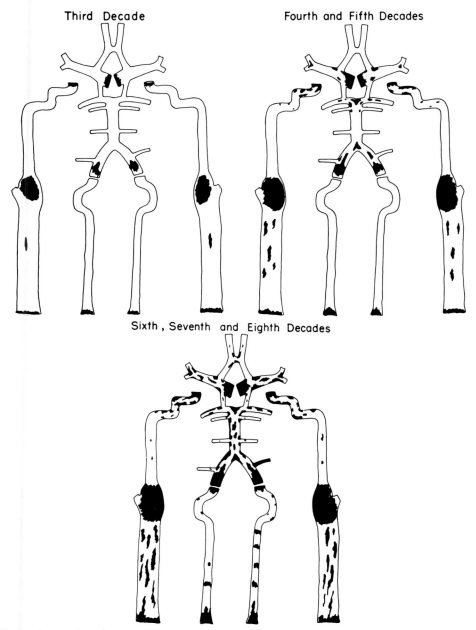

Third Decade

Fourth and Fifth Decades

Sixth , Seventh and Eighth Decades

Figure 9-1. The sites of atherosclerotic lesions in the carotid and vertebral systems illustrated for three different age groups are based on a large number of different studies (Moossy, 1966). Vertebral artery lesions first appear near the origin and termination of the artery. Later in life, lesions appear in the midcervical course of the vertebral arteries in association with osteoarthritic changes around the foramina transversaria of C3 to C6. From Moossy J: Morphology, sites and epidemiology of cerebral atherosclerosis, in Millikan CH (ed): Cerebrovascular Disease, Baltimore, Williams & Wilkins, 1966, pp 1–22. With permission.

structive surgery on stenoses. For the reasons considered in the previous section, such lesions are only slowly progressive and collateral flow through the other vertebral artery usually increases readily to compensate for flow reduction in the other. In cases of stenosis of the vertebral arteries, the surgeon usually prefers to rely upon the development of a collateral circulation via the other vertebral artery or the circle of Willis. Complete occlusion of the vertebral arteries at their origin, moreover, are inoperable. There are no branches of the vertebral arteries proximal to their entry into the transverse process of the sixth cervical vertebra through which collateral flow might develop; thus preserving blood flow through the artery. Occlusions, therefore, are accompanied by intravascular stasis and thrombosis usually extending into the upper neck just as an occlusion at the origin of the internal carotid artery is followed by clotting up to the origin of the ophthalmic artery.

The one exception to this limitation of surgical treatment is in those cases of stenosis or occlusion of the subclavian arteries just proximal to the origin of the vertebral artery. In such cases, the reduced pressure distal to the obstruction results in blood being stolen for the brachial artery from the ipsilateral vertebral artery, which in turn draws this blood from the contralateral vertebral artery. In such cases, symptoms of vertebrobasilar insufficiency with ischemia of the brain stem and posterior cerebra can occur and can readily be relieved by endarterectomy of the subclavian lesion. The detection of such surgically correctable steals is the major goal of nonintrusive vertebral artery investigations.

In summary then, the reasons for difficulty and relative neglect of the investigation of vertebral artery occlusive disease include the following: (1) The vertebral arteries are much less accessible than the carotid arteries, and commonly asymmetrical in size and, less commonly, subject to anomalous origin. (2) Because of their relatively deep course, the vertebral arteries are overlaid in the lower and upper neck, where they are most accessible for direct examinations, by other arteries with which they may be confused. (3) Because atherosclerosis of the vertebral arteries is less malignant than that of the carotid and basilar arteries, and because of the lesser accessibility of the vertebral arteries, radical surgical treatment has largely been confined to obstructions of the subclavian arteries causing steal syndromes. Diagnostic methods, including the noninvasive techniques, have largely been directed, therefore, toward the detection of reversed flow in the vertebral arteries in steal syndromes. Episodes of a nonspecific type of dizziness or unsteadiness, nevertheless, occur frequently and may result from vertebrobasilar ischemia. Any technique that identified such an etiology for these common symptoms and hence distinguished them from episodes of dizziness due to other causes, would be of great assistance to the physician.

Noninvasive Techniques for the Vertebral Arteries

Non-Doppler Systems

Although Moniz[8] first described the technique of angiography as long ago as 1927, it was not until after World War II that angiography became sufficiently safe to be used widely in the investigation of cerebral and cerebrovascular disease. It was not until angiography became a common procedure that the need to develop a less hazardous, less expensive and less unpleasant procedure became apparent, and this need coincided in time with the concurrent development of ultrasonic diagnostic techniques. Since ultrasonic Doppler techniques enjoy an advantage over all other procedures in the ease with which they can detect flowing blood, it was natural that the majority of such nonintrusive investigations made use of Doppler technology. Those that did not can be briefly summarized.

Kristensen[9] recorded reflections from the moving walls of the carotid and vertebral arteries in 1967 with both A-mode and M-mode pulse-echo techniques, but obviously this method was difficult and it must have been impossible to be certain that the wall motion recorded actually did originate from the desired artery. Voigt[10] also used a pulse-echo system to display the magnitude (in range and amplitude) of the motions of echoes obtained from the walls of the vertebral arteries during compression of the ipsilateral and contralateral vertebral artery at the root of the neck in seven proven cases of subclavian steal syndrome. This technique was also difficult and has not been widely used. The previous year Olinger[11] had used a pulse-echo technique with a storage display to make tomograms of the long axes of the carotid artery and had also displayed one segment of a normal vertebral artery. Once again, this manual scanning technique was obviously difficult, especially for imaging the vertebral artery. Such pulse-echo scanning techniques can now be made in real time and have come to play an important part in the diagnosis of early atheromatous lesions in the region of the carotid bifurcation. Strangely, despite the success of such real time pulse-echo techniques in the investigation of stenotic and occlusive disease at the carotid bifurcation and the plethora of publications that these have spawned, few attempts seem to have been made to apply the same techniques to the vertebral artery. Franceschi et al.[12] appear to have been the first to demonstrate that with real time B-mode systems, it is possible not only to display the whole of the carotid system in the neck but also the vertebral artery and the proximal connections of these systems to the aortic arch in the chest. Figure 9-2 is a photomosaic made by these authors through superimposition of scans made at different angles. The components of the mosaic can be recognized, and obviously such a composite picture does not need to be compiled in every case examined. However, it serves to show that with adequate skill and patience the cervical portions of the carotid and vertebral arteries and their intrathoracic origins can all be displayed with real-time pulse-echo methods. Instruments producing "pie-shaped" sector scans would appear to be advantageous for imaging the vertebral artery origin and the subclavian artery, *since these instruments have a small scan head amenable to imaging poorly accessible structures.* Baud et al.[13] used such scans to reproduce those made by Franceschi.[12] They try to identify the vertebral artery at its origin and separate it from the costocervical and thyrocervical trunks as well as from the jugular and vertebral veins. They admit however, that this is often difficult and is made more difficult by the frequent anatomical variations that occur in the site of the origin of the two vertebral arteries.

Duplex systems, as described in Chapter 7, offer distinct advantages over pure Doppler or B-mode methods, particularly in identification of the vertebral artery by its low resistance flow characteristics. Duplex instruments may be used to confirm that flow is present in the vertebral arteries and to determine the

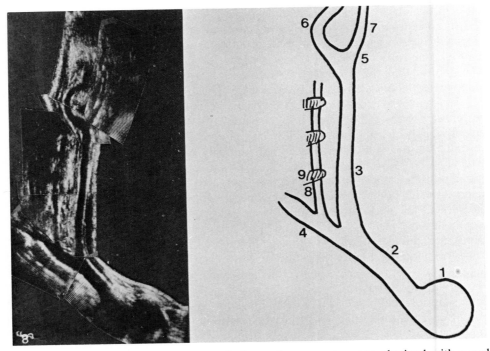

Figure 9-2. This photomosaic was made from nine separate scans obtained with a real time mechanical sector scanner with a water path, operating at a nominal frequency of 3.5 MHz. Included are the right carotid and vertebral arteries (8) in the neck as well as their intrathoracic orgins from the aortic arch (1) and innominate (2) arteries. Other arteries are: the subclavian artery (4), the transverse process of C6 (9), the common carotid, bifurcation and internal and external carotid arteries (3, 5, 6, and 7 respectively). From Franceschi C, Vadrot M, Lulzy F, et al: Echotomographic anatomy of the supra-aortic arterial trunks. Ultrason 2:57–61, 1981. With permission.

direction of flow. The duplex technique is considered further in the section of Doppler vertebral methods.

Doppler Vertebral Examination Techniques

All subsequent attempts to investigate the vertebral artery have been confined to the use of Doppler techniques and these can be broadly divided into those with and those without two-dimensional spatial displays (i.e., those that produce a two-dimensional image of the vasculature and those that do not). Historically, however, it is of note that the first use of Doppler techniques for the diagnosis of vertebral artery disease interrogated the brachial rather than the vertebral artery. Grossman[14] showed in 1970 that in cases of subclavian artery occlusion and a subclavian steal syndrome, there was a significant increase in the pulse-wave transit time to the brachial artery on the affected side.

Non-imaging Doppler techniques. Vertebral examination with nonspatial methods is hardly ever performed alone but is carried out in addition to the study

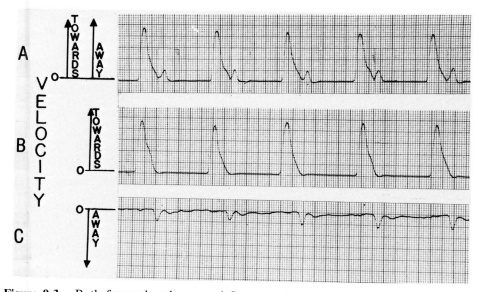

Figure 9-3. Both forward and reversed flow are shown as upward deflections in (A), recorded over a systemic artery with a nondirectional flowmeter. Traces (B) and (C) were made by a dual-channel directional discriminating flowmeter whereby flow is separately recorded in whichever direction is predominant at any one moment. These traces are characteristic of blood flowing in an artery feeding a high-resistance vasculature such as muscle or skin; during diastole, after an initial period of retrograde flow, very little flow occurs in either direction.

of the carotid system. As with the carotid examination, the artery is directly interrogated by holding the Doppler probe over the vertebral artery at whatever portal is chosen for the examination and orientating it until the audio Doppler signal is obtained and maximized. Much of the skill of the examination consists in listening to this audio signal and trying to determine from its characteristics, as well as the positioning of the probe, whether it does in fact arise from the vertebral artery.

A simple Doppler system with a zero crossing detector is usually considered quite adequate for the vertebral examination. The equipment necessary for the basic Doppler examination may, therefore, be any of the comparatively cheap Doppler flowmeters available on the market. However, the instruments should at least have a direction indicating facility, since the determination of the direction of flow is important for the detection of retrograde or oscillating flow in the vertebral arteries in cases of the subclavian steal syndrome. The display can either be on dual channels, as in the lower traces in Figure 9-3, where each channel displays flow in only one direction and the only channel activated is that in which flow is predominant at any one moment, or the display can be made in a single channel as in Figure 9-4 with forward and reversed flow being displayed above or below the zero baseline. Single channel displays such as those in Figure 9-4 are often believed, erroneously, to be direction-resolving but this is not the case and only the flow direction that is predominant at any one moment is manifest.

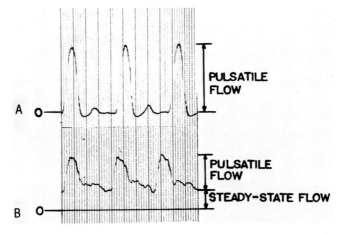

Figure 9-4. The velocity of blood flowing in a systemic artery such as the occipital (A), supplying a high-resistance vasculature, is contrasted with that in the vertebral artery (B) supplying the low-resistance vasculature of the brain. In the vertebral artery, as in the internal carotid artery, significant anterograde flow (above the zero) occurs throughout diastole so that flow is less pulsatile. These recordings were made with a single-channel directional discriminating flowmeter in which display flow is recorded in only one direction at a time, in whichever direction flow predominates at that moment.

Direction-resolving displays indicate flow in both directions simultaneously and not merely in the one predominant direction. Such displays can be made by processing the two quadrature detected signals in the phase domain. It is important, for the investigator to be aware of the problems inherent in such directional systems, especially when both forward and reversed flow are present simultaneously.

Recording from the vertebral artery suffers from two main restrictions. First, much of the artery is inaccessible to ultrasound, being obscured by bone, and second, the presence of numerous other vessels makes it difficult to be sure that Doppler signals being detected do in fact arise from the vertebral artery.

To overcome the first of these difficulties, workers have largely confined their efforts to examining the artery either low in the neck, before it enters the transverse process of C-6, or just below the base of the skull as it winds around the lateral mass of the atlas.

The latter portal has been the most popular and was first used by Pourcelot.[15–17] He positioned the Doppler probe behind the mastoid process and directed the beam medially (Fig. 9-5), but pointed out that from this position, because of the loop that the vertebral artery makes around the lateral mass of the atlas, the direction of blood flow recorded was of no help in identifying reversed flow in steal syndromes or in distinguishing the vertebral from other arteries. Both he and Mol and Rijcken[18] acknowledge that the technique was difficult and the

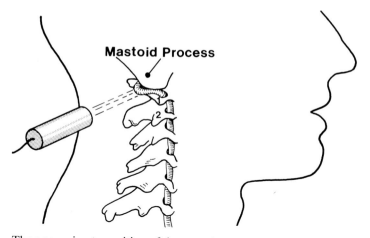

Mastoid Process

Figure 9-5. The approximate position of the transducer and its relationship to the C-1 loop of the vertebral artery is shown in vertebral examination from a posterior transducer position. Note that direction of flow cannot be assessed since it is impossible to determine which limb of the C-1 loop is being examined.

latter authors stated that recordings could "often" not be made, even in normal persons. Concerning the second difficulty, distinguishing the vertebral artery from other neighboring arteries, Pourcelot pointed out that such distinction could be made from systemic arteries that supply high-resistant vasculatures by the fact that the vertebral, like the internal carotid artery, has significant antegrade flow during diastole because it supplies the low-resistance vasculature of the brain (Fig. 9-4). Moreover, Muller and Gonzalez[19] suggested the identification of the vertebral artery could be improved if recordings were made only from arteries in which flow persisted during ipsilateral common carotid compression.

Despite the reservations expressed by Pourcelot, Barnes and Wilson[20] suggested that it was possible to record signals from the vertebral artery low in the neck if the overlying common carotid artery was manually displaced medially. This portal has obvious advantages if it is desired to record from the vicinity of stenoses, since most stenoses occur at the origin of the vertebral artery. Barnes noted, however, that the technique was also difficult.

Keller[21] proposed a transoral approach with the head of the transducer in the anesthetized lateral wall of the pharynx. Patient discomfort and swallowing of the artifacts have not made this a popular portal; moreover, the proximity of the internal carotid artery may well give rise to confusion.

Mol[22] endeavored to quantitate the time-velocity tracings that he made with his directional zero-crossing system. He calibrated his sytem by means of signals with known Doppler shifts and then measured the ratio between the peak systolic and mean diastolic flow. From these ratios Mol claimed to be able to diagnose most occlusive lesions of the carotid system as well as of the subclavian and innominate arteries.[23] In the vertebral arteries, however, he was only able to determine reversed or increased flow in subclavian steal syndromes and arterio-venous shunts, respectively.

In a study in 1978 De Bray et al.[24] using the postmastoid approach, studied the vertebral arteries with a time-velocity Doppler recorder in 25 patients who underwent subsequent angiography. He classified his cases according to the velocities he recorded during systole and diastole and claimed a satisfactory, but not very good, correlation between the two techniques. In a later study,[25] he found that the addition of cerebral gamma cineangiography, increased the information obtained by the Doppler examination alone.

Paludetti et al.[26] examined 54 normal subjects between the ages of 20 and 30 years. He recorded from the vertebral arteries both at their origin and from the postmastoid portal. By measuring the systolic and diastolic velocities and durations, these authors constructed curves that they considered to be normal for each portal of examination. However, their measurements showed large standard deviations, particularly during the diastolic portion of the flow curve, which might indicate marked variations in the vertebral arteries themselves or in the recording technique, or both. In the same year Morra et al.[27] studied 21 patients suffering mostly from "dizziness" but in a few cases from true vertigo. They found that two-thirds of these patients showed abnormalities in the time-velocity curves that they recorded from the vertebral arteries. More importantly, they found that all nine patients who developed nystagmus as a consequence of traction and lateral flexion of the neck, showed a significant reduction in flow in the contralateral vertebral artery. While it should be remembered that such a maneuver can partially occlude the vertebral artery of normal persons, the fact that they were able to record the reduction in flow in their nine cases suggests that their nonspatial imaging technique was truly recording from the vertebral artery. As will be described below, it is uncertainty regarding this matter that has caused many workers to abandon the nonspatial recording techniques despite their simplicity.

In a recent study, Ringelstein et al.[28] compared the performance of three graduate students in medicine at different times during a training period for the Doppler examination of the extracranial arteries. The students received instruction and supervision during their examination of 100 patients, half of whom had vascular disease. Their performance was also compared with that of the senior author who had trained himself by making 1700 Doppler examinations and comparing his results with the angiograms when these were also available. The students performance progressively improved during their training but, at the end, they still had difficulty, particularly with vertebral and subclavian lesions as well as patients with multiple vascular lesions. The authors concluded that 100 patients were insufficient adequately to train an operator in the nonspatial Doppler techniques. This study appears to show that, while a few experts in the field may achieve a commendable degree of accuracy, this accuracy is liable to be most difficult to achieve in the examination of the vertebral artery and also that not every worker may have achieved the highest possible accuracy.

It is difficult to ascertain the accuracy of the various reports of the vertebral examination by Doppler techniques without spatial imaging since only a few authors have reported their results in cases that subsequently received a satisfactory angiographic examination. With the exception of reversed or oscillating flow in cases of subclavian steal, which will be described separately, the only abnormalities that can be identified in the vertebral arteries are (1) absent flow due either to an occluded or an absent artery, (2) asymmetrical flow due either to hypoplasia or a severe stenosis proximal to the site of examination, or (3) the high frequency signals due to turbulence at a stenosis near the site of examination. Von Reutern[29] used both the postmastoid and supraclavicular portals for examination to identify normal vertebral flow in 27 patients, of whom 26 had normal vertebral angiograms while 1 had a 70 percent stenosis at the origin of the artery. Kaneda et al.[30] used the post mastoid approach only to identify correctly normal flow in 37 of 41 angiographically normal vertebral arteries. Of the four false positive results, no flow was detected by the Doppler examination in three vessels and reduced flow in the other. Of the 12 arteries shown by angiography to be hypoplastic or stenosed, they correctly showed asymmetrical flow in 11 but recorded normal flow in the 12th. Among 11 occluded or absent vertebral arteries, however, they correctly identified absent flow in only 6 and recorded reduced flow in the other 5. In the series reported from our laboratory,[31] of 259 angiography normal vertebral arteries the Doppler examination was also normal in 258, but in 1 case no flow could be recorded. Of 31 arteries that were hypoplastic, normal flow was found by the Doppler examination in 25 and absent flow in 6. In four arteries shown angiographically to be occluded or absent, normal flow was recorded in three and absent flow in only one. None of the eight stenoses angiographically, were detected by the Doppler examination.

Scanty as these reports are, the results reported both by Kaneda and ourselves clearly show that, in a significant number of cases, recordings must have been made erroneously from arteries other than the vertebral. Moreover, the results reported by all three investigators also emphasize another difficulty encountered in evaluating the accuracy of any technique where the majority of the examinations are normal. Under such circumstances there is a strong bias on the part of the operator to call any dubious result normal with a high probability of being correct. For these reasons it is suggested[31] that such operator bias can best be eliminated, and a more exact estimation of the accurancy of such techniques achieved, if only the abnormal cases are considered.

If such strict criteria are applied to the results summarized, it will be noted that of 59 angiographically abnormal vertebral arteries, the Doppler examination was correct in only 18 (30 percent).

Recently another difficulty has become apparent as a result of a study by Ringelstein[32] on a different population in which most of the patients studied had abnormal vertebral arteries. Ringelstein examined 151 patients all of whom were suspected of having vertebrobasilar disease. He also used the postmastoid and supraclavicular portals for his examinations. Although only 45 of his patients were subjected to vertebral angiography, 11 cases identified by the Doppler examination as having bilateral vertebral stenosis or occlusion were all confirmed angiographically. A further 9 cases identified by the Doppler examination as having unilateral vertebral stenosis or occlusion were also confirmed angiographically. Moreover, of 25 cases throught to be normal by the Doppler examination, 22 were also normal angiographically. Of the three false negative errors, two had elongation of the basilar artery and one had basilar stenosis, conditions that the Doppler examination could not be expected to identify. These are impressive results with a much higher accuracy than any of the previous studies described above. It should be noted however that all 20 cases found to be abnormal by the

Doppler examination were also suffering from severe neurological defects at the time of the examination resulting from vertebrobasilar disease. Of the 11 cases with bilateral vertebral disease on the Doppler examination, 5 subsequently died, 4 had resolving brain stem lesions, and 2 the "locked in" syndrome. These patients therefore had gross neurological deficits of a type known to be associated with basilar artery insufficiency and disease often associated with concurrent bilateral vertebral disease on the Doppler examination, 6 had Wallenberg's syndrome and the remaining 3 had other types of pontomedullary damage. The clinical picture in Wallenberg's and associated syndromes is also gross and characteristic and always results from thrombotic disease near the termination of the ipsilateral vertebral artery. It is possible that the increased accuracy achieved by Ringelstein in patients with gross neurological deficits usually resulting from basilar or bilateral vertebral artery disease or from unilateral vertebral artery disease may, in part, be due to clinical clues. These clues would suggest to the examiner the probable presence of unilateral or bilateral vertebral artery disease. In the same way, as will be described below, the accuracy of the diagnosis of the subclavian steal syndrome, with its characteristic clinical picture, is much greater than the diagnosis of vertebral artery occlusive disease not associated with obvious clinical defects.

In view of these serious reservations regarding the objective accuracy of the technique, it is probable that the nonspatial Doppler examination with its simple time-velocity recording would long ago have been abandoned were it not for the fact that the same safe, simple, quick and cheap technique has proven successful in the examination of the carotid system and particularly the anastomosis between the internal and external carotid arteries in the supraorbital region. It is easy to extend the carotid examination in an attempt also to include the vertebral system. The situation has been well summarized by Pourcelot, one of the leading proponents of the nonspatial imaging techniques for the carotid and vertebral systems. Pourcelot[33] states that, with the exception of the subclavian steal syndrome, the diagnosis of stenosis of the origin of the vertebral artery "is still difficult and the degree of accuracy needs to be improved." Further, he states that "it is often difficult to differentiate between occlusion and hypoplasia" and notes that the vertebral arteries are "often" asymmetrical.

In recent years the nonspatial Doppler techniques used for the examination of the carotid system have been extended to include a simultaneous spectral analysis of the Doppler signals in real-time which, it is claimed, improves the accuracy of the technique for the detection of minor degrees of stenosis. So far such additional spectral analyses do not seem to have been used in the nonspatial Doppler examinations of the vertebral arteries.

In 1978 Furuhata et al.[34] developed a combined A-mode reflection technique with a continuous wave Doppler device that used twin transducers to make it angle-independent, to measure quantitatively the volumetric flow in the carotid arteries. The system was described in more detail by Yoshimura et al. in 1981.[35] Furuhata et al.[36] later extended its application to measure volumetric flow in the vertebral arteries. No further studies appear to have been made on the vertebral arteries since that time, presumably indicating that it is very difficult to obtain an A-mode display of the short axis of the vertebral artery from a position perpendicular to the long axis of the artery in the neck at the same time as a

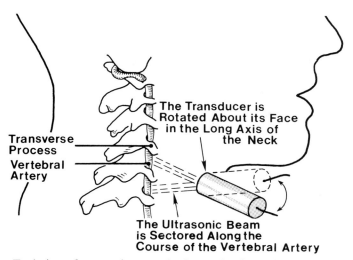

Transverse Process

Vertebral Artery

The Transducer is Rotated About its Face in the Long Axis of the Neck

The Ultrasonic Beam is Sectored Along the Course of the Vertebral Artery

Figure 9-6. Technique for anterior vertebral examination using a range-gated Doppler. [See text].

Doppler signal is received by the yoked A-mode and Doppler transducers. Moreover, the common asymmetry of the two vertebral probably largely negates the value of such volumetric measurements unless both vertebral arteries can be successfully interrogated in the same individual at the same examination.

Doppler imaging techniques. Since the great advantage of two-dimensional spatial displays in medical imaging is that they enable the organ being imaged to be identified unequivocally, and since it is obvious that much of the difficulty in the Doppler examination of the vertebral arteries results from uncertainty regarding the artery from which recordings are being made, it would be expected that Doppler scanning systems with spatial displays would be much more successful in examining the vertebral arteries. This expectation appears to be borne out in the case of real time pulse-echo spatial displays.

Spatial displays can be made with Doppler systems using either continuous wave or pulsed transmission. These devices do not image the artery walls as do pulse-echo techniques, but image instead the blood flowing through the arteries by means of the Doppler shifted energy backscattered by the moving red blood cells. The principals of operations of such instruments are described in Chapters 2 and 6, examples of Doppler vertebral images are shown in Figures 9-7 through 9-10.

There are only three continuous wave Doppler systems that make spatial displays. The Doppler imaging device developed by Coghlan and Taylor[37] does not appear to have been used to image the vertebral arteries. The first to have been developed, the DOPSCAN*[38] has been applied for this purpose, as has been the Echoflow†[39] (the latter instrument is color-coded to display increased flow velocities).

* Trademark, Carolina Medical Electronics, Inc., King, NC
† Trademark, Diagnostic Electronics Corp., Lexington, MA

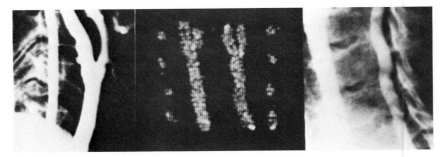

Figure 9-7. Both the carotid and vertebral arteries can be displayed in their midcervical course if they are scanned from the lateral surface of the neck with a continuous wave Doppler scanning system (Echoflow). From this scanning plane, only small portions of the vertebral artery can be insonated and visualized, however; the beaded appearance that results is completely characteristic. Angiograms of the two arterial systems appear on the corresponding sides of the scans.

The DOPSCAN appears to have been used only for imaging the vertebral artery low in the neck. Spencer[40] described the "down-imaging technique" whereby the origin of the vertebral artery can be displayed by reversing the normal upward inclination of the transducer used for carotid imaging. Spencer does not state how often this examination can be successfully performed nor give any figures for its accuracy as compared with angiography. White[41] first used the Echoflow system to image the vertebral artery in its midcervical course. In order to separate the artery from the overlying carotid system, the scans have to be made from a more lateral region of the surface of the neck (Fig. 9-7), from which scanning plane only small regions of the artery can be imaged between the transverse processes of the cervical vertebrae. More of the artery can be imaged

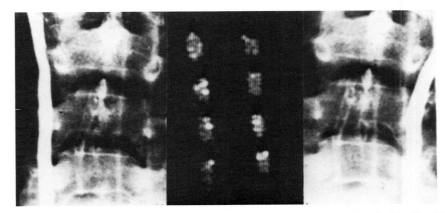

Figure 9-8. Larger portions of the vertebral artery can be insonated and visualized if the scan is made from the usual anterolateral surface of the neck. In such cases, however, because the overlying carotid artery must be time-gated out of the display, the system must be pulsed. Angiograms of the arteries are displayed on the corresponding sides of the scans.

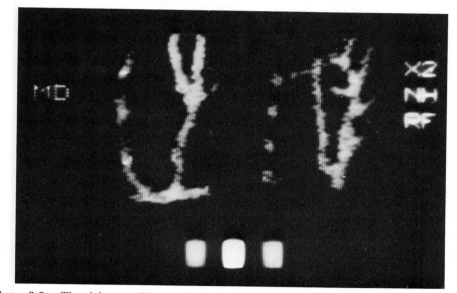

Figure 9-9. The right carotid and vertebral arteries displayed from their origins (left) low in the neck and continuing upward (right) to show the carotid bifurcation and numerous branches of the external carotid artery. The left-sided scan is made with the transducer pointed downward and the right-sided scan with it pointing upwards.

if the scan is made from the same anterolateral surface of the neck as is used for imaging the carotid artery (Fig. 9-8). In the latter case, however, the system must be pulsed so that the overlying carotid artery can be time-gated out of the display. While the images of the vertebral artery made by either of these two techniques are quite characteristic because of their "beaded" appearance, they cannot be made successfully in a significant number of the patients, and for this reason,

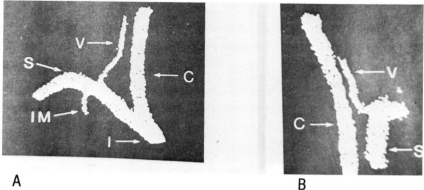

A B

Figure 9-10. Scans of the origins of the right (A) and left (B) carotid and vertebral arteries made by the MAVIS system show: C = common carotid artery, V = vertebral artery, S = subclavian artery, I = innominate artery, IM = internal mammary or internal thoracic artery. From Wood CPL, Meire HB: A technique for imaging the vertebral artery using pulsed Doppler ultrasound. Ultrasound Med Biol 6:329–339, 1980. With permission.

White et al. abandoned both techniques. Subsequently they adopted the down imaging technique, originally described by Spencer.[40] In this way they were able to image the origins of both the common carotid and vertebral arteries from the innominate and subclavian arteries high in the chest (left side, Fig. 9-9) and combine these images with those made higher up in the neck with their earlier continuous wave technique (Fig. 9-7 and right side of Fig. 9-9). Once again, however, the technique was difficult and it was impossible to complete a scan successfully in a significant number of patients. Moreover, the branches of the thyrocervical trunk often overlie the vertebral artery low in the neck and are difficult to distinguish from it. Although other workers claim more success with this technique, it would seem that, at the present time, continuous wave Doppler systems are incapable of providing spatial images of the vertebral arteries in a significant number of patients examined.

The first spatial displays made with Doppler techniques used a pulsed system[42] rather than the simpler continuous wave technique. Later Fish[43] developed a more complex multichannel Doppler system (MAVIS)* by means of which it was possible to make not only spatial displays of the blood vessels in three orthogonal planes, but also to display the velocity profiles of the blood flowing across the short axis of the vessel and also to calculate volumetric flow. Only the MAVIS system appears to have been used to make spatial images of the vertebral arteries[44] (Figs. 9-9 and 9-10) and these appear to be better than any other images made by Doppler scanning systems.

Preliminary results with the MAVIS technique[45] showed that, of 132 vertebral arteries scanned, 122 were successfully imaged. However angiographic confirmation of the arterial occlusion presumed present in these 10 cases was not obtained and some of these failures may have been due to the technique of examination rather than arterial occlusion. It is unfortunate that the development of this technique, which produces such excellent spatial images did not proceed beyond the manufacturer's clinical trial stage. The instrument was not produced commercially and its development has been suspended by the manufacturer.

It is interesting to speculate on the reasons why the spatial displays made with pulsed Doppler systems appear to give better images of the vertebral arteries than do continuous wave systems. Probably the most important reason is the narrower beam width of the pulsed systems that improves resolution in the lateral dimensions of the image. At the same time the range displayed by the pulsed system can be limited so that only the vessel of interest is displayed and signals from different depths are excluded. Moreover, when it is necessary to display two arteries simultaneously, the abilty to view them in the three orthogonal planes makes it easier to differentiate between the vessels and to direct the scan to the artery of interest.

Duplex Vertebral Examination

In view of the marked interest from a large number of different centers in the use of duplex scanning for the detection of carotid artery disease, it is surprising that few studies appear to have been directed at the vertebral arteries. Indeed Hennerici and Freund[46] stated only recently that duplex studies of the vertebral

---

* Trademark, GEC Medical Systems, London, England.

arteries "were impractical" because "reflections from the vessel wall are poor if the angle of the sound beam is not perpendicular" so that "examination of the tortuous, smaller and more deeply situated vertebral arteries in the neck can rarely be performed." However, in the same year, Ackerstaff et al.[47] reported that of 117 vertebral arteries studied they were unable to identify the artery with the duplex system in only 31 cases. In seven of these cases there was an occlusion of the artery concerned and in a further case it was congenitally absent. Of these 31 cases, 11 had normal vertebral arteries angiographically, though one of them had the left vertebral artery arising from the arotic arch. Of the remaining 13 cases, 3 had marked hypoplasia of the artery, another 3 had stenoses exceeding 50 percent of their lumen, and 5 had lesser degrees of stenosis. Reversed flow in one thyrocervical trunk was falsely identified on duplex scanning as reversed flow in the vertebral artery. In the subclavian artery, the duplex scan correctly identified 112 of 118 angiographically normal arteries. Of five occluded subclavian arteries, the duplex scan correctly showed the vertebral steal that was present in three cases and, in a forth case misidentified the stealing artery which was the thyrocervical trunk, as the vertebral artery. In the last case, where no steal was present, the occluded subclavian artery was correctly diagnosed by the duplex scan.

In addition, to the 31 sides on which the duplex system was unable to display the vertebral artery, there were a further 14 sides on which the duplex scan did not satisfactorily display the ostium or origin of the vertebral artery. Of the 72 arteries in which the ostium was satisfactorily displayed 49 were found to be normal on angiography and 45 of these had been correctly identified as normal in the preceding duplex scan. The other four cases were thought to have a stenosis as a result of the duplex examination. Of the 23 arteries shown to have an obstructive lesion at the ostium by angiography, the duplex scans had shown similar lesions in 18 cases. The remaining five cases had been considered normal on duplex scanning; two of these cases had an angiographic stenosis occluding over 50 percent of the arterial lumen.

More recently, in a personal communication to the author in 1985, Bendick and Jackson of the Indiana University School of Medicine[48] have reported upon 400 vertebral arteries examined with a 7.5- or 10-MHz real time imaging system coupled with a 3-MHz Doppler system. They examined the artery between two transverse processes and measured the diameter of the arteries as well as their flow characteristics. In 30 percent of their patients the artery could not be visualized and in a further 15 percent the images were suboptimal but adequate. They found enlarged arteries with high flow velocities in patients with carotid occlusive disease. Subsequent angiography confirmed the accuracy of the duplex examination in 186 of 187 normal arteries and in 10 of 19 abnormal arteries as well as reversed flow in all 4 cases of subclavian steal syndrome.

In summary, based on published reports of both nonimaging and imaging methods, it would appear that there is no single technique that so far successfully provides a noninvasive means for the detection of vascular disease in the vertebral arteries. At the one extreme there are the nonspatial time-velocity recordings made either from the postmastoid portal or from the supraclavicular region that successfully provide recordings in almost all the cases examined. However the accuracy of these recordings is suspect especially when steps are taken to eliminate the effects of operator bias on the interpretation given these recordings. At the other extreme, the techniques with spatial displays, whether made from the Doppler signal itself or from a concurrent pulse-echo display, largely eliminate errors due to the misidentification of arteries other than the vertebral. These spatial techniques suffer from two difficulties. The most important is that it is so difficult to make satisfactory displays with them that a significant number of examinations cannot be completed. In addition it is obvious that, even in those cases were the examination is successfully completed, they do not always reveal the vascular lesions that are present though the accuracy of the duplex technique, at least, is significantly greater than that of the nonspatial techniques.

The dismal situation concerning ultrasonic vertebral examination may be improved by the introduction of simultaneous B-mode and flow imaging. Based on preliminary clinical experience, it appears that vertebral artery identification may be considerably easier with this type of instrumentation than with other devices. It is possible that simultaneous B-mode and flow imaging may reduce the technical problem of vertebral sonography to a point that will permit the acquisition of useful flow information.

SUBCLAVIAN STEAL SYNDROME

It will be remembered that, when the accuracy of all the published reports is assessed but using only those cases that were reported as being abnormal in order to eliminate any operator bias toward normality in a series of patients who were mostly normal, only 18 (30 percent) of 59 angiographically identified lesions were successfully identified by the Doppler examination. In marked contrast to this degree of inaccuracy are the results reported by various investigators in the diagnosis of the subclavian steal syndrome. These all approximate toward 100 percent accuracy.

Keller et al.[21] correctly diagnosed reversed vertebral flow in 11 of 12 patients with a subclavian steal syndrome; they also only made a false diagnosis of reversed flow in 1 of 20 patients subsequently shown to have anterograde flow in the vertebral arteries. Von Reutern et al.[29] correctly identified the direction of flow by Doppler techniques in all 27 cases examined with anterograde flow and all 5 cases of retrograde flow. Nikitin[49] correctly diagnosed reversed flow due to a subclavian steal syndrome in 24 of 25 cases, while Corson et al.[50] correctly identified reversed flow in 2 cases as did Yoneda et al.[51] in 5 cases. Reversed flow thus was correctly identified by these workers with their nonspatial Doppler techniques in 47 of 49 cases. This is an error rate of only 4 percent in contrast to the 70 percent error rate for other types of vertebral artery abnormality.

The subclavian steal syndrome results from stenosis or occlusion of the subclavian or innominate arteries proximal to the origin of the ipsilateral vertebral artery. If the stenosis is sufficiently severe, the pressure distal to it in the region from which the vertebral artery arises is reduced below the pressure at the junction of the two vertebral arteries at the base of the brain (which is maintained by the contralateral vertebral artery). As a result, blood may flow retrograde down the vertebral artery on the side of the stenosis, the blood being "stolen" from the contralateral vertebral artery to supply the upper extremity and subclavian branches on the side of the subclavian obstruction. Reversal of flow in the vertebral artery evolves through stages of oscillating flow as the subclavian stenosis increases in severity, and these stages have been well described by von Reutern and Pourcelot.[52] At first there is deceleration of anterograde flow during systole, followed by a stage of oscillating flow, with retrograde flow occurring during systole and reduced anterograde flow continuing during diastole. Finally, with the fully developed syndrome, retrograde flow occurs during the whole of the pulse cycle. They explain this sequence as the consequence of (1) the reduced pressure differential across the length of the affected vertebral artery, causing reduction of anterograde flow or reversal of flow during systole, and (2) the difference in vascular resistance between the blood flowing into the basilar artery and that flowing into the brachial artery, which results in the pressure at the basilar end of the artery exceeding that at the subclavian end throughout the period of diastole.

Somewhat similar pressure changes occur between the origin and termination of the vertebral artery in cases of severe stenosis of the artery near its origin. In these cases, the normal acceleration of anterograde flow during systole is replaced by deceleration. It should be noted, however, that steady or oscillating reversal of flow does not occur in cases of vertebral artery stenosis and anterograde diastolic flow is always present.

The direct imaging, by ultrasonic means, of the causal stenosis or occlusions of the subclavian artery or the origin of the vertebral artery is difficult. The ultrasonic diagnosis of a subclavian steal syndrome or stenosis of the origin of the vertebral artery depends, therefore, not upon the display of the causal lesion, but upon the detection of the hemodynamic effects of such a lesion.

The ultrasonic diagnosis of a subclavian steal syndrome thus requires the demonstration of retrograde flow in the ipsilateral vertebral artery either during systole or throughout the pulse cycle. The display of oscillating flow with a Doppler technique may be difficult, so the ultrasonic examination should include ipsilateral brachial compression, which will result in reduced retrograde and increased anterograde flow. Such brachial compression is best carried out with a sphygmomanometer cuff inflated above the central systolic blood pressure. During the period of inflation, when the retrograde flow is reduced, the muscle of the forearm are exercised to that, when the cuff is deflated, there is reduced pressure in the brachial artery vasculature as a result of reactive hyperemia. As a result, the duration and amount of reversed flow in the ipsilateral vertebral artery, which decreased during the inflation period, will markedly increase following deflation.

The accuracy of such an ultrasonic diagnosis will obviously largely depend, as it does for the ultrasonic diagnosis of other vertebral artery lesions, upon the correct identification of the vertebral artery and the ability to record from it continuously during the manipulations with the sphygmomanometer cuff. In identifying the vertebral artery, it must be remembered that the operator will no longer be able to obtain assistance from the marked anterograde flow during diastole that normally characterizes flow in the vertebral arteries. Because the retrograde flow is now supplying the high-resistance vasculature of the arm, the flow pattern in the ipsilateral vertebral artery will be the same as in other systemic arteries. It would appear, therefore, that the ultrasonic diagnosis of the subclavian steal syndrome is at least as difficult as the ultrasonic diagnosis of stenosed, hypoplastic, or occluded or absent vertebral arteries. Yet the accuracy achieved by investigators appear to be much higher for the reversed flow of the steal syndrome.

We believe that the reason for this discrepancy lies in the fact that the subclavian steal syndrome can also be diagnosed on clinical grounds, which is not the case for vertebral stenoses, asymmetries or occlusions. The clinical diagnosis of the subclavian steal syndrome consists of the elicitation of a loud supraclavicular bruit or the presence of a reduced pulse and blood pressure in the ipsilateral arm. These are relatively easy physical signs to elicit. Not only is the clinical diagnosis of the steal syndrome reasonably accurate, but is has been usually made before the patient is referred for ultrasonic diagnosis. Even if this is not the case, the careful ultrasonographer usually conducts a clinical examination before the ultrasonic test from which a clinical diagnosis may be made suggesting the presence or absence of a steal syndrome. Finally there is some preselection of the cases referred for ultrasonography and most such cases are sent for the ultrasonic examination with the information that a steal syndrome is suspected and the request that it be confirmed or excluded.

Thus the ultrasonic examination for reversed flow in the vertebral arteries is not a truly blind examination as it is in the case of stenoses, asymmetries and occlusions where previous clinical examination cannot indicate the probable presence of such abnormalities. In the case of subclavian steal, the sonographer is already alerted to the fact the clinician suspects that reversed flow may be present and has clinical evidence to support such an opinion. As a result, the sonographer may search more diligently for an artery with caudad rather than cephalad flow. In this way, increased accuracy is achieved in the diagnosis of subclavian steal syndromes, but it would be a mistake to ascribe this accuracy to the ultrasonic examination alone. It results from a combination of the ultrasonic and clinical diagnoses, and is due to operator bias during the ultrasonic examination, which results from the previous clinical examination.

That such operator bias may indeed play a part in the ultrasonic examination is illustrated by two reports. The first by Wood and Meire[53] concerns a 9-year-old girl known to have Takayasu's arteritis who lost the pulses in her right arm followed five months later, by the development of vertigo. The blood pressure in both arms was lower than it had been a year earlier. Clinically her arteritis was considered to have progressed and she now had bilateral subclavian steal syndromes. The authors stated that "to confirm the clinical diagnosis we performed pulsed Doppler ultrasonic arteriograms of the cervical part of the subclavian arteries and the origins and proximal portions of both vertebral arteries," using the MAVIS system described previously. They were able to confirm that reversed flow was intermittently present in both vertebral arteries being precipitated by reactive hyperemia of the ipsilateral arm. In this case the authors document in more detail than is usually the case, the clinical information that they had received before commencing the Doppler examination that was used to confirm their well based clinical diagnosis. Such a situation appears to be fairly typical of all cases referred for Doppler examination to confirm a clinical diagnosis of subclavian steal syndrome.

The second report originates from our laboratory. The patient had a loud left supraclavicular bruit, a diminished arterial pulse in the left wrist and brachial artery, and systolic blood pressure in the left arm 20 mmHg lower than in the right. The ultrasonic Doppler examination confirmed that the flow velocities in the left brachial artery were lower than in the right, and retrograde flow was found in the left vertebral artery that apparently was reduced by brachial artery compression. The reactive hyperemia response was not performed but a diagnosis of subclavian steal syndrome was made and accepted by the clinicians. No angiogram was performed until the patient was readmitted several months later, when the clinical and ultrasonic examinations gave the same results. An angiogram performed on this second occasion showed, however, that while a subclavian artery stenosis was indeed present, the stenosis was distal to the origin of the left vertebral artery so that no vertebral steal could occur nor had occurred nor was occurring.

It would seem reasonable, therefore, to conclude that, while the diagnosis of the subclavian steal syndrome is reasonably accurate, this is not due only to the ultrasonic examination but also to the bias that results from the additional clinical examination.

SUMMARY

The present situation concerning vertebral artery ultrasonography reminds the author strongly of the situation of midline echoencephalography two decades ago. Midline echoencephalography enjoyed a considerable vogue at that time because of the clinical importance of a noninvasive technique to diagnose deforming cerebral disease in the days before computed axial tomography. The accuracy of the ultrasonic technique as reported by various investigators varied widely, when their results were validated by means of pneumoencephalography or cerebral angiography.[54] One group was able to achieve a positive predictive accuracy of 98.3 percent and a negative predictive accuracy of 99.7 percent on aproximately 1000 cases in each cohort. Other workers, including the writer, were unable to achieve such an excellent accuracy. It took many years before it became apparent that such accuracy was only achieved by the application of the two types of bias described above. The echoencephalographic studies reported had fallen into two main groups. On the one hand were surveys of the apparently normal population in which it was hoped that the echoencephalographic technique would identify the very occasional case of unsuspected deforming cerebral disease. On the other hand were studies of neurological and neurosurgical patients, a large percentage of whom had deforming neurological disease. When surveying the apparently normal population, almost all patients had an undisplaced cerebral midline, so that a very high degree of negative predictive accuracy could have been achieved even if every examination had been said to be normal. Thus the operator was strongly influenced to call all cases normal, particularly the dubious or difficult cases. If, as a result, the occasional case of deforming cerebral disease was not identified such cases would be rare and would little reduce the negative predictive accuracy of the technique below 100 percent. When a neurologically damaged group of patients were examined the echoencephalographic technique only achieved acceptable accuracy if it was performed by a neurologist or neurosurgeon, especially one involved in that patient's case. The neurologist or neurosurgeon, therefore, was in an excellent position to know, prior to the ultrasonic examination, whether deforming cerebral disease was likely to be present and, if so, to which side the cerebral midline would be displaced. Without such bias from the clinical knowledge of the patient, it was easy for the operator to misidentify echoes from non-midline structures as the M-echo and thus give rise to error.

In the same way, it now seems evident that, in vertebral ultrasonography without a spatial display, the Doppler examination is unsatisfactory because of the difficulty in identifying the vertebral artery with certainty.

Ultrasonic examinations of the vertebral arteries with two-dimensional spatial displays overcome the difficulty in identifying the artery that have made the nonspatial techniques unsatisfactory. However, all of these spatial techniques appear to be difficult to perform satisfactorily, and in a significant number of cases the examination cannot be completed. It was for these reasons that we abandoned our attempts to examine the vertebral arteries either with a pulsed technique or with a continuous wave spatial display. If one in every ten or so patients referred for examination cannot have a satisfactory examination completed, clinicians soon lose patience with the waste of time and money involved and stop sending patients for such examinations. Moreover, even in those patients in whom a satisfactory examination can be completed with a spatial display, the accuracy with which vascular lesions can be diagnosed, while better than that of the nonspatial displays, remains far from satisfactory. To date only the duplex technique has received any study validating the accuracy it achieves.[47] It is to be hoped that further studies and the development of new instrumentation will show improvement both in accuracy and the percentage of examinations that can be satisfactorily performed.

It is unfortunate that the multichannel pulsed Doppler systems that make such excellent spatial scans of both the carotid and vertebral systems have, so far, received no adequate validation of their accuracy in identifying vascular lesions. It is possible that those investigators who have access to such systems have appreciated that the accuracy achieved with these systems is insufficient to justify the time and trouble necessary to undertake the validation of an adequate series of cases with concurrent vertebral angiography. If so, this is unfortunate, since negative information is as valuable as positive data and it prevents other workers from wasting time pursuing an unfruitful approach.

However, overriding all the strengths and weaknesses of the various systems that have been developed to date and that will, no doubt, be developed in the future, must always be the consideration of the worth of developing a successful technique balanced against its cost in time and money that might have been directed more fruitfully towards other projects. In view of the variations in the anatomy of the vertebral artery, its common asymmetry in size, its depth and proximity to many other blood vessels, it would seem that recordings from it are never going to be made with ease. These difficulties are magnified by the fact that for much of its course the vertebral artery is hidden within bone. Atherosclerotic disease of the vertebral arteries moreover, is not so serious a problem as it is in the carotid, cerebral, and basilar systems, and when atheromatous disease does occur, it usually is so near to the vertebral origin that numerous other vessels in its vicinity favors the development of a collateral circulation that may retard the onset of symptoms of brainstem ischemia. In the same way the twin vertebral arteries, each separately supplying the basilar artery, safeguards the brainstem against the development of crippling ischemic lesions until both arteries become equally diseased. Finally, even in the presence of known vascular lesions in the vertebral arteries, surgical intervention, except near their origin, rarely appears to be easy or indicated. The only exception being the surgical treatment of brainstem ischemia due to a steal syndrome. In this latter case however, since the surgery of the occluded subclavian artery can usually be decided on the basis of the clinical signs alone, the ultrasonic test seems largely superfluous.

Denis N. White, M.D., F.R.C.P.
Professor Emeritus
Queens University
230 Alwington Place
Kingston, Ontario
Canada K7L498

REFERENCES

1. Scheinberg P: Cerebral blood flow, in Towers DB (ed): The Nervous System 2. New York, Raven Press, 1975
2. Wang C: Mortality rate of cardiovascular disease in Dong Changzhi neighbourhood of Hong Kong District, Shanghai. Chinese J Cardiol 9:83–84, 1981
3. Meyer JS, Lobe C: Strokes due to Vertebro-Basilar Disease. Charles C Thomas, Springfield, IL, 1965
4. Stopford JSB: The arteries of the pons and medulla oblongata. J Anat 50:131, 1916
5. Fields WS, Brustman ME, Weibel J: Collateral Circulation of the Brain. Baltimore, Williams & Wilkins, 1965
6. Wissler RW: Overview of problems of atherosclerosis, in Scheinberg P (ed): Cerebrovascular Disease. New York, Raven Press, pp 59–75, 1976
7. Crompton MR: Pathology of degenerative cerebral arterial disease, in Russell RW Ross (ed): Cerebral Arterial Disease. London, Churchill Livingstone, London. pp 40–56, 1976
8. Moniz E: L'encephalographie arterielle, son importance dans la localisation des tumeurs cerebrales. Rev Neurol 34:72, 1927
9. Kristensen JK: Ultrasonic pulse detection applied to the carotid and vertebral arteries. Scand J Thor Cardiovasc Surg 1:178–180, 1967
10. Voigt K, Kendel K, Sauer M: Subclavian steal syndrome: zur unblutigen diagnose des syndroms mit ultraschall-puls-echo und vertebralis kompression. Fort Neurol Psychiat 38:20–33, 1970
11. Olinger CP: Ultrasonic carotid echoarteriography. Am J Roentgen Rad Ther Nucl Med 106:282–295, 1969
12. Franceschi C, Vadrot M, Luizy F, et al: Echotomographic anatomy of the supra aortic arterial trunks. Ultrasons 2:57–61, 1981
13. Baud JM, Gras C, De Crepy B, et al: Apport de l'echotomographie en temps reel dans le bilan de la maladie atheromateuse cervico-encephalique. J Mal Vasc (Paris) 8:239–244, 1983
14. Grossman BL, Brisman R, Wood EH: Ultrasound and the subclavian steal syndrome. Radiology 94:1–6, 1970
15. Planiol Th, Pourcelot L: Doppler effect study of the carotid circulation, in deVlieger M, White DN, McCready VR (eds): Ultrasonics in Medicine. Excerpta Medica, Amsterdam, pp 104–111, 1974
16. Pourcelot L: Applications cliniques de l'examine Doppler transcutane in Ultrasonic Doppler Velocimetry. INSERM, Paris, pp 213–240, 1974
17. Pourcelot L: Diagnostic ultrasound for cerebral vascular diseases in Donald I, Levi S (eds): Present and Future of Diagnostic Ultrasound. London, Wiley, pp 141–147, 1976

18. Mol JMF, Rijcken WJ: Doppler haemato-tachographic investigation in cerebral circulation disturbances, in Reneman RS (ed): Cardiovascular Applications of Ultrasound. Amsterdam, Elsevier North-Holland, pp 305–314, 1974

19. Muller HR, Gonzalez RR, Jr: Evaluation of cranial blood flow with ultrasonic Doppler techniques, in deVlieger M, White DN, McCready VR (eds) Ultrasonics in Medicine. Amsterdam, Excerpta Medica, pp 89–96, 1974

20. Barnes RW, Wilson MR: Doppler Ultrasound Evaluation of Cerebrovascular Disease. Ames, IA, University of Iowa Press, 1975

21. Keller HM, Muller A, Meier WE, et al: Transorale Dopplersonographie unter schleimhautanasthesia zur beurtilung der stromungsverhaltrisse in den Aa. verte-brales (Vertebrales-Doppler). Deutsch Med Wochenschr 100:943–946, 1975

22. Mol JMF: Doppler-haematotachografisch onderzoek bij cerebrale circulatiestoornis-sen. Thesis, University of Utrecht, 1973

23. Mol JMF: The clinical use of Doppler haematographic investigation in cerebral circulation disturbances, in Reneman RS (ed): Doppler Ultrasound in the Diagnosis of Cerebrovascular Disease. London, Research Studies Press, 1982

24. De Bray JM, Dauzet M, Teisseire-Girod F, et al: L'effet Doppler applique a l'etude des arteres vertebrales. Nouv Presse Med 7:39–42, 1978

25. De Bray JM, Dauzet M, Pouplard F, et al: Etude comparee de la circulation vertebrale basilaire par l'effet Doppler, la cineangi-ogammagraphie (delai carotido basilaire) et l'angiographie. Rev Otoneuroophtalmol 51:333–339, 1979

26. Paludetti G, Mannarino E, Tassoni A, et al: Ultrasonografia Doppler delle arterie vertebrali del giovane: definizione dei parametri normali. G Clin Med (Bologna) 64:167–181, 1983

27. Morra B, Albera R, Poli L, et al: Rapporti fra ultrasuonografia Doppler e prove vestibolari nella insufficienza vertebro-basilare. Acta Otorhinol Ital 2:231–243, 1982

28. Ringelstein EB, Kolmann H-L, Kruse L: Dopplersonographie der extrakraniellen Hirnarterien: in erster Linie ein didak-tisches Problem. Ultraschall 4:182–187, 1983

29. Reutern GM von, Budingen HJ, Freund HJ: Dopplersonographische diagnostic von stenosen und verschlussen der vertebral-arterien und des subclavian-steal syndroms. Arch Psychiat Nervenkr 222:209–222, 1976

30. Kaneda H, Irino T, Miname T, et al: Diag-nostic reliability of the percutaneous ultra-sonic Doppler technique for vertebral arte-rial occlusive disease. Stroke 8:571–579, 1977

31. White DN, Ketelaars CEJ, Cledgett PR: Non-invasive techniques for the recording of vertebral artery flow and their limita-tions. Ultrasound Med Biol 6:315–327, 1980

32. Ringelstein EB, Zeumer H, Hundgen R, et al: Angiologische und prognostische Beurteilung von Hirnstamminsulten. Dtsch Med Wochenschr 108:1625–1631, 1983

33. Pourcelot L: Continuous wave Doppler techniques in cerebral vascular distur-bances, in Reneman RS (ed): Doppler Ultra-sound in the Diagnosis of Cerebrovascular Disease. London, Research Studies Press, 1982

34. Furuhata H, Kanno R, Kodiara K, et al: Development of ultrasonic volume flow meter. Proc Jpn Soc Med Eng Biomed Eng 2 D 33, 1978

35. Yoshimura S, Kodaira K, Fujishiro K et al: A newly developed non-invasive technique for quantitative measurement of blood flow: with special reference to the measurement of carotid arterial blood flow. Jikeikai Med J 28:241–256, 1981

36. Furuhata H, Suzuki N, Yoshimura S, et al: Non-invasive and quantitative measure-ment of volume flow-rate at internal and external and vertebral arteries, in Lerski RA, Morley P (eds): Ultrasound '82. Pergamon Press, Oxford, pp 239–242, 1983

37. Coghlan BA, Taylor MG: A carotid imaging system utilizing continuous wave Doppler-shift ultrasound and real-time spectrum analysis. Med Biol Eng Comput 16:739–744, 1978

38. Reid JM, Spencer MP: Ultrasonic Doppler technique for imaging blood vessels. Sci-ence 176:1235–1236, 1972

39. Curry GR, White DN: Color coded ultra-sonic differential velocity arterial scanner (Echoflow). Ultrasound Med Biol 4:27–35, 1978

40. Spencer MP: An over-view of non-invasive cerebrovascular evaluation using Doppler ultrasound, in Spencer MP, Reid JM (eds): Cerebrovascular Evaluation with Doppler

Ultrasound. The Hague, Matinus Nijhoff, pp 1–22, 1981

41. White DN, Curry GR, Stevenson RJ: Recording vertebral artery blood flow, in White DN, Lyons EA (eds): Ultasound in Medicine 4. New York, Plenum Press, pp 377–381, 1978

42. Hokansen DE, Mozersky DJ, Sumner DS, et al: Ultrasonic arteriography: a new approach to arterial visualization. Bio Med Eng 6:420, 1971

43. Fish PJ: Multichannel, direction-resolving Doppler angiography, in Kazner E, deVlieger M, Muller HR, McCready VR (eds): Ultrasonics in Medicine. Excerpta Medica, Amsterdam, pp 153–159, 1975

44. Wood CPL, Meire HB: A technique for imaging the vertebral artery using pulsed Doppler ultrasound. Ultrasound Med Biol 6:329–339, 1980

45. Wood, Cal: Personal communication, 1982

46. Hennerici M, Freund H-J: Efficacy of CW-Doppler and duplex system examination for the evaluation of extracranial carotid disease. JCU 12:155–161, 1984

47. Ackerstaff RGA, Hoeneveld H, Slowikowski JM, et al: Ultrasonic duplex scanning inatherosclerotic disease of the innominate, subclavian and vertebral arteries: a comparative study with angiography. Ultrasound Med Biol 10:409–418, 1984

48. Bendick PJ and Jackson VP. Indiana University School of Medicine. Personal Communication. 1985

49. Nikitin IuM: Ultrasound Dopplerography in the diagnosis of the subclavian steal syndrome. Zh Neuropat Psikhiatr 83:1295–1299, 1983

50. Corson JD, Menzoian JO, LoGerfo FW: Reversal of vertebral artery blood flow demonstrated by Doppler ultrasound. Ann Surg 112:715–719, 1977

51. Yoneda S, Kukuda T, Tada K, et al: Subclavian steal in Takayasu's arteritis: a haemodynamic study by means of ultrasonic Doppler flowmetry. Stroke 8:264–268, 1977

52. Reutern GM von, Pourcelot L: Cardiac cycle dependent alternating flow in vertebral arteries with subclavian artery stenoses. Stroke 9:229–236, 1978

53. Wood CPL, Meire HB: Intermittent bilateral subclavian steal detected by ultrasound angiography. Br J Radiol 53:727–730, 1980

54. White DN: Ultrasonic investigation of the brain, in Wells PNT (ed): Ultrasonics in Clinical Diagnosis, 2nd Ed, London, Churchill Livingstone, pp 35–61, 1977

Eugene F. Bernstein M.D., Ph.D.

10

Additional Noninvasive Techniques for Cerebrovascular Diagnosis

Noninvasive testing for arterial occlusive disease of the cerebrovascular system is still in an early stage of development; none of the current technology existed 15 years ago. One spectrum of techniques has been aimed at identifying the presence of hemodynamically significant stenoses at the origin of the great vessels from the aortic arch and in the carotid bifurcation area. Other methods are directed at the detection of shallow ulcerative lesions and simple atherosclerotic plaques. Such techniques also should be able to routinely distinguish internal carotid artery occlusion from very severe stenosis. At present, however, the technology is not able to successfully meet all of these requirements, but available techniques can detect hemodynamically significant lesions with a very high degree of accuracy. Currently, noninvasive cerebrovascular diagnosis is primarily used to screen patients who may be uncertain candidates for angiography, to follow patients who have undergone carotid artery surgery, to search for recurrence or progression of the disease and to evaluate patients in scientific studies involving the natural history of the disease, with and without intervention modalities.

Older techniques still in use in many noninvasive cerebrovascular laboratories include carotid phonoangiography, at least one variant of oculoplethysmography and the supraorbital Doppler evaluation. A second generation of more sophisticated techniques is currently available, including quantitative spectral analysis of the carotid phonoangiogram and/or the carotid velocity profile and the duplex scanner, which includes both B-mode imaging and pulsed Doppler velocity waveform analysis. Other new approaches include supraorbital photoplethysmography, carotid compression tomography, and several new forms of angiographic assessment, including radionuclide angiography with MTC-pertechnetate, computerized enhancement of intravenous or intraarterial contrast angiography (digital subtraction angiography) and transvenous xeroarteriography.

This chapter familiarizes the reader with important noninvasive or semi-invasive methods for cerebrovascular diagnosis that are not the principle subject of this textbook. Ultrasound methods presented in other chapters of this textbook will not be considered herein, except to compare ultrasound results with those of other techniques.

Carotid Phonoangiography

Carotid phonoangiography (CPA) simply involves the electronic amplifcation of sounds heard over the carotid artery, usually at the low, mid-, and high neck.[1] The sound waveforms are displayed on an oscilloscope and photographed. Although simple, the technique is of considerable value in differentiating sounds of carotid origin from transmitted bruits from the chest, which constitute approximately 50 percent of the arterial sounds observed clinically that stimulate requests for laboratory clarification.

There is an empiric correlation of the duration of the bruit with the degree of stenosis: sounds that persist throughout systole and enter diastole are almost invariably associated with a hemodynamically significant stenosis. Unfortunately, the technique cannot distinguish external from internal carotid artery lesions, and in addition fails to detect extremely high-grade stenosis or occlusion of the internal carotid artery, since the bruits disappear when stenosis is very severe, or when the vessel has been completely thrombosed.

Quite valuable as a simple and inexpensive screening device, CPA has provided valuable information regarding the importance of a bruit in the prognosis of a patient with carotid disease. Kartchner has demonstrated that those patients in whom a pansystolic bruit was confirmed by a positive oculoplethysmographic test had a greater than 20 percent likelihood of experiencing a stroke, although the disease was originally detected as an asymptomatic carotid bruit.[2] Further, this technique demonstrated that 7 percent of the patients studied following surgery had residual or recurrent carotid stenosis. It should be clear that a negative CPA test is no assurance that serious carotid disease does not exist, since severe stenosis and occlusion often are unassociated with detectable bruits.

Quantitative Spectral Phonoangiography

Within the past several years, Lees has developed technology for further analysis of the carotid phonoangiogram.[3] Basically, the amplified audio signal is passed through a spectrum analyzer for frequency analysis. A plot of the amplitude versus frequency is made in an effort to obtain the break frequency, or frequency at which the amplitude is highest (Fig. 10-1). This information can then be factored in an equation (which includes an empirical constant) to estimate the narrowest diameter of the internal carotid artery. Lees has obtained correlations with 170 carotid angiograms and is able to identify the diameter within 1 mm of the angiographic lumen in 93 percent of the patients.[4] Quantitative spectral phonoangiography has the advantage of being a very simple and rapid test; it is directed at the carotid bifurcation, the area of greatest surgical interest. To this extent, it represents an important advantage over those techniques that simply identify a hemodynamically significant stenosis at some point between the heart and the ophthalmic artery.

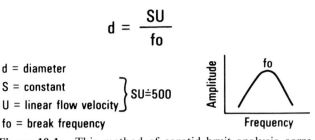

$$d = \frac{SU}{fo}$$

d = diameter
S = constant
U = linear flow velocity $\left.\right\}$ SU≐500
fo = break frequency

Figure 10-1. This method of carotid bruit analysis correlates the break frequency of the audio signal with the smallest internal diameter of the internal carotid artery.

Oculoplethysmography (OPG-K)

The earliest oculoplethysmograph was developed by Kartchner and McRae: water-filled transducers were used in both eyes and one ear, with analysis of the arrival time of the arterial pulse in the orbit as a method of detecting stenosis at any point between the heart and eye.[1] The ear was used as a monitor for the external carotid artery, which is less frequently involved in stenotic lesions. A differential circuit was used to amplify the difference between the right and left eye pulse arrival times (Fig. 10-2). The advantages of oculoplethysmography (OPG-K) are that it is simple, fast, inexpensive, and technician operated. In addition, there is a very large database available with OPG-K information. On the other hand, the disadvantages of the device are that it is not quantitative, that its sensitivity depends on relative criteria selected for diagnosis and that bilateral disease is not as easy to detect as one would like.

Table 10-1 details the criteria for a positive diagnosis listed by a number of investigators and summarizes the accuracy of the device as detailed in their reviews in comparison with angiography.[5-13] Fortunately, both the OPG-K system and an air-filled digitized system manufactured by Zira* have been evaluated by several investigators in addition to the developers, and a consistent picture of their ability to detect hemodynamically significant lesions is available. It is clear that the devices are highly sensitive, but not perfect, in detecting 50–60 percent stenotic lesions, and appear to have 100 percent sensitivity in detecting complete occlusion. Oculoplethysmography is one of the most widely used methods of cerebrovascular diagnosis, and several commercial variants of the machine have been developed to facilitate or automate the technique.

Oculopneumoplethysmography (OPG-GEE)

The Gee technique of oculoplethysmography must be clearly differentiated from the Kartchner approach. Gee uses an eye transducer with relatively high suction to measure ophthalmic artery pressure.[15] By increasing suction on a cup applied to the eye, the ocular pulse is first obliterated (Fig. 10-3). Then the eye cup

---

* Zira International Inc., 3872 East Lizard Rock, Tucson, Ariz. 85718.

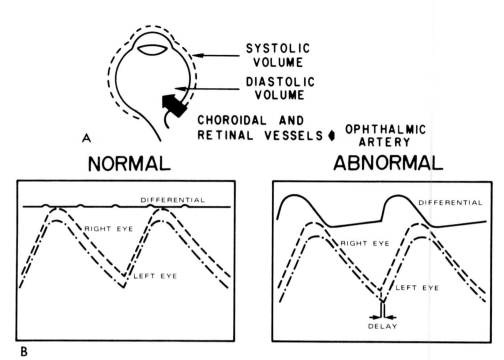

Figure 10-2. (A) The ocular pulse originates in the choroidal and retinal vessels. (B) Schematic representation of the OPG-K system demonstrates the arrival time of the arterial pulse wave in both orbits, and amplifies any delay between them (or in comparison with arrival time in the ear lobe) in a differential tracing.

Table 10-1
Comparison of Oculoplethysmography-K Accuracy Rates

	Angiographic Stenosis Criteria (%)	Sensitivity (%)	Overall Accuracy (%)
Kartchner et al.[23]	40	76	91
Sumner et al.[38]	40	64	78
House et al.[21]	40	75	—
Satiani et al.[36]	50	72	86
Hobson et al.[19]	50	—	87
Blackshear et al.[5]	50	52	68
McDonald et al.[29]	60	76	87
Baker et al.[1]	60	—	94
House et al.[21]	70	90	—
Egan et al.[9]	80	—	90
Strandness[37]	100	100	100

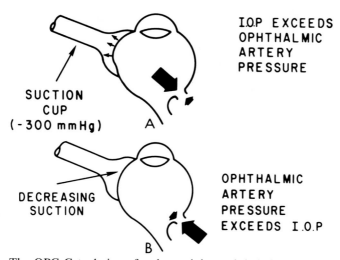

Figure 10-3.   The OPG-G technique for determining ophthalmic artery pressure is schematically represented. (A) A suction cup is applied to the orbit, and suction increased to −300 mm Hg. with disappearance of pulsation. (B) Suction is gradually decreased and the negative pressure at which orbital pulsations return is noted and empirically correlated with the ophthalmic artery systolic pressure.

suction is gradually reduced until the pulse returns. Correlations between the OPG-measured ophthalmic artery pressure and the actual ophthalmic artery pressure are excellent;[16] in Gee's experience, the accuracy is ± 7.4 mm Hg.[17]

The original OPG-Gee criteria for the diagnosis of a hemodynamically significant lesion required an ophthalmic systolic pressure less than 0.66 of the brachial pressure or documentation of a 2-mm pressure difference between ophthalmic arteries. The more recent modification of this device extends its range to 500 mm of negative pressure on the orbit, which permits the accurate detection of ophthalmic systolic pressures to 150 mm Hg.[17] In addition, the technique is now more sensitive in the detection of bilateral disease. It also can be used to demonstrate the adequacy of collateral circulation in situations involving proposed carotid artery resection or ligation by using preoperative carotid compression with measurements of the resulting ophthalmic artery pressure. When carotid artery pressure is 60 mm Hg or more, carotid artery resections and ligations have not been associated with postoperative strokes. In the range of 50 to 60 mm Hg, several strokes have been observed. Table 10-2 details the experience of several investigators with the OPG-GEE technique, including the angiographic criterion of stenosis employed in each study.[13,18–20] These data confirm the accuracy of the OPG-GEE device, which must be considered one of the most sensitive noninvasive methods currently available.

The OPG-GEE system is excellent for the detection of hemodynamically significant carotid artery occlusive disease. Therefore, its main application has been as a screening device for patients with carotid bruits, or for patients about to undergo surgery for peripheral arterial disease, abdominal aortic aneurysms, or

Table 10-2
Comparison of Oculoplethysmography (OPG-GEE)
Accuracy Rates

		Angiographic Stenosis Criteria (%)	Sensitivity (%)	Specificity (%)
Gee	1976–1982	50	92	96
Eikelboom	1979–1981	65	87	84
Gross	1977	—	—	—
Baker/Machleder	1977–1981	60	87	96
McDonald	1978–1979	60	87	100
O'Hara	1980	70	—	—
Kempczinski	1979	50	93	93
Berkowitz	1980	60	81	80
Archie	1980	50	70	96
Lynch	1981	50	92	95
Marck	1982	60	91	93
Raviola	1982	55	75	91
Wiebers	1982	75	85	97
Riles	1983	50	91	89
Mean:			86	92

From Eikelboom BC: Ocular pneumoplethysmography, in Bernstein FD (ed), Non-invasive Diagnostic techniques in Vascular Disease (3rd Ed). St. Louis, CV Mosby, 1985. With permission.

coronary artery bypass. In each of these situations, a positive OPG-GEE has been an indication for angiography.

In addition, the OPG-GEE is an excellent device for the exploration of the incidence, prevalence, and progression of carotid artery disease. Although it does not identify the site of obstruction between the heart and the eye (in contrast to the direct carotid diagnostic methods), it provides a reliable and reproducible measure of the presence and degree of such obstruction.

Performance of an OPG-GEE with carotid compression (low in the neck) provides information regarding the adequacy of the cerebral collateral circulation from the vertebrobasilar and contralateral carotid systems. Such information has important predictive value for potential future stroke. Further, the preoperative performance of this test with carotid compression provides an ophthalmic artery pressure equivalent to that measured with common carotid cross-clamping in the operating room—and therefore can be used as a measurement of internal carotid backflow, or "stump" pressure—and an indication of the need for placement of intraoperative shunts. Most surgeons, however, rely upon the intraoperative pressure measurement, or an EEG, or both, as the indication for shunting.

In the postcarotid endarterectomy patient, routine follow-up with the OPG-GEE permits identification of recurrent carotid stenosis and contralateral disease progression, although direct techniques (especially duplex scanning) are used more frequently for this purpose.

Limitations of Indirect Tests

The indirect tests for cerebrovascular diagnosis (periorbital Doppler and oculoplethysmography) are only useful to detect hemodynamically significant stenoses, but do not localize the lesions anatomically, and cannot distinguish between high-grade stenoses and occlusion. Of the indirect tests, only the OPG-GEE provides accurate quantitation of the effects of stenoses.

Integration of B-Mode and Doppler Systems with Other Approaches

In most laboratories, it is recognized that several tests, using different physical or physiological principles, are supplementary. Any positive test is considered a positive screen, and an indication for angiography. Thus, a test based on hemodynamics (so-called indirect tests, such as the OPG or supraorbital Doppler) will be supplemented by one or more direct tests, such as carotid imaging and spectral analysis of the audio or carotid velocity signal. The data indicate the relative value of the separate tests, but it must be remembered that the advantage of a battery of tests is increased sensitivity, which is paid for by an increasing incidence of false-positive studies. Further, none of the tests described will demonstrate shallow, ulcerating lesions. It is hoped that the newer approaches of radioactive platelet labeling techniques currently under development will help identify and characterize these important sources of atheroemboli.

DIGITAL SUBTRACTION ANGIOGRAPHY

The introduction of digital subtraction angiography (DSA) in 1981 promised a semi-invasive, low risk, outpatient graphic screening procedure of the entire cerebrovascular circulation from the aortic arch to the intracerebral vasculature.[21] Early reports suggested that intravenous subtraction arteriography (IV-DSA) was safe, inexpensive, and usually diagnostic.[21,22] However, continuing experience has identified some significant deficiencies of the method that appear to limit its usefulness and applicability.

Intravenous DSA (Fig. 10-4) requires the rapid injection of 40–100 ml of contrast material into a large peripheral or central vein by a power injector. Multiple video images are obtained with an image intensifier and then converted to a digital format by a videodigital computer. A preinjection control image is digitally subtracted from the postinjection views, and the resulting angiogram is then improved with computer enhancement techniques.

The major problems with IV-DSA have been (1) resolution and image quality, (2) motion artifact, and (3) vessel overlap. Poor image quality in 17 percent of cases was reported by Chilcote (Cleveland Clinic),[23] and at least one view was deficient in 25 percent of studies tabulated at the Mayo Clinic by Earnest.[24] At the University of California at Los Angeles (UCLA), only 58 percent of the studies were considered to be of diagnostic quality,[24] and the likelihood of a completely useless study has ranged from 6 to 16 percent in several reports.[14,21–23,25–27,28]

A principle reason for unsatisfactory IV-DSA studies is motion artifact between the time the "mask" image is obtained and the final postinjection views.

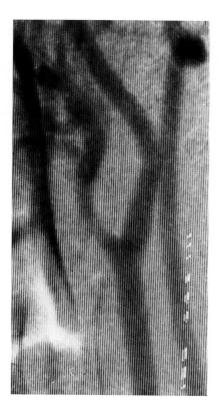

Figure 10-4. Intravenous digital subtraction angiogram of the carotid bifurcation.

Swallowing is a frequent cause of this problem, which is exaggerated in the anxious and uncooperative patient. It seems unlikely that technological advances will significantly reduce difficulties caused by motion artifacts. Poor circulation, as seen in congestive heart failure or other low cardiac output states, dilutes the contrast bolus, accentuating difficulties with resolution and motion artifacts.

Vessel overlap is also a common and difficult problem with IV-DSA, since the intravenously injected dye simultaneously fills all of the patient cerebrovascular inflow vessels. Superimposition of carotid bifurcations by overlying vertebral vessels can usually be eliminated by obtaining views at other oblique angles. Each view requires the injection of additional contrast material, and even with multiple projections, the best view for visualizing the arterial area of interest may be compromised by artifacts.

Finally the resolution of the video technique itself is limited by the video and fluoroscopic equipment, which is currently not nearly as sensitive as conventional angiography. Thus, 0.5-mm resolution is about the best that can be expected, and shallow ulcerating lesions will frequently escape detection.

Data regarding the accuracy of IV-DSA in detecting and classifying carotid bifurcation disease are presented in Tables 10-3 through 10-6. In Russell's report, 14 percent of the IV-DSA studies were deemed inadequate for interpretation.[14] If these were included in the analysis, 80 percent of the DSA studies were within one category (plus or minus) of the conventional angiogram, and only 61 percent

Table 10-3
Comparison of DSA and Conventional Arteriography

DSA—Percent Stenosis	Conventional Arteriography—Percent Stenosis					
	0	25	25–49	50–74	75–99	100
0	38	5	2	4	1	—
<25	1	3	3	1	—	—
25–49	2	2	8	3	3	—
50–74	2	—	2	10	5	—
75–99	—	—	—	2	19	3
100	—	—	—	—	—	9
Uninterpretable	6	—	3	2	3	—

From Russell et al: Digital subtraction angiography for evaluation of extracranial carotid occlusive disease: comparison with conventional angiography. Surgery 94:604, 1983. With permission.
$K = 0.588 \pm 0.053$ ($n = 128$)

agreed with the precise category of the conventional study (Table 10-3). An analysis of the predictive value (Table 10-4) indicates that the negative predictive value of IV-DSA was only 76 percent when the conventional angiogram indicated no obstructive disease (e.g., zero percent stenosis).[14] Thus, in 24 percent of the IV-DSA studies interpreted as normal, a stenosis was actually present. Further, when greater than 50 percent stenosis was the angiographic criterion, negative predictive value for IV-DSA was only 84 percent, so the method failed to diagnose 16 percent of the hemodynamically significant lesions. These results do not compete with the screening capability of ultrasonic diagnosis (Tables 10-7) or pressure dependent (OPG) methods (Table 10-2) for detecting significant stenoses. On the other hand, a positive IV-DSA report of a greater than 50 percent stenotic lesion proved to be highly reliable (PPV 91–94 percent). (Additional data is summarized in Tables 10-5 and 10-6). Thus, the IV-DSA method can logically be applied to confirm the presence of hemodynamically significant lesions identified by other noninvasive tests, but is a poor screening method for such pathology. Should an IV-DSA study fail to confirm a stenosis documented by other methods,

Table 10-4
Ability of DSA to Detect Internal Carotid Artery Disease
Compared with Conventional Angiography

Degree of Stenosis Considered Positive (%)	Prevalence (%)	Sensitivity (%)	Specificity (%)	Positive Predictive Value (%)	Negative Predictive Value (%)	Accuracy (%)
>0	66	86	88	94	76	87
≥25	56	85	89	91	81	87
≥50	47	80	94	92	84	88

From Russell et al: Digital subtraction angiography for evaluation of extracranial carotid occlusive disease: comparison with conventional angiography. Surgery 94:604, 1983. With permission.

Table 10-5

Accuracy of Diagnostic Quality DSA for Detecting
Hemodynamically Significant Internal Carotid Artery
Stenoses Compared with Conventional Arteriograms

Author	Positive Criterion	Prevalence (%)	Sensitivity (%)	Specitivity (%)	Positive Predictive value (%)	Negative Predictive value (%)	Accuracy (%)
Chilcote, et al., 1981[23]	≥40%	39	87	88	82	91	88
	≥60%	24	95	92	79	98	93
Turnipseed, et al., 1982[22]	≥50%	63	98	100	100	96	99
Eikelboom, et al., 1983[26]	≥50%	56	95	92	93	94	94
Wood et al., 1983[28]	≥40%	40	95	96	95	96	96
	≥60%	32	93	94	88	96	94
Kempczinski, et al., 1983[27]	≥50%	43	93	93	90	94	93
	50%	43	93	93	90	94	93

Table 10-6

Comparison of Diagnostic Quality DSA and Conventional
Internal Carotid Arteriography

	Uninterpretable studies excluded	Perfect Agreement	Agreement ± 1 Category	K ± O	Normalized K ± O
Chilcote et al., 1981[23]	11%	65%	91%	0.572 ± 0.044	0.718 ± 0.43
Turnipseed, et al.,1983[26]	?	96%	99%	0.942 ± 0.030	0.943 ± 0.032
Eikelboom et al., 1983[26]	12%	81%	94%	0.739 ± 0.051	0.778 ± 0.049
Wood et al., 1982[28]	8%	58%	99%	0.497 ± 0.061	0.690 ± 0.062
Earnest et al., 1983[24]	6%	73%	95%	—	—
Celesia et al., 1983[25]	9%	84%	?	—	—

From Sumner DS, Russell JB, Ramsey DE, et al: Noninvasive diagnosis of extracranial carotid arterial
disease. Arch Surg 114:1222–1229, 1979. With permission.

254

Table 10-7

Comparison of Pulsed-Doppler Imaging Accuracy Rates With
Spectrum Analysis

	Angiographic Stenosis Criteria (%)	Sensitivity (%)	Accuracy (%)
Sumner et al.[13]	40	86	89
Barnes et al.[29]	50	88	96
Blackshear et al.[30]	50	92	92
Hobson et al.[31]	50	89	85
Blackshear et al.*[30]	50	100	97

* Duplex scanner with spectrum analysis.

a conventional arteriogram should be obtained without hesitation. In our experience, such studies usually confirm the vascular laboratory data.

IV-DSA techniques are usually quite effective in identifying lesions of the great vessels at their origin from the aortic arch. Therefore, such diagnoses as subclavian steal and Takayasu's arteritis are readily demonstrated. In addition, major intracranial vessels may be visualized with IV-DSA. However, problems with resolution, motion artifact and vessel overlap limit the ability of IV-DSA to identify specific lesions in the smaller vessel with predictable regularity.

Clinical applications of IV-DSA may be summarized as follows. IV-DSA may be used for certain screening applications, when a technically satisfactory study has been obtained, although it would not be our technique of choice. If IV-DSA is positive for a significant (greater than 50 percent) stenosis or occlusion, the positive predictive value is well over 90 percent. On the other hand, a negative IV-DSA is not nearly as accurate as a positive test, missing 16–24 percent of existing lesions. If the purpose of a screening technique is to identify every patient with the condition screened for, and it is, then IV-DSA fails in comparison with the best noninvasive laboratory methods. In addition IV-DSA is not a cost effective method for screening in comparison with the noninvasive laboratory. Therefore, we believe the vascular laboratory should be used as the primary approach to the identification and quantitation of carotid artery disease in asymptomatic and postendarterectomy patients. If a significant stenosis is documented intravenous or intra-arterial DSA are good methods to confirm its location, and usually are adequate to justify surgery. For symptomatic patients, this algorithm is also reasonable, although it is equally appropriate and cost effective to proceed directly to formal contrast angiography. Thus, the availability of each of these modalities increases the logical options for good patient management.

In the discussion of DSA, it is important to distinguish between intravenous and intra-arterial DSA techniques. Intra-arterial injection eliminates or limits many of the technical problems that plague IV-DSA, and intra-arterial DSA has become an accepted method of intracranial and extracranial arteriography. With advanced DSA systems, spacial resolution is satisfactory for the great majority of intracranial and extracranial examinations.[32]

SUMMARY

The noninvasive detection of carotid bifurcation lesions has emerged from the laboratory to widespread clinical application within the past 10 years, and remains an exciting area of medical progress. In placing these advances in perspective, we must remember that the major goal of any noninvasive detection system is to identify suspected lesions routinely. That is, the sensitivity, or ability to detect every positive lesion is most important, even at the price of some false negatives. None of the devices is perfect, (i.e., there is none that has 100 percent sensitivity and yields no false positives) at present. Therefore, the best current strategy for the clinician is to accept the relative imperfections in each device and compensate for them by using a battery of instruments. In so doing, the investigator must agree that a positive result with any single test must be considered a positive screen. In our laboratory such a battery of tests does provide 100 percent sensitivity, but it also yields a relatively high rate of false positives (about 40 percent).[1]

Eugene F. Bernstein, M.D., Ph.D.
Division of Vascular and Thoracic Surgery
Scripps Clinic and Research Foundation
10666 No. Torrey Pines Rd
La Jolla, California 92037

REFERENCES

1. Kartchner MM, McRae LP, Morrison FD, et al: Noninvasive detection and evaluation of carotid occlusive disease. Arch Surg 106:528–535, 1973
2. Kartchner MM, McRae LR: Oculoplethysmography and carotid phonoangiography, in Bernstein EF (ed): Noninvasive Diagnostic Techniques in Vascular Disease (2nd Ed). St. Louis, CV Mosby, 1981
3. Lees RS, Kistler JP: Carotid phonoangiography, in Bernstein EF (ed): Noninvasive Diagnostic Techniques in Vascular Disease (1st Ed). St. Louis, CV Mosby, 1978
4. Lees RS, Kistler JP, Miller A: Quantitative carotid phonoangiography, in Bernstein EF (ed): Noninvasive Diagnostic Techniques in Vascular Disease (2nd Ed). St. Louis, CV Mosby, 1982
5. Baker JD, Barker WF, Machleder HI: A clinical evaluation of ocular pneumoplethysmography. Proceedings, Symposium on Noninvasive Techniques in Vascular Disease, San Diego, CA, September 1979, p 33
6. Blackshear WM Jr: Comparative review of OPG-K&M, OPPG-G and pulsed Doppler ultrasound for carotid evaluation. Vasc Diag Ther 1:43–48, 1980
7. Egan R, Herrman JB: Accuracy of the LSI-PVR-OPG in detecting carotid occlusive disease in 100 consecutive patients undergoing cerebral angiography. Proceedings, Symposium on Noninvasive Techniques in Vascular Disease, San Diego, CA, September 1979, p 30
8. Hobson RW, Berry SM, O'Donnell JA: Improved accuracy in noninvasive diagnosis of extracranial carotid arterial disease. Proceedings, Symposium on Noninvasive Techniques in Vascular Disease, San Diego, CA, September 1979, p 35
9. House SL, Mahalingam K, Hyland LJ, et al: Noninvasive flow techniques in the diagnosis of cerebrovascular disease. Surgery 87:696–700, 1980
10. McDonald PJ, Rich NM, Collins GJ, et al: Doppler cerebrovascular examination, oculoplethysmography, and ocular pneumoplethysmography. Use in detection of carotid disease: A prospective clinical study. Arch Surg 113:341–349, 1978

11. Satiani B, Cooperman M, Clark M, et al: An assessment of carotid phonoangiography and oculoplethysmography in the detection of carotid artery stenosis. Am J Surg 136:618–621, 1978

12. Strandness DE: Results of prospective evaluation of the OPG-CPA. Proceedings, Symposium on Noninvasive Techniques in Vascular Disease, San Diego, CA, September 1979, p 23

13. Sumner DS, Russell JB, Ramsey DE, et al: Noninvasive diagnosis of extracranial carotid arterial disease. Arch Surg 114:1222–1229, 1979

14. Russell JB, et al: Digital subtraction angiography for evaluation of extracranial carotid occlusive disease: comparison with conventional arteriography. Surgery 94:604, 1983

15. Gee W, Mehigan JR, Wylie EJ: Measurement of collateral cerebral hemispheric blood pressure by ocular pneumoplethysmography. Am J Surg 130:121–127, 1975

16. Johnston GG, Bernstein EF: Quantitation of internal carotid artery stenosis by ocular plethysmography. Surg Forum 26:290–297, 1975

17. Gee W: Ocular pneumoplethysmography, in Bernstein EF (ed): Non-invasive Diagnostic Techniques in Vascular Disease (2nd Ed). St. Louis, CV Mosby, 1982

18. Berkowitz HD: Diagnostic accuracy of oculopneumoplethysmography attachment for pulse volume recorder. Arch Surg 115:190–193, 1980

19. Eikelboom BC: Ocular pneumoplethysmography, in Bernstein EF (ed), Non-invasive Diagnostic Techniques in Vascular Disease (3rd Ed). St. Louis, CV Mosby, 1985

20. Kempczinski RF: A combined approach to the noninvasive diagnosis of carotid artery occlusive disease. Surgery 85:689–694, 1979

21. Turnipseed WD, Sackett JF, Strother CM, et al: Computerized arteriography of the cerebrovascular system. Arch Surg 116:470–473, 1981

22. Turnipseed WD, Sackett JF, Strother CM, et al: A comparison of standard cerebal arteriography with noninvasive Doppler imaging and intravenous angiography. Arch Surg 117:419, 1982

23. Chilcote WA, Modic MT, Paulicek WA, et al: Digital subtraction angiography of the carotid arteries: a comparative study in 100 patients. Radiology 139:287, 1981

24. Earnest F IV, Houser DW, Forbes GS, et al: The accuracy and limitations of intravenous digital subtraction angiography in the evaluation of atherosclerotic cerebrovascular disease: an angiographic and surgical correlation. Mayo Clin Proc 58:735–746, 1983

25. Celesia GG, Strother CM, Turski PA, et al: Digital subtraction arteriography. A new method for evaluation of extracranial occlusive disease. Arch Neurol 40:70, 1983

26. Eikelboom BC, Ackerstaff RGA, Ludwig JW, et al: Digital video subtraction angiography and duplex scanning in assessment of carotid artery disease: Comparison with conventional angiography. Surgery 94:821, 1983

27. Kempczinski RF, Wood GW, Berlatzky Y, et al: A comparison of digital subtraction angiography and noninvasive testing in the diagnosis of cerebrovascular disease. Am J Surg 146:207, 1983

28. Wood GW, Lukin RR, Tomsick TA, et al: Digital subtraction angiography with intravenous injection: assessment of 1,000 carotid bifurcations. AJNR 4:125, 1983

29. Barnes RW, Bone GE, Reinertson J, et al: Noninvasive ultrasonic carotid arteriography: Prospective validation by contrast arteriography. Surgery 80:328–335, 1976

30. Blackshear WM, Phillips DJ, et al: Detection of carotid occlusive disease by ultrasonic imaging and pulsed Doppler spectrum analysis. Surgery 86:698–706, 1979

31. Hobson RW, Berry SN, Katocs AS, et al: Comparison of pulsed Doppler and real-time B-mode echo arteriography for noninvasive imaging of the extracranial carotid arteries. Surgery 87:286–293, 1980

32. Brant-Zzwadski M, Gould R, Normal D, et al. Digital subtraction cerebral angiography by intra-arterial injection: Comparison with conventional angiography. AJR 140:347–353, 1983

SECTION III

EXTREMITY VASCULAR DIAGNOSIS

The noninvasive vascular laboratory came into existence with the development of methods for arterial and venous diagnosis in the extremities, and the performance of such techniques continues to be an important function of the vascular laboratory. In this section, we are particularly honored to present chapters by three pioneers of extremity vascular diagnosis, Drs. Barnes, Strandness, and Sumner.

We begin with techniques for upper-extremity vascular evaluation (Chapter 11) by Drs. Pearce, Ricco, and Yao. In Chapter 12, Dr. Strandness succinctly describes the clinical relevance of noninvasive lower-extremity arterial diagnosis. This material is followed, in Chapter 13, by description of the anatomy and collateral routes of the lower-extremity arterial system, as presented by Drs. Crummy and Stieghorst. Chapters 14, 15 and 16 contain the essential elements of lower-extremity vascular diagnosis. In Chapter 14, Drs. Zierler and Strandness present methods for lower-extremity arterial evaluation. Techniques for venous evaluation are presented by Dr. Barnes in Chapter 15, and important new methods for extremity vascular diagnosis using B-mode and duplex instrumentation are described by Mr. Talbot in Chapter 16. Although B-mode techniques are not in widespread use as of this writing, the editor assumes that they will enjoy broad clinical application during the lifetime of this textbook. Finally, in Chapter 17, Dr. Sumner succinctly describes the application of plethysmography for extremity vascular diagnosis. This subject is somewhat outside the scope of this textbook, but it is included because plethysmography is an important and commonly used procedure for extremity vascular evaluation.

William H. Pearce, M.D.
Jean-Baptiste Ricco, M.D.
James S.T. Yao, M.D., Ph.D.

11

Upper Extremity Vascular Diagnosis Using Doppler Ultrasound

Symptomatic vascular disease involving the upper extremities is uncommon. Unlike occlusive disease affecting the lower extremities, where the etiology is either atherosclerotic or embolic, a wide variety of systemic and neurogenic diseases may cause ischemia of the hands. Because of this, evaluation of upper-extremity ischemia requires a thorough history-taking and a careful physical examination. Even so, the diagnosis may be difficult, and various tests may be needed to establish an accurate diagnosis.

In order to supplement the clinical examination, several noninvasive tests have been introduced to aid in diagnosis of arterial or venous occlusion. These are strain-gauge plethysmography and photoplethysmography, the transcutaneous Doppler ultrasound flow detection technique, and B-mode ultrasound scanning of the peripheral arteries. The Doppler flow detection technique is of particular use in evaluation of the ulnar and digital arteries, which, in general, are not accessible to physical examination.

In the past, arteriography was required to establish the diagnosis when arterial occlusion was suspected, yet arteriography gave no information regarding the hemodynamic abnormality present. Doppler ultrasound has not only improved diagnostic capabilities but has also provided important hemodynamic data needed for surgical decisions.

This chapter considers Doppler techniques for evaluation of arterial and venous disease in the upper extremities. Doppler methods are the mainstay of upper-extremity diagnosis, but B-mode sonography may also be used to evaluate upper-extremity vascular disorders. The reader is directed to Chapter 16 for consideration of the B-mode techniques being developed.

For full appreciation of the material in this chapter, the reader should be familiar with the primary and secondary manifestations of arterial venous obstruction, as described in Chapter 3.

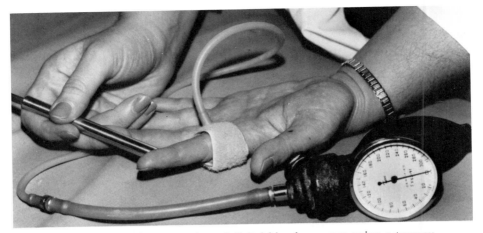

Figure 11-4. Demonstration of digital blood pressure using a transcutaneous Doppler.

Arterial Evaluation

Segmental Limb and Digital Pressure Measurements

Methods. For segmental pressure measurements in the upper extremity, pneumatic cuffs are placed at the arm* (brachial artery), proximal forearm, and wrist levels. Each cuff is independently inflated above systolic pressure and slowly deflated. The return of the Doppler signal, as monitored at the wrist, designates the segmental pressure. Segmental pressures are obtained in both extremities to serve as a reference and to detect asymptomatic disease in the opposite extremity. In many diabetic patients the arterial wall may be calcified and incompressible, invalidating this technigue.

Arterial obstruction distal to the palmar arch is detected by systolic pressure measurements. Here a small cuff (2.5 cm) is placed around the proximal phalange, and the sytolic pressure is recorded at the finger tip either with the Doppler flow probe (Fig. 11-4) or with photoplethysmography. In those patients in whom further distal occlusive disease exists within the digits, the cuff may be moved to the middle phalanx.

Interpretation. A low brachial systolic pressure implies obstruction of the ipsilateral innominate, subclavian, axillary, or proximal brachial artery.[14] Bilateral obstruction is implied if brachial pressures are reduced in both arms and ankle systolic pressure is normal. A difference of 20 mm Hg between right and left brachial pressure indicates a proximal arterial obstruction on the side with reduced pressure. Similarly, a pressure gradient greater than 20 mm Hg between any two levels of one extremity signifies obstruction located between these levels. In the forearm, a difference in ulnar and radial pressures will locate the obstructive process to the vessel with the lower pressure. A subcritical stenosis

---

* The "arm" is the portion of the upper extremity between the shoulder and elbow. The "forearm" is the portion between the elbow and wrist.

may not be evident with segmental pressure measurements in a resting patient; such lesions may be manifested only in the presence of reactive hyperemia. Therefore, in patients with upper-extremity claudication who show normal segmental limb pressures, the arm should be exercised and the measurements repeated.[6] If the values do not change, the pain is of musculoskeletal or neurologic, rather than vascular, origin.

Patency of the Palmar Arch and the Digital Arteries

The palmar arch. The palmar circulation is best assessed by searching the hypothenar and thenar eminences for signals from the palmar arches (Fig. 11-5). Patency of the palmar arch is evaluated by a modified Allen test.[18] The Doppler probe is placed over the radial artery while the ulnar artery is compressed. Should the waveform be obliterated with compression, the arch depends on the ulnar artery for supply. If the pulse remains present during compression, the arch is complete. The procedure is repeated by listening over the ulnar artery while compressing the radial artery. To determine the source of flow to the digital arteries, the Allen test can be repeated while listening at the base of each digit or along the proper digital vessel of each finger. Even though the arch appears patent, the pulsatile flow will sometimes be lost to the digits with radial or ulnar compression. In these patients, the digital vessels originate not from the palmar arch but directly from the radial or ulnar artery. Arterial obstructiondistal to the palmar arch is detected by diminished digital pressure measurement. Becuase of the dual blood supply to the fingers, disease in a single common or proper digital artery may be missed because of compensating flow in collateral arteries.

The digital arteries. Arterial obstruction distal to the palmar arch is defined by a pressure difference between the fingers of greater than 15 mm Hg or a wrist-to-digit gradient of 30 mm Hg. If all digital pressures are equally reduced, and the wrist-to-digit gradient is normal, the palmar circulation is intact. However, if the digital pressures are significantly lower in several digits, disease within the palmar and digital circulation is implied. There is good correlation between these Doppler criteria and angiography[15-17]; nonetheless, because of the anatomic variability in the palmar circulation, patency of the palmar arch is difficult to assess with pressure measurements alone. One should exercise caution in interpreting digital pressures if the wrist pressure is reduced because of a proximal arterial stenosis. Overall lowering of the arterial pressure may obscure pressure gradients between the forearm and wrist or between the wrist and digits.

Distal arterial obstructions affecting the palmar and digital circulations may be due to emboli, Buerger's disease, artherosclerosis, arthritis, or vasospasm.

Doppler Flow Studies

Technique. Direct Doppler examination of the upper extremity is a simple and rapid method for evaluating arterial and venous diseases. The examination must be performed in a warm environment to prevent cold-induced vasospasm. The Doppler probe is placed over the vessel to be examined, usually at an incident angle of 60°C. To avoid technical errors, the examiner should be well aware of the

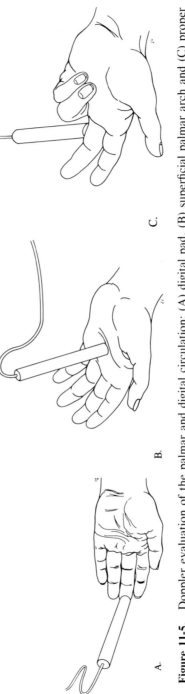
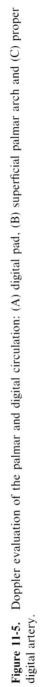

Figure 11-5. Doppler evaluation of the palmar and digital circulation: (A) digital pad, (B) superficial palmar arch and (C) proper digital artery.

A.

B.

C.

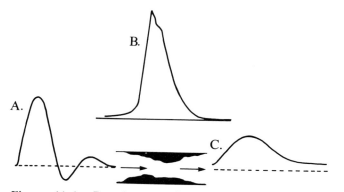

Figure 11-6. Doppler waveform analysis: (A) normal triphasic arterial waveform, (B) increased flow velocity and loss of the reverse component, and (C) monophasic waveform distal to an area of stenosis.

anatomy of the veins and arteries of the arm. The Doppler waveform may be abnormal when only a portion of an artery is examined or when a major branch, rather than the arterial truck, is insonated. Dense scar tissue, hematoma, and obesity may influence the waveform locally, while normal signals are found elsewhere in the same vessel.

The upper-extremity Doppler waveform bears a close resemblance to that observed with an electromagnetic flowmeter. Normal arterial Doppler signals in the extremities exhibit three distinct components (Fig. 11-6). Blood velocity (frequency shift) rapidly rises to a peak during systole (first component) and then falls abruptly during early diastole, where transient reversal of flow occurs (second component). The final component is forward flow in late diastole. In young healthy adults, a fourth sound may be audible over the brachial artery; it appears to emanate from vibratory movements of the arterial wall. Arterial Doppler waveform may be obtained in the upper extremity at the following locations: (1) the distal axillary artery, (2) the brachial artery, (3) the ulnar and radial arteries at the wrist, (4) the palmar arch, and (5) the digital arteries.

Interpretation. The specific waveform alterations observed in connection with arterial obstruction depend on the location at which Doppler signals are pained, i.e., proximal to the stenosis, distal to the stenosis, or in the stenotic zone. Characteristic waveform findings in these three areas have been described in detail in Chapter 3, and only a brief discussion is warranted here. Proximal to an obstruction lesion (occlusion of severe stenosis) arterial velocity may be diminished with increased pulsatility. One or the other of these findings may predominate, depending on the location of Doppler sampling in relation to the point of obstruction and the origin of collateral vessels. Stenotic-zone Doppler findings are dominated by increased velocity, loss of the reversed systolic component (Fig. 11-6B), and, in very severe stenoses, the development of continuous forward flow throughout both systole and diastole. Turbulent flow may be observed immediately distal to a stenotic lesion. Further downstream from a severe stenosis, the systolic waveform component may be damped, and forward flow may continue

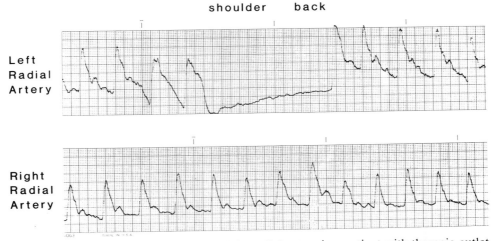

Figure 11-7. Flow velocity recording of the radial artery in a patient with thoracic outlet compression on the left side. Note cessation of flow when the shoulder was placed in an exaggerated military position.

throughout diastole (Fig. 11-6C) because of reactive hyperemia. With very severe obstruction and marked reactive hyperemia, continuous flow may produce a flat "waveform" with little or no systolic/diastolic differentiation.

Tests for Thoracic Outlet Compression

Since thoracic outlet compression is not primarily a vascular disorder, this diagnosis cannot be made with Doppler ultrasound alone. The Doppler examination will only suggest compression of the vascular structures within the thoracic outlet, and a negative test does not necessarily exclude thoracic outlet syndrome. Arterial waveforms and pressures are first obtained in the resting position. Brachial or radial artery waveforms are then monitored during the following series of maneuvers (Fig. 11-7). The patient is asked to assume an exaggerated military position with the shoulders back, closing the costoclavicular space. Next, the arm is placed across the chest in full 90° abduction, stretching the subclavian artery over the clavicle. Finally, the Adson maneuver is performed by abduction and external rotation of the arm with the patient's head turned first toward the arm and then away. Here, the subclavian artery is stretched while the tone of the scalene muscles changes. Because it is often difficult to obtain a continuous tracing with the Doppler probe during these maneuvers, photoplethysmography is more convenient.

Clinical Applications

Major arterial occlusions. Subclavian artery occlusion is recognized by a monophasic waveform high in the axilla and a brachial pressure gradient of greater than 20 mm Hg between the arms. The occlusion is usually atherosclerotic although, in younger patients, this may be the first manifestation of Takayasu's disease.[20] In most patients, subclavian artery occlusion is entirely asymptomatic.

However, patients with this lesion may present with cerebral symptoms (subclavian steal) or arm claudication. When the proximal subclavian artery is occluded, blood flow to the arm is reconstituted by way of the ipsilateral vertebral artery, stealing blood from the cerebral circulation. The reversal of flow in the vertebral artery may be detected with directional probes.[21-23] An alternative approach is to measure the delay in pulse arrival in the affected arm. A delay of 30 ± 10 msec between the arm is characteristic of subclavian stenosis with reconstitution through the vertebral artery.[21] In the patient with chronic ischemia and arm claudication, exercise testing will reproduce the symptoms and enhance the pressure differential, similar to the effects of exercise testing in the lower extremities.

Major vessel occlusion may also be the result of emboli from the heart or from a proximal atheromatous lesion.[24-26] Since embolic occlusion occurs suddenly, collaterals are poorly developed, and systolic pressure measurements in the affected extremity will generally be lower with emboli than with arteriosclerotic obstruction. If the embolus lodges in the axillary or brachial artery, its location will be easily detected by direct Doppler examination of the involved artery. Abrupt cessation of flow or alteration of the Doppler arterial signals, as discussed above, will reveal the location of the obstruction. Since portions of the ulnar and radial arteries lie deeply within the tissues of the forearm, direct Doppler localization of occlusion in these vessels is not always possible. Occlusion of the ulnar and radial arteries, however, will be manifested at the wrist by a pressure drop across the forearm and by a damped waveform appearance.

Thoracic outlet syndrome. The thoracic outlet syndrome is a symptom complex consisting of forearm, shoulder, and hand discomfort often characterized as a dull ache.[12] Pain is usually associated with upper-extremity activities in which the hand is raised above the shoulder. Paresthesias are usually present in the distribution of the C8–T1 dermatomes. However, the paresthesias may affect all the dermatomes of the upper extremity. These symptoms result from irritation of the brachial plexus in the thoracic outlet and are usually not caused by arterial insufficiency.

Diminution or loss of the arterial waveform with the thoracic outlet maneuvers previously described is evidence of vascular compression in the thoracic outlet[27,28] (Fig. 11-8). Before treatment is recommended, however, a chest X-ray film, cervical spine series, and peripheral nerve conduction studies are necessary. Depending on the patient's symptoms, the surgeon may choose either an exercise program or a first-rib resection. The Doppler study is used primarily to diagnose vascular complications of the disease.

Intimal damage or aneurysms of the subclavian artery may occur as a direct result of thoracic outlet compression (Fig. 11-9). These complications may be a source of emboli that occlude major distal arteries or digital branches.[10,29,30] Segmental pressures or direct Doppler investigation may be used to localize arterial obstruction in such cases. The aneurysm itself may be detected with B-mode ultrasound scanning of the subclavicular region. When an aneurysm is found, it should be resected to prevent embolic complications. The subclavian artery may also become stenosed or thrombosed in response to repeated trauma in the thoracic outlet. In such cases, an abnormal arterial waveform will be

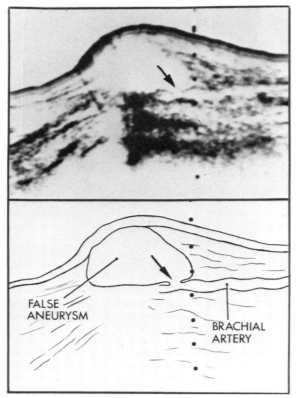

Figure 11-10. B-mode ultrasound scan of a brachial artery
with a false aneurysm. Note the communication of the false
aneurysmal sac with the defect in the brachial artery.

pitch and may be pulsatile. It is important to compare the involved extremity with
the opposite extremity to avoid mistaking a superficial artery for an arteriovenous
malformation. When surgical repair is indicated, a sterile Doppler probe may be
used intraoperatively to localize the exact site of the arteriovenous communication.

In acute arterial trauma, resuscitation and restoration of the patient's blood
volume are most important. Once the arterial injury is defined, there should be no
delay in transporting the patient to the operating room for repair. Only in the
stable patient with controlled blood loss is there time to perform ultrasonography
or angiography. Doppler techniques are particularly useful in diagnosing vascular
trauma associated with orthopedic injuries. For example, dislocation of the elbow
or shoulder may fracture the intima of the axillary or femoral arteries, producing
flaps that obstruct flow.[34,35] An abnormal waveform or pressure measurement in
these instances mandates arteriography. Despite its usefulness in diverse trauma
situations, Doppler ultrasound unfortunately has no value in the diagnosis or
monitoring of the compartment syndromes that may follow crush injuries or
prolonged periods of extremity ischemia.

Iatrogenic arterial injuries infrequently occur after radial artery cannulation for monitoring blood pressure or brachial artery catheterization for coronary angiography.[36-39] Forearm ischmia may develop after these procedures from either an intimal flap or an improper arterial closure. Doppler ultrasound is a convenient way to localize the arterial injury and provides accurate assessment of the viability of the extremity.[40] If a brachial artery injury occurs during cardiac catheterization, early exploration and repair are recommended.[36,41]

Hand and digital ischemia.   One of the most challenging problems in the upper extremity is management of severe hand and digital ischemia. In the lower extremity, ischemia is invariably the result of atherosclerotic or embolic disease. In the upper extremity, however, vasomotor diseases are very common. In all patients with hand or digital ischemia, both angiography and noninvasive evaluation should be performed to rule out proximal arterial disease.

The most frequently encountered vasospastic condition of the upper extremity is Raynaud's phenomenon, consisting of periodic episodes of vasospasm in the samll arteries and arterioles of the hand in response to cold or emotional stimuli. Patients exhibit a characteristic syndrome of color changes in the hand consisting first of pallor, followed by cyanosis and then rubor. More than 50 percent of patients with Raynaud's phenomenon eventually develop scleroderma,[47] but the onset of vasospastic symptoms may precede other manifestations of the underlying disease by many years. A wide variety of other disorders may underlie Raynaud's phenomenon, including collagen vascular diseases other than scleroderma, atherosclerosis, neurogenic injury or entrapment, immunoglobulin disorders, myeloproliferative disorders, and systemic malignancies. Raynaud's syndrome also occurs in patients with occupational trauma from prolonged use of pneumatic tools or hammers.[5]

Terms used in discussing Raynaud's phenomenon are quite confusing. Authors frequently use the term *Raynaud's disease* and *Raynaud's phenomenon* without indicating that they are discussing a primary occlusive disorder or a secondary vasospastic phenomenon. It is useful to think of Raynaud's phenomenon in terms of two etiologies. *Primary* Raynaud's phenomenon is a benign vasospastic disorder in which arterial occlusion results from *abnormal* vasospasm in extremity arteries that are histologically *normal*. *Secondary* Raynaud's phenomenon is also a vasospastic condition, but the involved arteries are histologically abnormal. Arterial occlusion in secondary Raynaud's phenomenon results from *normal* or *abnormal* degrees of vasospasm in *diseased* arteries. Even though Raynaud's phenomenon is primarily a vasospastic disorder, underlying proximal arterial occlusion and diffuse distal small artery occlusion may be present. The diagnostic dilemma, then, is to differentiate between vasospastic and fixed organic obstruction. The presence of fixed digital artery occlusion as detected by Doppler examination indicates intrinsic arterial disease rather than vasospasm,[1] i.e., secondary versus primary Raynaud's phenomenon. If a single digit is involved with the occlusive process, localized trauma (see Fig. 11-2) or proximal embolic source can be suspected. Likewise, ischemia of only the fourth and fifth fingers may represent a hypothenar hammer injury with damage to the ulnar half of the palmar arch.[5] If all digits are affected by fixed occlusion, however, including the asymptomatic hand, a systemic disease (scleroderma) or Buerger's disease should be suspected. When a fixed arterial obstruction is present, cold-induced vasospasm may be severe.[48] In such cases, noninvasive testing will help determine the relative contribution of fixed obstruction and vasospasm to the patient's symptoms.

In all patients with a fixed arterial obstruction and hand ischemia, complete arch, upper extremity, and magnification hand arteriography are mandatory. An abnormal cold-stimulation test with a normal arterial examination suggests primary Raynaud's phenomenon.[1,48–50] Armed with anatomic information from arteriography and physiologic data from noninvasive studies, the vascular surgeon may select the appropriate management strategy for the disease process and follow it objectively. Doppler examination is frequently useful in evaluating patients after treatment.[51]

Postoperative monitoring.   Doppler ultrasound plays an important role in defining the success or failure of arterial reconstructions. A successful reconstruction is manifested by the return of palpable pulses or an improvement in pressure. Since pulses may be present even when there is an obstruction in the upper extremity, improvement in wrist pressure must be documented quantitatively. Initially the improvement may be modest; however, once the hand is rewarmed and the effects of anesthesia are dissipated, blood pressure should improve. This improvement typically occurs within 24 to 48 hours. If the wrist pressure is less than the preoperative pressure, repair is a hemodynamic failure and reinvestigation is usually required.

In many extra-anatomic bypasses, the subclavian artery or axillary artery is used as a donor vessel. The vessel is examined preoperatively to detect underlying stenosis. Following surgery, it is important to assess the result of the bypass and also to evaluate the effect of the procedure on the donor artery. Technical problems with the anastomosis or a significant steal will lower the arm pressure and alter the arterial waveforms. A significant pressure drop diagnosed by Doppler examination may require angiography or reexploration.

Venous Examination

Techniques

Venous flow signals may be obtained from many upper-extremity veins. However, only obstructions of the axillary and subclavian veins are of any clinical importance. The examiner identifies the vein by first listening to the arterial signal and then moving the probe until the venous signal is heard. Venous signals are low pitched with a wide spectrum of frequencies that are phasic with respiration. In contrast to the lower extremity, upper-extremity venous flow increases with inspiration and decreases with expiration (Fig. 11-11). In patients with congestive heart failure, the venous signals may even be pulsatile.[19]

Deep Venous Thrombosis

Deep venous thrombosis of the upper extremity is an uncommon event and accounts for less than 2 percent of all episodes of deep venous thrombosis.[42] With prolonged central venous catheterization for hyperalimentation and hemodynamic monitoring, however, deep venous thrombosis of the upper extremity is a more

Peak
Inspiration

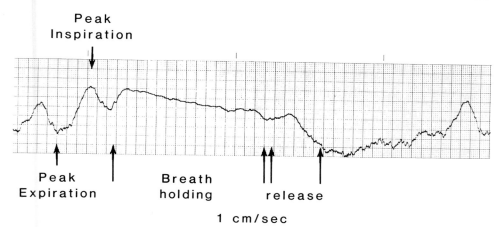

Peak   **Breath**
Expiration   **holding**   **release**

1 cm/sec

Figure 11-11. Demonstration of normal venous velocity waveforms from the axillary vein. Note the increase in forward flow with inspiration and decrease with expiration (phasic variation). Flow ceases when the breath is held and augments when the breath is expelled. Absense of phasic variation and loss of augmentation following breath holding indicate venous obstruction.

frequent occurrence. Upper-extremity deep venous thrombosis also may occur spontaneously or as a result of trauma. Stress or effort thrombosis may occur in muscular young patients after vigorous physical exertion. The etiology of effort thrombosis is thought to be related to entrapment of the subclavian vein as it passes between the clavicle and the first rib. The subclavian vein is subjected to repeated trauma and intermediate obstruction at this point, and it is believed that exacerbation of such trauma by vigorous exercise precipitates the thrombotic process. In some patients, various arterial, muscular, or skeletal abnormalities may contribute to the development of effort thrombosis.[10,43] Venous symptoms may also occur as part of the thoracic outlet syndrome. Other traumatic causes of upper-extremity deep venous thrombosis include fractures of the clavicle, infusion of caustic intravenous fluids, repeated venapuncture, and the chronic presence of transvenous pacemaker leads. Spontaneous deep venous thrombosis of the upper extremity may develop in association with malignant disorders (local or distant), congestive heart failure, hypercoagulability, or other systemic illnesses. The right arm is more frequently affected in cases of effort thrombosis, while the left arm predominates in cases of spontaneous thrombosis. This difference in etiology probably occurs as a result of the anatomic differences between the venous drainage of the two upper extremities.[42]

The clinical implications of upper-extremity deep venous thrombosis are several. First, fatal pulmonary emboli may occur. Adams reported a 12 percent incidence of pulmonary embolie associated with upper-extremity deep venous thrombosis.[42] Second, although recanalization of axillary and subclavian veins is frequent, long-term disability is common in the affected extremity. Early recognition of venous occlusion and treatment with either heparine or streptokinase appears to be beneficial, but the data on this subject are inconclusive.[42] Finally,

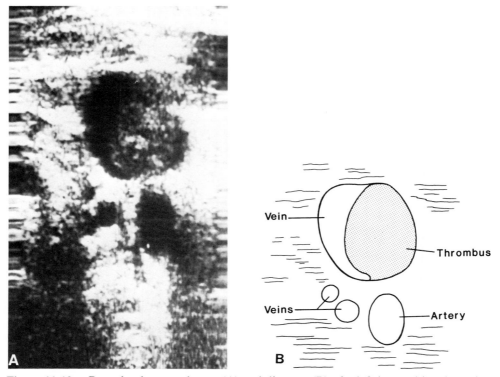

Figure 11-12. B-mode ultrasound scan (A) and diagram (B) of a left internal jugular vein thrombosis in a patient with prolonged central venous hyperalimentation.

untreated upper-extremity or cervical thrombophlebitis may lead to fatal cerebral sinus thrombosis through extension of the thrombotic process.[45]

Deep venous thrombosis of the upper extremity should be suspected in any patient presenting with recent onset of arm or hand swelling with tenderness in the axillary or infraclavicular region and a prominent venous pattern over the arm or anterior chest. The diagnosis can be made accurately at bedside with Doppler auscultation of the venous system.

In a comparative study involving venography and utlrasound, Towner reported a 100-percent sensitivity and specificity for Doppler ultrasound in detecting acute venous obstruction in the arm.[46] B-mode scanning will also delineate the thrombus, particularly in silent areas such as the internal jugular (Fig. 11-12). B-mode venous examination techniques are presented in Chapter 16.

SUMMARY

Because upper-extremity ischemia is an uncommon disorder with many etiologies, the Doppler ultrasonic examination is a logical first step in evaluating patients with signs and symptoms of ischemia in the upper extremity. Noninvasive assessment with Doppler ultrasound provides objective hemodynamic information. Although this information may not be diagnostic, it serves as a basis for deciding whether further workup is neccessary. In addition, Doppler evaluation is safe and painless, allowing for serial examination to follow the disease progression and to assess the result of medical and surgical therapies. Doppler techniques, when combined with other noninvasive methods, may accurately distinguish between fixed organic obstruction and vasospasm in the upper extremity. Doppler techniques also fascilitate prompt diagnosis of arterial and venous occlusion and are particularly valuable following orthopedic injuries to the upper extremity.

William H. Pearce, M.D.
Assistant Professor of Surgery
University of Colorado Sciences Center and
VA Medical Center
1055 Fairmont Street
Denver, Colorado 80220

Jean-Baptiste Ricco, M.D.
#2 BisRue Ste. Opportune
Poitiers, France

James S.T. Yao, M.D., Ph.D.
Professor of Surgery and
Director, Blood Flow Laboratory
Northwestern University Medical School
303 East Chicago Avenue
Chicago, Illinois 60611

REFERENCES

1. Sumner DS: Noninvasive assessment of upper extremity ischemia, in Bergan JJ, Yao JST (eds): evaluation and treatment of upper and lower extremity circulatory disorders. Orlando, FL, Grune & Stratton, 1983, pp 75–97
2. Sullivan ED, Reece CI, Cranley JJ: Phleborheography of the upper extremity. Arch Surg 118:1134, 1983
3. Gray B, Williams LR, Flanigan DP, et al.: Upper extremity deep venous thrombosis, diagnosis by Doppler ultrasound and impedance plethysmography. Bruit 7:30–34, 1983
4. Sotturai VS, Towner K, McDonnell AE, Zarius CK: Diagnosis of upper extremity deep venous thrombosis using noninvasive techniques. Surgery 91:582–585, 1982
5. McNamara MF, Takaki HS, Yao JST, Bergan JJ: A systematic approach to severe hand ischemia. Surgery 83:1–11, 1978
6. Kempczinski RF, Penn I: Upper extremity complications of axillofemoral grafts. Arch Surg 136:209–211, 1978
7. Whitehouse WM: Direct Revascularization for Forearm and Hand Ischemia, in Bergan JJ, Yao JST (eds): Evaluation and Treatment of Upper and Lower Extremity Circulatory Disorders. Orlando, FL, Grune & Stratton, 373–378 1983
8. Edwards EA: Organization of the small arteries of the hand and digits. Am J Surg 99:837–846, 1960
9. Little JM, Zylstra PL, West J, et al.: Circulatory patterns in the normal hand. Br J Surg 60:652–655, 1973
10. Wellington JL, Martin P: Poststenotic subclavian aneurysms. Angiology 16:566–572, 1965
11. Roos DB: Congenital anomalies associated with thoracic outlet syndrome. Am J Sur 132:771–776, 1976
12. Roos DB: Experience with first rib resection for thoracic outlet syndrome. Ann Surg 173:429–435, 1971
13. Yao JST: In discussion of Erlandson EE, et al.: Discriminant arteriographic criteria in

D. Eugene Strandness, Jr., M.D.

12

The Role of Noninvasive Procedures in the Management of Lower Extremity Arterial Disease

Nearly all the diseases that affect the arterial supply to the lower limbs interfere with tissue perfusion by obstruction of the involved segment(s). Thus, the degree to which the disease produces symptoms or signs depends on both the location and extent of arterial involvement. If the collateral circulation available is adequate and is given time to respond to the occlusive event, limb survival can be expected. However, it is uncommon for the patient to be entirely free of symptoms in most cases of acute and chronic arterial occlusion.

It is important to recognize that the clinical manifestations of arterial obstruction are the same regardless of the cause. It then becomes mandatory in approaching a patient with suspected arterial disease to establish that a stenosis or occlusion is indeed present and proceed to identify not only the sites of involvement but the nature of the underlying disease.

Atherosclerosis is by far the most common cause of chronic occlusive disease in the Western world. The terminology used to describe this entity is *arteriosclerosis obliterans* (ASO). Lagging far behind in terms of prevalence is *thromboangiitis obliterans* (TAO). In this country, TAO accounts for less than 1 percent of all chronic vascular diseases involving the large and medium-sized arteries.

In order to apply noninvasive diagnostic tests properly, it is essential to have an understanding of the more common disease entities and their clinical expression. If these tests are to be used intelligently, it must be understood that they complement the usual diagnostic workup. In this chapter, some of these considerations will be reviewed briefly.

PATHOLOGY AND SITES OF INVOLVEMENT

It is important, both from a clinical standpoint and with regard to noninvasive testing procedures, to review briefly the important relationship between pathology and sites of involvement. The atherosclerotic plaque, in its evolution, undergoes pseudoclaudication syndromes that may produce symptoms similar to those observed with chronic arterial occlusion. These include such diseases as herniated nucleus pulposus, degenerative joint disease, spinal canal stenosis, and spinal cord tumors. These disorders may be suspected by noting in the history that the walk-pain-rest cycle varies from day to day. With true claudication, this relationship is relatively constant from day to day. In addition, the pain of pseudoclaudication may occur while the patient is standing—something never observed with arterial disease.

While the distinction between true claudication and pseudoclaudication may be suspected on clinical grounds, the ankle blood pressure response to exercise can be very helpful. As will be discussed in Chapter 14, patients with claudication secondary to arterial disease *always* have a fall in their ankle systolic pressure when exercised to the point of pain. It is a simple matter to verify this fact and direct the patient into the proper channel for further workup and therapy.

Where is the disease located?

Although the level at which the pulses can be palpated is of use in estimating the most proximal level of occlusion, further information is desirable because it can have important therapeutic implications. Determining the level of occlusion is possible without arteriography by using a combination of noninvasive tests at the time of the patient's first visit. These include the measurement of segmental pressure gradients, screening of all large and medium-sized arteries with an ultrasonic duplex scanner, and waveform analysis of signals obtained from regions of suspected disease.

To what extent is the patient disabled?

Physicians traditionally use city blocks as a frame of reference in documenting the patient's disability. This is at best a very crude estimate, since the length of city blocks varies even within the same community. Further, claudication is influenced by a variety of other factors such as walking speed, grade, and walking patterns. Although the use of city blocks as the index of disability is pleasing to some physicians, a more objective assessment is possible with exercise testing. The use of the treadmill permits not only measurement of the physiologic response but the detection of other problems, such as shortness of breath and angina, which affect both walking time and subsequent therapeutic decisions.

Is collateral artery function stable?

Documentation of either improvement in limb perfusion or worsening secondary to disease progression is extremely difficult unless the change is dramatic. Further, when the patient is first seen, it is often relatively close in time to the event that led to the arterial occlusion. It is generally unwise at the time of the initial visit to proceed with a more vigorous workup, since collateral artery flow may increase and result in marked improvement in the patient's status. This fact can now be determined objectively by repetitive measurements of ankle blood pressure and assessment of the response to treadmill exercise.

What is the potential for limb loss?

One of the major roles for the physician is to inform the patient fully of future prospects for limb loss. If the patient has ischemia at rest, it is not difficult to assess the prospects, but frequently this is not the case. The measurement of ankle or digit pressure is extremely useful in providing a clue for the physician that the circulation is precarious and that the patient should not only be followed more closely but also should be cautioned to watch for trouble signs indicating rapid deterioration of the circulation. If the perfusion pressure is low, then frequent evaluations become of increasing importance.

Is impotence secondary to arterial insufficiency?

The problem of impotence in the male patient is demanding increasing attention. It has become clear that this problem has been neglected for too long, and it is necessary to evaluate this symptom complex by objective methods. The history can be helpful but clearly does not provide the definitive answer to this difficult dilemma. Noninvasive tests and their interpretation are becoming more sophisticated and widely applied as one step in evaluating this problem.

Has arterial surgery been successful?

The correction of arterial perfusion problems by direct arterial surgery is commonplace. In practice, verification of the immediate result has been by the return of pulses. The long-term assessment has relied on patient testimony and retention of peripheral pulses.

The noninvasive tests have come to occupy an important place in this area for a host of reasons: (1) pulses may not always return particularly early, and some independent method of verification is desirable; (2) detection of failure, particularly in the first 24 hours, may be difficult on clinical grounds alone; and (3) it is now known that problems within an arterial reconstruction may be detected during followup before the patient becomes symptomatic and the graft is totally occluded. Therefore, it is possible to salvage arterial reconstructions at a stage when a simple procedure may be used to correct the defect.

SUMMARY

In this chapter, those areas where noninvasive procedures may have an impact have been reviewed. The details concerning how this might be done will be covered in Chapter 14. For many physicians, these areas may appear to be self-evident, but such is not the case. Those who doubt the efficacy of noninvasive vascular tests feel these are wasteful of time, energy, and money. This is true only if the tests are improperly used or performed. It is time that those of us in this field accept the fact that more information can in fact be useful to both patient and physician.

D. Eugene Strandness, Jr., M.D.
Professor of Surgery
University of Washington
School of Medicine
Department of Surgery
RF25
Seattle, Washington 98195

Michael F. Stieghorst, M.D.
Andrew B. Crummy, M.D.

13

Lower-Extremity Arterial Anatomy and Collateral Routes

The first step in correct assessment of lower-extremity arterial disease is a thorough knowledge of vascular anatomy, which is important both for assessing symptomatology and for interpreting noninvasive test results. A sound understanding of potential collateral circuits is equally important, since the development of collateral flow can vastly affect the outcome of arterial occlusion. There is tremendous potential for development of collaterals throughout the vascular system, both collateral development may take some time. Therefore, the clinical manifestation of vascular occlusion is often related to the rapidity of its onset. If the onset is relatively slow, allowing for the formation of collaterals, occlusion of major vessels may occur with a minimun of symptomatology. However, abrupt occlusion of even a relatively small distal vessel may cause profound symptoms.

It is our purpose in this chapter to outline the anatomy of the vascular supply of the lower extremities and to describe the major potential collateral circuits that may appear in response to vascular occlusion. Numerals inserted parenthetically throughout the chapter identify vessels illustrated in Figures 13-1, 13-2, and 13-3. The reader is encouraged to refer frequently to these figures while studying the normal anatomy and collateral routes described herein.

ABDOMINAL AND LOWER-EXTREMITY VASCULAR ANATOMY

The Abdominal Aorta

The abdominal aorta (Figs. 13-1 and 13-2) begins at the level of the diaphragmatic hiatus and terminates by division into the common iliac arteries (41) at the L4 vertebral body. The aorta lies just to the left of midline and describes a ventral convex course over the lumbar spine with the apex of the curve at the

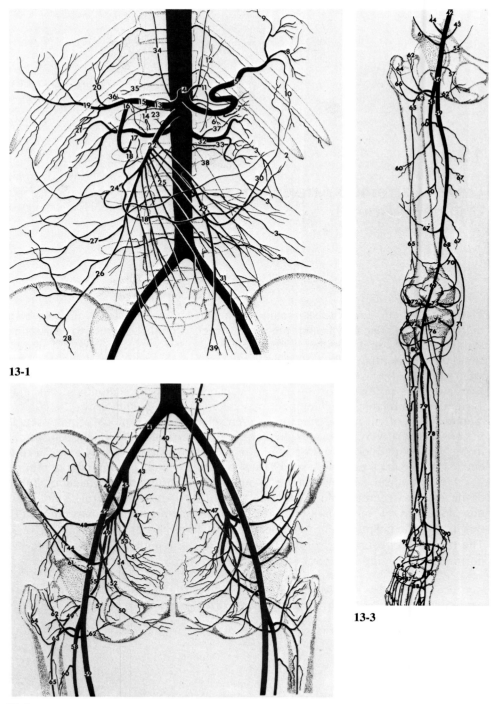

13-1

13-2

13-3

Figures 13-1 to 13-3. Normal abdominal, pelvic, and lower extremity arterial anatomy. (From Muller RF, Figler MM, Rogoff SM, et al.: Arteries of the Abdomen, Pelvis, and Lower Extremity. Rochester, NY, Eastman Kodak Company. With permission.)

288

L3 vertebral body. In its course throughout the abdomen, the ventral surface of the aorta contacts the stomach, splenic vein, pancreas, left renal vein, third duodenum, and mesentery.

The celiac axis (4), the first major aortic branch, arises ventrally at the L1 level. Although it is the principal source of blood flow to the liver, stomach, and spleen, it is not an important collateral vessel in lower-extremity arterial disease. The superior mesenteric artery (SMA) (22) arises 1 cm below the celiac axis and supplies the small and large bowel. It is frequently an important lower-extremity collateral, as discussed below. Proceeding distally, the renal arteries (32, 33) are the next major aortic branches. The renal arteries are most often single, paired vessels but may be multiple in a small percentage of individuals. They originate from the anterolateral aspect of the aorta slightly below the SMA, most frequently between the midbodies of L1 and L2. Because the renal arteries receive 25 percent of cardiac output, the caliber of the aorta decreases rather abruptly below their origin. The most commonly employed vascular reconstructive procedure for "inflow" disease (disease proximal to the level of the inguinal ligament) is an aortobifemoral or aortobiliac graft. This graft is anastomosed with the aorta just below the renal arteries, and its placement requires an adequate segment of nonaneurysmal aorta below the renal arteries; therefore, the localization of atheromatous disease of the distal aorta in relation to the origin of the renal arteries is of considerable clinical importance.

Paired lumbar arteries (3) originate posterolaterally from the aorta throughout its length near the midbody of each lumbar vertebra. Each lumbar artery passes dorsolaterally (those on the right traveling retrocavally) and gives off a posterior and anterior ramus, or branch. The posterior ramus supplies the skin and muscles of the back and gives off a branch to the contents of the spinal canal. The anterior ramus continues laterally and then ventrally into the abdominal wall, providing twigs for adjacent muscles. The anterior lumbar branches often form collateral routes in cases of inflow disease. The inferior mesenteric artery (IMA) (29), which is the final *visceral* aortic branch, arises ventrally near the midbody of L3. This level corresponds to the most caudal extent of the third portion of the duodenum and is 3–4 cm above the aortic bifurcation. The IMA descends parallel to and just to the left of the aorta, crosses the left iliac artery, and then passes into the pelvis. After giving off left colic (30) and sigmoid (31) branches, which supply the descending and sigmoid colon, it terminates in superior rectal branches (39) supplying the rectum. The IMA and its branches may provide an important collateral route in aortic and iliac obstruction. Just proximal to the aortic bifurcation and near the midbody of L4, the aorta gives rise to its final branch, the middle sacral artery (40), which is the only branch to arise dorsally. It descends near the midline, over L4, L5, the sacrum, and the coccyx. Its branches may serve as primarily collateral channels, as discussed below.

The Iliac System

At the midbody of L4, the aorta bifurcates into the common iliac arteries (41), which extend for approximately 5 cm before dividing at the lumbosacral junction into external (42) and internal (45) iliac branches (Fig. 13-2).

The external iliac artery (42) gives off two branches dorsally, which provide important collateral routes, the inferior epigastric (43) and deep iliac circumflex (44) arteries. From its origin, just cephalad to the inguinal ligament, the inferior epigastric artery (43) gives off a pubic branch, which ramifies along the back of the pubic symphysis. After ascending obliquely toward the midline along the medial margin of the deep inguinal ring, it ends in numerous subcutaneous anterior abdominal branches. The deep iliac circumflex artery (44) originates from the lateral aspect of the external iliac just above the inguinal ligament. It ascends deep to the inguinal ligament, obliquely and laterally, to the region of the anterior iliac spine. It then follows the inner aspect of the iliac crest, gives an ascending branch near its midpoint, and terminates in several dorsally directed subcutaneous terminal branches.

The internal iliac (hypogastric) artery divides shortly beyond its origin into an anterior and posterior division. Extensive collaterals may develop between the branches of the anterior and posterior divisions as well as to branches that originate from the aorta, the external iliac, and the superficial and deep femoral system. The anterior division includes the umbilical (not shown), obturator (52), internal pudendal (50), middle rectal (51), and inferior gluteal (49) arteries. The posterior division gives rise, consecutively, to the iliolumbar (46), lateral sacral (47), and superior gluteal (48) arteries. Because of the complexity and importance of internal iliac collaterals, we will describe the two divisions in greater detail.

The Posterior Internal Iliac Division

The iliolumbar artery (46) arises dorsally from the posterior division but then ascends ventral to the sacroiliac joint to the iliac fossa, where it gives off an iliac branch to supply pelvic musculature and a lumbar branch that ascends and supplies the psoas major and quadratus lumborum muscles and the contents of the spinal canal. The lateral sacral artery (47) arises dorsally but parallels the anterior surface of the sacrum and supplies the contents of the sacral canal and pelvic musculature. The posterior division trunk continues as the superior gluteal artery (48), which leaves the pelvis through the upper part of the greater sciatic foramen. Upon leaving the pelvis, it divides into superficial and deep branches, both of which may provide collaterals.

The Anterior Internal Iliac Division

The first visceral branch of the anterior hypogastric division is the umbiliac artery, an unimportant collateral. The second visceral branch, the obturator artery (52), follows the lateral pelvic wall to reach the obturator foramen where it pierces the obturator membrane and divides into terminal branches. Just before exiting the pelvis, it gives off a pubic branch, which ramifies on the posterior surface of the pubis. Beyond the obturator artery origin, the anterior trunk essentially trifurcates into the inferior gluteal (49), internal pudendal (50), and middle rectal (51) vessels. The inferior gluteal artery (49) leaves the pelvis through the greater sciatic foramen just below the piriformis muscle and descends deep to the gluteus maximus, which it supplies. It terminates in a muscular and cutaneous coccygeal branch and an anastomotic branch (discussed below in further detail). The internal pudendal artery (50) also leaves the pelvis through the greater sciatic foramen. It then crosses the ischial spine and enters the pudendal canal, where it branches into an inferior rectal vessel, a perineal vessel, and many other branches supplying genitourinary structures. The final discrete branch of the anterior division, the middle rectal artery (51), passes medially to the midportion of the rectum, which it supplies. It may, at times, give rise to an inferior vesical artery, although that vessel may also arise separately.

The Femoral System

The common femoral artery (56) is a continuation of the external iliac artery (42) and assumes its name as it passes beneath the inguinal ligament lateral to the femoral vein (Fig. 13-3). Since aortofemoral, femoral–femoral, and femoropopliteal grafts all have a surgical anastomosis at this level, it is an important site of pseudoaneurysm formation, should this complication occur. It is also a very common site of atherosclerotic obstruction. Aneurysmal disease may occur in the common femoral artery but is a somewhat unusual finding.

Between its origin and bifurcation, the common femoral artery gives off one branch directed laterally, the superficial iliac circumflex (61), and two branches medially, the superficial epigastric (55) and superficial external pudendal (57) arteries, all of which are subcutaneous vessels. About 4 cm below the inguinal ligament, the common femoral artery divides into superficial (59) and deep (58) femoral vessels. The superficial femoral artery continues distally in the thigh without the division to the level of the adductor hiatus in the tendon of the adductor magnus muscle (Hunter's canal). Upon leaving the canal, the superficial femoral artery gives off the descending genicular artery (68) and becomes the popliteal artery (69). Small muscular branches arise from the superficial femoral artery, especially in its distal segment.

The deep femoral artery (58) is directed posterolaterally at its origin. It continues distally in the thigh just medial to the femur, and ends in the distal third of the thigh as the fourth perforating artery (60) supplying the hamstring muscles. Along its course, it gives off the lateral femoral circumflex artery (63) with its ascending (64), transverse (66), and descending (65) branches, the medial femoral circumflex artery (62), and three perforating arteries (60). There are also muscular branches (67), which can serve as a critical collateral route in instances of superficial femoral artery obstruction.

The Popliteal System

The vessels included in the popliteal system are the popliteal (69), anterior tibial (77), posterior tibial (78), and peroneal (79) arteries and their branches (Fig. 13-3). The popliteal artery (69) can be the site of atheromatous obstruction as well as aneurysmal disease. It is the recipient of femoral–popliteal grafts and so is subject to the complications of these procedures. As the superficial femoral exits the adductor hiatus and gives off its descending genicular branch (68) it becomes the popliteal artery, which descends with a slight lateral deviation and ends at the border of the popliteus muscle. There it divides into the anterior tibial artery (77) and the tibioperoneal trunk. In its descent, the popliteal artery gives off two or three muscular branches, as well as the medial (73) and lateral (72) superior genicular arteries, the medial and lateral sural arteries (76), the middle genicular artery (not illustrated), and medial (75) and lateral (74) inferior genicular branches.

The muscular branches of the popliteal artery arise proximally and supply the adductor magnus and hamstring muscles. The sural arteries (76) supply the gastrocnemius, soleus, and plantaris muscles, while the middle genicular pierces the joint capsule to supply the synovium and ligaments. The paired superior and inferior geniculars supply the bones and soft tissue about the knee joint and provide important collaterals.

The first branch at the termination of the popliteal artery is the anterior tibial artery (77). It passes anterolaterally just above the proximal extent of the interosseous membrane and then descends along the anterior surface of this membrane. In its distal extent, the anterior tibial artery approaches and finally comes to overlie the tibia. Thereafter, it crosses the ankle joint and ends as the dorsalis pedis artery (81). As the anterior tibial crosses the interosseous space, it gives off the anterior tibial recurrent artery (80), which ascends and ramifies over the knee joint. Numerous branches are then given off to supply adjacent muscles as it courses distally. Several centimeters above the ankle joint, it gives rise to anterior medial (90) and anterior lateral (91) malleolar branches to supply structures of the ankle joint. These branches provide collateral routes around the joint.

The second terminal branch of the popliteal artery is the tibioperoneal trunk, which descends over a variable length before dividing into the posterior tibial (78) and peroneal (79) arteries. The posterior tibial artery (78) inclines medially on an oblique course and comes to lie posterior to the tibia. In this location, it descends to the ankle, where it rests just medial to the lateral malleolus. After crossing the ankle, it terminates as medial (86) and lateral (84) plantar arteries in the foot. At times, the posterior tibial is a small vessel or totally absent, its supply being replaced by an enlarged peroneal artery. Before its terminal bifurcation, it gives rise to muscular branches to adjacent musculature, to a communicating branch to the posterior tibial artery, the posterior medial malleolar artery, which ramifies over the medial malleolus, and to medial calcaneal branches, which supply the deeper soft tissues of the medial side of the heel.

The peroneal artery (79), the other branch of the tibioperoneal trunk, is inclined laterally in its proximal portion and comes to lie adjacent to the posteromedial border of the fibula. At the level of the ankle, it lies posterior to the tibiofibular syndesmosis and terminates as posterior lateral malleolar and lateral calcaneal arteries. The latter vessel supplies deep soft tissues about the heel laterally, while the former ramifies over the lateral malleolus. Branches given off in its descent are muscular twigs to adjacent muscles, a perforating branch, which pierces the interosseous membrane to lie anteriorly and provide anastomotic channels, and a communicating vessel to the posterior tibial artery.

The Foot

The posterior tibial artery continues into the plantar aspect of the foot (Fig. 13-3) and divides into a small medial plantar branch (86) and a larger lateral plantar branch (84), which joins with the deep plantar branch of the dorsalis pedis (88) artery to form the plantar arch. The plantar metatarsal branches, which provide the major supply to the digits, arise from the plantar arch.

The dorsalis pedis artery (81) is the continuation of the anterior tibial artery at the ankle. It passes medially on the dorsal surface to the first intermetatarsal space and divides into deep plantar (88) and first dorsal metatarsal arteries. Along its course it gives off the lateral tarsal artery (85), which originates over the navicular bone and is directed laterally to anastomose with lateral plantar (84) and lateral malleolar branches (81), as well as with the perforating branch of the peroneal. The medial tarsal (83) is unimportant as a collateral pathway except for communication with medial malleolar branches. The arcuate artery (87) is given off at the level of the metatarsal bases and is directed laterally with a slight caudal convex curve that ends by anastomosis with lateral tarsal (85) and plantar (84) branches forming the dorsal arcade. In its course, it gives off dorsal metatarsal branches to the digits, which are less important than their plantar counterparts.

COMMON LOCATIONS OF SEVERE ATHEROSCLEROTIC INVOLVEMENT

Although atherosclerosis is a diffuse disease, there is a distinct predilection for some portions of the circulations to be more severely affected than others. Thus, certain arterial segments are extremely prone to severe atheromatous involvement and consequent obstruction, while other regions are seldom affected to that degree. Sharply curved segments and bifurcations are typical areas of severe involvement. The cause for enhanced plaque development at these locations is not understood, although turbulence and pressure from jet effects may be influential.

In the aorta, the infrarenal segment is a common location of severe occlusive involvement or aneurysm formation, whereas occlusion is almost unheard of above that point. Severe atheromatous disease occurs frequently at any point in the common or external iliac arteries but is especially frequent at or just below the origin of the common iliac artery and at its bifurcation into external and internal iliac branches. In the lower extremities, the common femoral artery is a common site of major obstructive involvement, as is the origin of both the deep and superficial femoral arteries. More distally, the superficial femoral artery is prone to occlusion at its entry into the adductor canal, and the popliteal artery is prone to severe involvement immediately behind the knee. In the leg, the origin of any of the major popliteal branches is a common location of significant stenosis or occlusion.

AORTIC AND FEMORAL COLLATERAL ROUTES

From the previous discussion of arterial anatomy, it can be surmised that the vascular branches of the abdomen, pelvis, and lower extremities offer potential for a great number of collateral circuits at any level of obstruction. In a given patient, one or another collateral circuit will frequently predominate and contribute a major source of blood flow about an obstructed segment. Which route comes to supply the majority of flow is frequently determined by the absence of atherosclerotic disease in the components of one potential collateral and its presence in another. The number of possible collateral routes is generally greater in the abdomen and pelvis than it is in the lower extremities proper. Accordingly, it is easier to describe succinctly the major collateral routes below the inguinal ligament and much more difficult to be concise in this task above that level. The following discussion will therefore attempt to describe and illustrate major representative collateral circuits in the abdomen and pelvis as well as in the thigh and leg. The reader should be aware that myriad other pathways are available for each level of arterial obstruction.

Through knowledge of vascular anatomy, it is relatively easy to deduce the potential collateral circuits that might bypass a specific obstruction. Before proceeding with each of the following sections in which collateral circuits are described, the reader would do well to review Figures 13-1, 13-2, and 13-3 and envision the potential collateral routes that might span the level of obstruction in question. This procedure will make it easier for the reader to follow and understand the collateral described.

Collateral Routes Circumventing Distal Aortic or Common Iliac Obstruction

Collateral flow bypassing severe infrarenal aortic or common iliac blockages may follow visceral or somatic channels. The visual pathways may be very direct, as is the case in the SMA (22), right or middle (24) colic, left colic (30), or IMA (29) collateral, which may occur with aortic obstruction above the IMA. The route

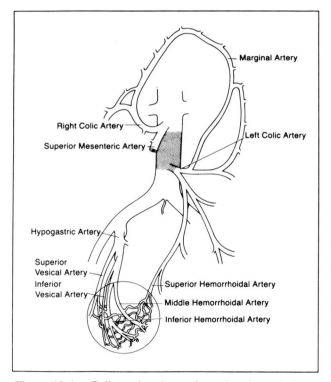

Figure 13-4. Collateral pathway from the visceral circulation to the hypogastric bed. From Krupski WC, Svonchai A, Effeney DJ, et al.: The importance of abdominal wall collateral blood vessels. Arch Surg 119:854–857, 1984. With permission.

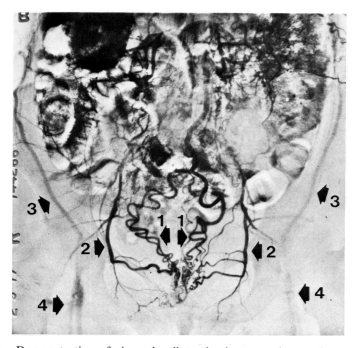

Figure 13-5. Demonstration of visceral collaterals circumventing aortic occlusion. This patient had complete atherosclerotic occlusion of the infrarenal aorta. Although not demonstrated on this film, the inferior mesenteric artery was obstructed at its origin; however, it filled through the middle colic–left colic anastomosis from the superior mesenteric artery. The superior rectal branch (1) filled in an antegrade manner. The internal pudendal arteries (2) filled retrograde through the rectal anastomoses and superficial iliac circumflex collaterals. The femoral system (4) was reconstituted primarily through the superficial iliac circumflex arteries (3).

requires patency of both the SMA and IMA. More often than not, however, the IMA is severely stenosed or occluded. Moreover, aortic obstruction is prone to occur below the level of IMA origin rather than above it. Even if the IMA is occluded or the aorta is obstructed at the bifurcation, visceral collaterals may still develop between the proximal aorta and the internal iliac system. The collateral route in this case is as follows: SMA → right/middle colic (24) → left colic (30) → IMA (29) → rectal, hemorrhoidal (39, 51) and vessical (54) branches. This collateral circuit is diagrammed in Figure 13-4 and illustrated by Figure 13-5. Flow in this circuit may also proceed through anastomotic branches between the inferior rectal arteries and middle sacral artery (40) directly to the distal aorta.

Somatic collaterals are equally important routes bypassing distal aortic or common iliac occlusion (Figs. 13-6 and 13-7). Inflow into this system is often through lumbar (3) or lower intercostal (1, 2) arteries, which anastomose through muscular branches with the iliolumbar artery (46) of the internal iliac system. Flow therefore proceeds as follows: lumbar/intercostal → iliolumbar → internal iliac → common iliac, and so on. Lumbar or iliolumbar flow may also extend to

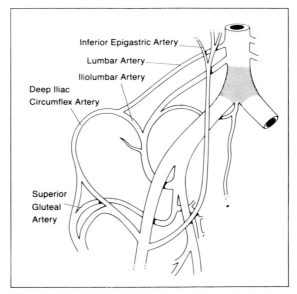

Figure 13-6. Collateral pathway from the lumbar hypogastric arteries to the deep iliac circumflex and external iliac arteries. From Krupskiw et al.: The importance of abdominal wall collateral blood vessels. Arch Surg 119:854–857, 1984. With permission.

anastomosis with the deep iliac circumflex (44) and inferior epigastric (43) branches of the distal external iliac artery.

The collateral route bypassing aortic and common iliac occlusion that spans the greatest distance is that involving the epigastric arteries (Figure 13-8). In this circuit, blood flows from the subclavian artery to the internal thoracic artery and then to the superficial epigastric artery (55), which anastomoses with branches of the inferior epigastric artery (43). Blood then flows retrograde in the inferior epigastric branches to the external iliac artery (42). The pubic branches of the inferior epigastric also ramify with terminal branches of the internal pudendal artery (50), offering an additional route of flow into the internal iliac artery (45).

In the event of unilateral internal iliac occlusion, collateral flow may develop across the pelvis between branches of the posterior division of the internal iliac system, including lateral sacral (47), internal pudendal (50), middle rectal (51), and inferior vesical (54) arteries. The middle sacral artery (40) may also contribute to this network.

Collateral Routes Circumventing External Iliac and Common Femoral Obstructions

External iliac blockage may be circumvented by the previously mentioned lumbar/intercostal → superficial iliac circumflex (44) route or by communications with the superficial epigastric (55), the inferior epigastric (43), and the deep iliac

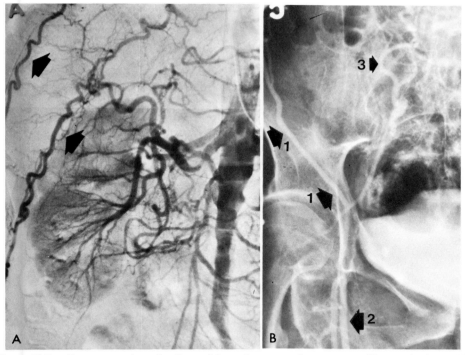

Figure 13-7.   Demonstration of collateral flow circumventing common iliac occlusion. This patient had an occlusion of the right common iliac artery. The lumbar arteries were also involved in the atherosclerotic occlusion. (A) Large intercostal arteries (arrowheads) are an important proximal collateral. (B) The superficial and deep femoral arteries (2) are filled by deep iliac circumflex (1) and iliolumbar (3) collaterals.

circumflex (61) arteries. A number of other collateral circuits of importance are possible and are frequently seen. For example, flow may proceed by an ipsilateral internal iliac to external iliac collateral circuit as follows: internal iliac (45) → iliolumbar (46) and superior gluteal (48) → communications with deep iliac circumflex artery (44) →external iliac (Figs. 13-9 to 13-11).

Blood flow distal to an external iliac or common femoral blockage is also frequently reconstituted through collaterals to the superficial and deep femoral arteries, with hypogastric branches being an important source of supply. Specifically, the upper and lower divisions of the superior gluteal artery (48) and the terminal branches of the inferior gluteal artery (49) anastomose freely with the lateral circumflex branch (63) of the deep femoral system. An internal iliac (45) →gluteal (48, 49) →lateral circumflex (63) →deep femoral (58) →superficial femoral route is thereby established. The inferior gluteal artery (49) also communicates with the first perforating and medial circumflex (62) branches of the deep femoral (58), forming an additional collateral pathway. Furthermore, the medial circumflex branch (62) of the deep femoral (58) may also receive blood from the obturator branch (52) of the hypogastric system through an anastomotic network.

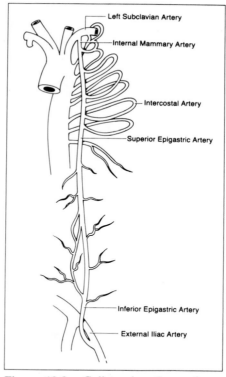

Left Subclavian Artery

Internal Mammary Artery

Intercostal Artery

Superior Epigastric Artery

Inferior Epigastric Artery

External Iliac Artery

Figure 13-8. Collateral pathway from the thoracic and upper-extremity circulation to the lower extremity. From Krupskiw et al.: The importance of abdominal wall collateral blood vessels. Arch Surg 119:854–857, 1984. With permission.

Collateral Routes Circumventing Deep Femoral, Superficial Femoral, and Popliteal Obstruction

Obstruction of the deep femoral artery is almost always at its origin. Collateral flow can occur from the common femoral artery through the superficial iliac circumflex (61) →lateral femoral circumflex (63) pathway. Flow may also be reconstituted from several superficial femoral sources, as described below. These same pathways may operate in reverse to supply deep femoral–superficial femoral flow if the superficial femoral is obstructed in either its proximal or distal segments (Fig. 13-9).

Deep femoral–superficial femoral collaterals include anastomotic networks between the descending branch (65) of the lateral femoral circumflex and the superior medial (73) and lateral (72) geniculars. Muscular branches of the superficial and deep femoral arteries (67) may also form anastomotic pathways. Finally, the perforating branches of the deep femoral (60) freely anastomose with

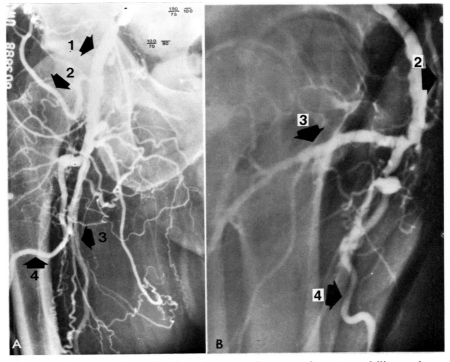

Figure 13-9. Demonstration of collateral routes circumventing external iliac and superficial femoral artery obstructions. (A) This patient has a high-grade atherosclerotic obstruction of the external iliac artery (1). A large superficial iliac circumflex artery (2) serves as the major collateral route. The gradient at the iliac obstruction is indicated by the pressure measurements. The superficial femoral artery also is occluded as well. Distal flow is provided by a large descending branch (4) of the lateral femoral circumflex artery. (B) The lateral projection in the femoral region demonstrates collaterals circumventing the superficial femoral artery, including the superficial circumflex iliac artery (2), the profunda femoral artery (3), and the descending branch of the lateral femoral circumflex artery (4). Note the high-grade stenosis at the origin of the profunda femoral, which is not well appreciated on the frontal film (A).

each other, and the fourth perforating branch communicates with the muscular branches of the popliteal system (Fig. 13-12).

When the superficial femoral is occluded at the adductor canal, or the popliteal artery is occluded, a vast array of collateral possibilities exist. Deep femoral–popliteal collaterals are possible through the descending lateral femoral circumflex (65) and the geniculars (72–75) or through muscular communication between the deep femoral and popliteal arteries (Fig. 13-13). The deep femoral routes are important when the superficial femoral is obstructed near its origin or throughout much of its length. If femoral obstruction is distal (near or in the adductor canal) or the popliteal artery is blocked, an anastomotic network about the knee consisting of ten arteries comes into play. Contributing to this network are two arteries from above (the descending branch of the lateral femoral circumflex [65] and the descending genicular [68]), five from the popliteal artery

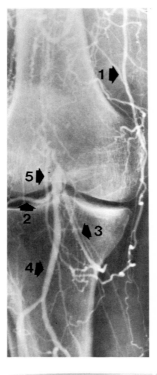

Figure 13-13. Demonstration of collateral channels about the knee. Flow in the popliteal artery (4) is reconstituted through multiple channels including the descending genicular artery (1), the lateral inferior genicular artery (2), the medial inferior genicular artery (3), and sural branches (5).

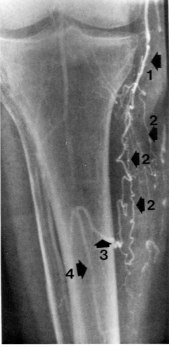

Figure 13-14. Demonstration of genicular collaterals to the posterior tibial artery. The descending genicular artery (1) fills through muscular branches (2), which communicate with the posterior tibial recurrent artery (3) and thereby reconstitute the posterior tibial artery (4).

302

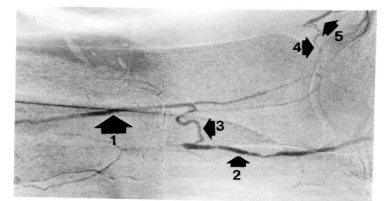

Figure 13-15. Demonstration of collateral channels at the ankle. The large peroneal artery (1) provides flow to the posterior tibial artery (2) through the communicating artery (3). In addition, the dorsalis pedis artery (5) fills through the anterior malleolar collaterals (4).

on the pattern of disease in the primary and potential collateral channels as well as the patient's level of activity. Knowledge of the anatomy and collateral routes is important for assessing symptoms and interpreting noninvasive test results.

Michael F. Stieghorst, M.D.
Department of Medical Imaging (Radiology)
St. Mary's Hospital Medical Center
707 South Mills Street
Madison, Wisconsin 53715

Andrew B. Crummy, M.D.
Professor of Radiology
University of Wisconsin Clinical Science Center
600 Highland Avenue
Madison, Wisconsin 53792

REFERENCES

1. Abrams HL (ed): Angiography (2nd ed.) Boston, Little, Brown, 1971
2. Gray H, Goss CM (eds): Anatomy of the Human Body (28th ed.) Philadelphia, Lea and Febiger, 1966
3. Johnsrude IS, Jackson DC: A Practial Approach to Angiography. Boston, Little, Brown, 1979
4. Krupski W, Svonchai A, Effency DJ, et al.: The importance of abdominal wall collateral blood vessels. Arch Surg 119:854–857, 1984
5. Muller RF, Figley MM, Rogoff SM, et al.: Arteries of the Abdomen, Pelvis, and Lower Extremity. Rochester, NY, Eastman Kodak Company.
6. Woodburne RT: Essentials of Human Anatomy (4th ed). New York, Oxford University Press, 1969

R. Eugene Zierler, M.D.
D. Eugene Strandness, Jr., M.D.

14

Doppler Techniques for Lower-Extremity Arterial Diagnosis

Although a careful history and physical examination are often adequate to establish the diagnosis of arterial occlusive disease affecting the lower extremity, noninvasive tests can provide objective confirmation of the clinical impression and quantify the degree of abnormality. It is well recognized that patient testimony is not completely reliable, since some patients with claudication may unconsciously compensate for their disability by walking more slowly or for shorter distances. Thus, patients may be unaware of their own limitations, particularly if the occlusive process occurs gradually. In addition, a variety of disorders produces symptoms in the legs that can simulate true intermittent claudication. The physical signs of lower-limb ischemia, such as the character of peripheral pulses, presence of bruits, and trophic skin changes, are subjective and provide only a crude assessment of the location and severity of disease. In a prospective study of 458 diabetic patients, 31 percent of those who gave no history of claudication and 21 percent of the group with a normal physical examination had arterial occlusive disease documented by objective noninvasive tests.[1]

Contrast arteriography remains the standard method for investigating patients with suspected arterial disease; the precise anatomic information provided is essential in planning reconstructive arterial operations. There are certain limitations with arteriography, however, particularly in estimating the hemodynamic significance of stenoses. Single-plane views may underestimate the severity of disease whenever plaques do not produce concentric narrowing. The addition of multiple views may improve accuracy somewhat, but even then the problem of interpretation is considerable.[2–5] Furthermore, when there is occlusive disease at multiple levels, it may be difficult to predict which segment is most responsible for the patient's symptoms.[6, 7]

The limitations of contrast arteriography, together with its inherently invasive nature, have stimulated the development of noninvasive physiologic methods for studying the lower-limb circulation. Although many devices and techniques have been described,[8] those that employ Doppler ultrasound are the most widely applied and thoroughly evaluated.

INSTRUMENTATION

Doppler Flowmeters

The transmitting frequency of Doppler ultrasonic instruments used for peripheral arterial studies is in the range of 2–10 MHz. Since the depth in tissue to which the ultrasound beam penetrates is inversely proportional to the transmitting frequency, lower frequencies are best suited for examining deeply located vessels, such as those in the thigh. As discussed in Chapter 2, the Doppler effect refers to the shift in frequency that occurs when sound is reflected from a moving object. The Doppler shift in vascular diagnosis varies from a few hundred to several thousand cycles/second, and this signal can be amplified to provide an audible signal with a pitch (or frequency) that is directly proportional to blood velocity.

The simplest Doppler instruments used in peripheral vascular diagnosis are pocket-sized units with the audio output presented through earphones or a small loudspeaker. These are quite satisfactory for a rapid bedside arterial or venous examination. For more elaborate studies, a direction-sensing Doppler flowmeter is necessary to separate the forward- and reverse-flow components normally present in peripheral arteries.[9] The output of directional Dopplers can be conveyed either through stereo headphones, by deflections on a pair of meters, or as an analog waveform on a strip chart recorder.

Pocket-sized Doppler devices and many directional instruments operate in the continuous-wave mode. Because these instruments provide no information regarding distance from the ultrasound source, Doppler shifts resulting from motion in superimposed vessels will be summed in the audible or analog output. However, arterial and venous signals are easily distinguished by their different directions and flow characteristics: venous flow produces low-frequency signals that vary with respiration, while arterial flow is associated with relatively high-frequency signals having pulsatile components that correspond to the cardiac cycle. Failure to obtain a Doppler signal from an artery usually indicates occlusion; however, extremely low flow rates (less than 2 cm/sec) will not produce a detectable Doppler shift.[10]

With pulsed wave ultrasound, it is possible to detect flow at discrete points along the sound beam.[11] This technique eliminates the problem of superimposed signals and permits characterization of flow patterns at specific sites in the arterial lumen. Pulsed wave Dopplers have been employed in two imaging systems: the ultrasonic arteriograph for flow visualization[12] and the duplex scanner, which combines B-mode imaging and Doppler flow detection.[13,14] These devices have been used extensively in the detection of carotid artery stenosis. Duplex scanning with spectral analysis of pulsed Doppler signals has also been used to assess the aortoiliac and femoropopliteal arteries. A more detailed discussion of basic principles and instrumentation in Doppler ultrasound is given in Chapter 2.

Imaging Systems

Tissue imaging with B-mode ultrasound is a rapid, noninvasive method for diagnosing aneurysmal disease of the aortoiliac segment.[17-19] The common femoral and popliteal arteries can also be assessed by this technique (see Chapters 16 and 18). Since noncalcified plaque and thrombus often have an acoustic impedance similar to that of flowing blood, it may be difficult to estimate the degree of stenosis from a B-mode image. As previously mentioned, arteriographic images can also be difficult to interpret. To avoid these problems, the noninvasive tests for lower-extremity arterial disease are based on physiologic parameters, namely, indirect measurements of blood pressure and flow.

Non-Doppler Devices for Flow Detection

Although this chapter emphasizes ultrasonic techniques, other methods have been developed for measuring blood flow in the extremities. The plethysmographic devices (see Chapter 17) include the mercury-in-Silastic strain gauge, the photoplethysmograph, and the pulse volume recorder (PVR). When ultrasonic evaluation is hampered by arterial-wall calcification or low flow, plethysmography provides an alternative method for assessing the lower-limb circulation.

Recording Devices

The routine lower-extremity arterial evaluation is based on the noninvasive measurement of systolic blood pressures, the audible characteristics of arterial Doppler signals and analog waveforms derived from the Doppler signal. Although it is not usually necessary, the Doppler signals may be recorded on audiotape for subsequent analysis and review.

A simple device for generating an analog waveform on a strip chart recorder is the zero crossing detector described in Chapter 2. Although this instrument is subject to errors and artifacts related to signal-to-noise ratio, amplitude dependency, and transient response,[20] it provides a graphic representation of the Doppler signal suitable for qualitative interpretation. Spectral analysis, as discussed in Chapter 3, is an alternative method for Doppler signal processing that overcomes the inherent limitations of the analog waveform. This technique has been widely used in the diagnosis of carotid artery disease, but its role in lower-extremity arterial diagnosis has not been established.

Vascular Laboratory Equipment

For the qualitative assessment of arterial flow patterns, a direction-sensing Doppler and strip chart recorder with zero crossing detector are needed. The measurement of segmental systolic blood pressures in the lower extremity requires pneumatic cuffs of appropriate size, a manometer to measure cuff pressure, and a means for detecting distal flow. Any continuous-wave Doppler or one of the plethysmographic devices can be used as a flow detector. A standard mercury or aneroid manometer is used to measure cuff pressure. Although cuff inflation can be accomplished manually, the examination is facilitated by using a

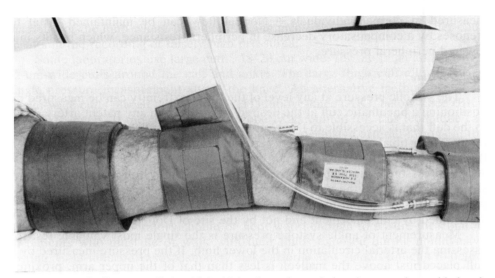

Figure 14-1. Cuffs are applied at high-thigh, above-knee, below-knee, and at ankle levels for measurement of segmental pressures.

able bladders, are used on each leg. The cuffs are applied at HT, AK, BK, and ankle levels. Systolic pressure is determined at each level using the Doppler technique outlined previously. The Doppler probe can be placed over the posterior tibial (PT) or dorsalis pedis (DP) arteries for all measurements (Fig. 14-1).

The systolic pressure in the proximal thigh as measured by the cuff method normally exceeds brachial systolic pressure by 30–40 mm Hg. Direct intra-arterial pressure measurements have shown that the actual pressures in the brachial and common femoral arteries are identical;[31] however, the use of a relatively small cuff on the thigh results in a significant cuff artifact. The ratio of HT systolic pressure to brachial systolic pressure (thigh pressure index) is normally greater than 1.2.[32] An index between 0.8 and 1.2 suggests aortoiliac stenosis, while an index less than 0.8 is consistent with complete iliac occlusion. Although the thigh pressure index usually reflects iliac inflow to the common femoral artery, the combination of superficial femoral occlusion and profunda femoris stenosis also may result in reduced HT pressure.

The difference in systolic pressure between any two adjacent levels in the leg should be less than 20 mm Hg in normal individuals.[27] Gradients in excess of 20 mm Hg usually indicate significant occlusive disease in the intervening arterial segment: an HT–AK gradient reflects superficial femoral disease; an AK–BK gradient reflects popliteal disease; and a BK–ankle gradient reflects disease in the tibial and peroneal arteries.[10] In addition to vertical gradients down a single leg, the horizontal gradients between corresponding segments of the two legs may also indicate the presence of occlusive lesions. The difference in systolic pressures measured at the same level in both legs normally should not exceed 20 mm Hg.

Toe Pressure

Measurement of toe pressure can be used to identify obstructive disease involving the pedal arch and digital arteries. Toe pressures are also valuable when ankle pressures are found to be spuriously high because of arterial calcification. Normal systolic toe pressure is approximately 80–90 percent of the brachial systolic pressure.[33] Because of the smaller size and lower flow rates of digital arteries, flow detection by ultrasonic methods may be difficult. The plethysmographic techniques described in Chapter 17 are better suited for blood-flow measurement at the digital artery level.

Penile Pressure

The measurement of penile systolic pressure has been useful in the evaluation of male impotence.[34] The technique is analogous to that used for pressure measurements in the lower limb and employs a small, digit-sized pneumatic cuff and a Doppler device for monitoring flow in a penile artery distal to the cuff. Alternatively, a strain-gauge plethysmograph or photoplethysmograph can be used to detect flow.[35] Reduced pelvic blood flow and vasculogenic impotence are usually associated with occlusive arterial disease affecting the lower extremity. In young potent males, the ratio of penile to brachial systolic pressure is greater than 0.8; a ratio of less than 0.6 is consistent with penile arterial insufficiency. Because of the wide variability in penile systolic pressure among potent and impotent males, a multidisciplinary diagnostic approach to the problem of impotence is necessary.[34]

Exercise and Reactive Hyperemia Testing

Lower-extremity exercise and reactive hyperemia both increase limb blood flow by causing vasodilation of peripheral resistance vessels. In limbs with normal arteries, this increased flow occurs with little or no drop in ankle systolic pressure. When occlusive lesions are present in the main lower-limb arteries, blood is diverted through high-resistance collateral pathways. Although the collateral circulation may provide adequate flow to the resting extremity with only a modest reduction in ankle pressure, the capacity of collateral vessels to increase flow during exercise is limited. Pressure gradients, which are minimal at rest, may be accentuated by increasing flow rates with exercise. Thus, stress testing provides a method for detecting less severe degrees of arterial disease.

Treadmill Exercise

Standard treadmill exercise at 2 miles/hr on a 12-percent grade is the simplest way to stress the lower-limb circulation. Treadmill testing is advantageous because it simulates the activity that produces the patient's symptoms and determines the degree of disability under controlled conditions. It permits an assessment of nonvascular factors that may affect performance, such as musculoskeletal or cardiopulmonary disease. The ability to perform treadmill exercise is also determined by patient effort, motivation, and pain tolerance.

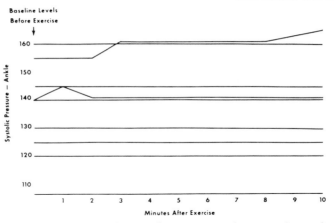

Figure 14-2. Ankle systolic pressure values are shown for eight normal subjects after walking on the treadmill for 5 minutes at 2 mph on a 12-percent grade. In each case the ankle pressure either remained at the preexercise level or increased slightly. (From Strandness DE: Abnormal exercise responses after successful reconstructive arterial surgery. Surgery 59:329–333, 1966. With permission.)

Walking on the treadmill is continued for 5 minutes or until symptoms occur and the patient is forced to stop. The walking time and nature of any symptoms are recorded, and the ankle and arm systolic pressures are also measured before and immediately after exercise. Two components of the response to exercise are evaluated: (1) the magnitude of the immediate drop in ankle systolic pressure and (2) the time for recovery to resting pressure. Changes in both these parameters are proportional to the severity of arterial occlusive disease.

A normal response to exercise is a slight increase or no change in the ankle systolic pressure compared with the resting value (Fig. 14-2). If the ankle pressure is decreased immediately after exercise, the test is considered positive, and repeat measurements are taken at 2- to 3-minute intervals for up to 10 minutes or until the pressure returns to preexercise levels. When a patient is forced to stop walking because of symptomatic arterial occlusive disease, the ankle systolic pressure in the affected limb is usually less than 60 mm Hg. If symptoms occur without a significant fall in the ankle pressure, a nonvascular cause of leg pain must be considered.

The postexercise pressure changes in patients with symptomatic arterial disease can be divided into three groups.[29] Ankle pressures that fall to low or unrecordable levels immediately after exercise and then rise toward resting values in 2–6 minutes suggest occlusion or stenosis at a single level such as the superficial femoral artery. When ankle pressures remain decreased or unrecordable for up to 12 minutes, lesions involving multiple arterial levels are almost always present. Rarely, this pattern may occur with an isolated iliac artery occlusion. In patients with ischemic rest pain, postexercise ankle pressures may remain unrecordable for 15 minutes or more.

Reactive Hyperemia Testing

Reactive hyperemia is an alternative method for stressing the peripheral circulation.[36] Inflating a pneumatic cuff at thigh level to suprasystolic pressure for 3–5 minutes produces ischemia and vasodilation distal to the cuff. The changes in ankle pressure that occur upon release of cuff occlusion are similar to those observed in the treadmill test. Although normal limbs do not show a drop in ankle systolic pressure after treadmill exercise, a transient drop does occur with reactive hyperemia.[37] This decrease in ankle pressure is in the range of 17–34 percent. In patients with arterial disease, the response to reactive hyperemia is usually more prominent, and there is a good correlation between the maximum pressure drop with reactive hyperemia and the maximum pressure drop after treadmill exercise. However, there may be considerable overlap in the ankle pressure response to reactive hyperemia among normal subjects and patients with arterial disease.[38] As a general rule, patients with single-level arterial disease show less than a 50-percent drop in ankle pressure with reactive hyperemia, while patients with multiple-level arterial disease show a pressure drop greater than 50 percent.[37] Reactive hyperemia testing is useful for those patients who are unable to walk on the treadmill because of amputations or other physical disabilities. Treadmill exercise is generally preferred over reactive hyperemia, since the former produces a physiologic stress which reproduces a patient's ischemic symptoms.

Doppler Signal Waveform Analysis

A qualitative analysis of the arterial flow pattern can be performed by simply listening to the Doppler audio output. An experienced examiner learns to recognize the high-pitched, harsh character and the changes in phasic components of the Doppler signal that are associated with stenoses. A graphic display of the velocity waveform permits a more objective analysis. The previously described zero crossing detector is a convenient method for generating an analog waveform on a strip chart recorder, and the output of this device closely resembles that of an electromagnetic flowmeter (Fig. 14-3).

The Analog Waveform

The flow pattern in the main arteries of the lower extremity normally has three components or phases during each cardiac cycle. The first phase has the highest frequency and is the large forward-velocity peak produced by cardiac systole. This is followed by a second, brief phase of flow reversal in early diastole and a third, low-frequency phase of forward flow in late diastole (Fig. 14-4). The triphasic flow pattern is modified by a variety of factors, one of the most important being peripheral vascular resistance. For example, body heating, which causes vasodilation and decreased resistance, will abolish the second phase of flow reversal; the opposite will occur on exposure to cold.

When a waveform is obtained from an arterial site *distal* to a stenosis or occlusion, a single forward-velocity component is observed, with flow remaining above the zero line throughout the cardiac cycle. The peak systolic frequency is lower than normal, and the waveform becomes flat and rounded (Fig. 14-4). These

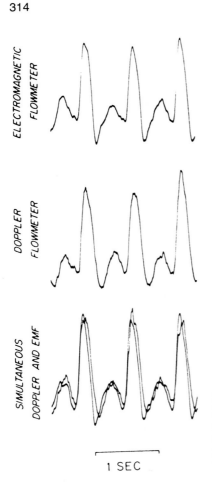

Figure 14-3. Comparison of electromagnetic and Doppler flow tracings obtained from the carotid artery of a dog shows their similarity. (From Strandness DE, Sumner DS: Hemodynamics for Surgeons. New York, Grune and Stratton, 1975. With permission.)

changes result from decreased velocity of flow as well as the compensatory fall in peripheral resistance that occurs in limbs with arterial occlusive disease.

If the Doppler probe is placed *directly over* a stenotic lesion, the signal will have an abnormally high peak systolic frequency. This reflects the increased flow velocity in the stenotic segment. The character of Doppler signals obtained *proximal* to an arterial obstruction depends on the capacity of the collateral circulation. If there are well-developed collaterals between the Doppler probe and the point of obstruction, the waveform will be normal. The flow signal obtained immediately proximal to an obstruction, when there is no collateral outflow, has a harsh quality and has been described as a "thumping" sound.[39] Failure to obtain a flow signal over a vessel indicates occlusion or, rarely, a flow velocity too low to produce a detectable Doppler frequency shift.

Parameters Derived from the Velocity Waveform

Since the magnitude of the Doppler shift is directly proportional to the cosine of the beam/vessel angle, θ, as discussed in Chapter 2, a direct quantitative analysis of the velocity waveform requires a value for this angle. Measurement of

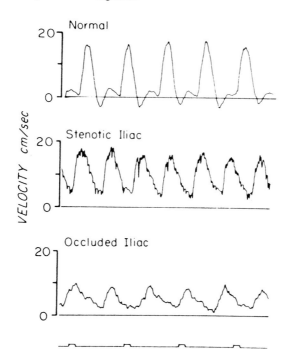

Figure 14-4. Velocity patterns obtained with a directional Doppler flowmeter from the femoral artery of a normal subject, a patient with a stenotic external iliac artery, and a patient with an occluded common iliac artery. The triphasic pattern in the normal artery includes a brief phase of flow reversal. Flow velocity is proportional to Doppler frequency. (From Strandness DE, Sumner Ds: Hemodynamics for Surgeons. New York, Grune and Stratton, 1975. With permission.)

beam angle is difficult with currently available equipment for lower-extremity diagnosis; however, quantitative data can still be obtained by using ratios of Doppler shifts that are independent of beam/vessel angle.

One such ratio is the pulsatility index (PI), which is calculated by dividing the peak-to-peak frequency difference by the mean frequency (Fig. 14-5). Measurements for calculating PI can be based on either analog waveforms or the output of a spectrum analyzer. The use of analog waveforms has been criticized on the grounds that they may contain errors and artifacts.[20] Nonetheless, there is a close correlation between reduction in PI and severity of arterial occlusive disease as assessed by arteriography and ankle pressure measurement.[40] The PI of the normal common femoral artery has a mean value of 6.7. More distally, the PI increases to 8 in the popliteal and 14.1 in the posterior tibial artery.[41] These values are decreased in the presence of proximal occlusive lesions. In a study that compared common femoral artery PI with intra-arterial pressure measurement, a PI value greater than or equal to 4 was highly predictive of a hemodynamically normal aortoiliac segment.[42] The predictive value of a PI less than 4 depended on

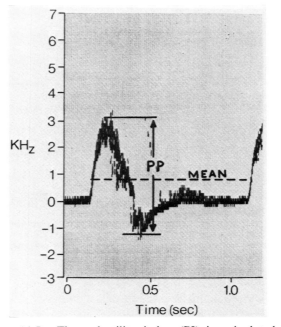

Figure 14-5. The pulsatility index (PI) is calculated by dividing the peak-to-peak frequency difference (PP) by the mean frequency. The waveform was produced by a spectrum analyzer. (From Knox RA, Strandness DE: Ultrasound tehniques for evaluation of lower extremity arterial occlusion. Semin Ultrasound 2:264–275, 1981, with permission.)

the condition of the superficial femoral artery. When the superficial femoral artery was patent, a PI less than 4 indicated a hemodynamically significant aortoiliac lesion, but a low PI value with an occluded superficial femoral artery was not diagnostic.

Another approach to velocity waveform analysis is the Laplace transform (LT) method.[43,44] For LT analysis, the waveform shape is expressed mathematically by a curve-fitting technique, and a damping coefficient that indicates lumen size is calculated. A comparison of common femoral artery PI and LT damping values indicated that the LT method was more sensitive in the detection of iliac artery stenoses.[43] Furthermore, the LT damping results were not affected by the presence or absence of occlusive disease in the superficial femoral artery. Thus, LT damping would be a more useful diagnostic test than PI in patients with multiple-level arterial occlusive disease.

Although quantitative methods for waveform analysis, such as PI and LT damping, provide information of diagnostic value, they are currently too complicated and time-consuming for routine clinical use. When devices for automatic quantitative waveform analysis become available, these methods may be more widely applied.

A summary of the measurements and indexes used in lower extremity arterial diagnosis is given in Table 14-1.

Table 14-1
Summary of Measurements and Indexes

Ankle Systolic Pressure	Normally > brachial systolic pressure; absolute pressure <40 mm Hg consistent with severe occlusive disease and ischemic rest pain.
Ankle pressure Index	Normally >1.
High-thigh Systolic Pressure	Normally 30–40 mm Hg > brachial systolic pressure.
Thigh pressure Index	Normally >1.2.
Segmental Pressure Gradients	Normally <20 mm Hg between adjacent levels on the same leg or the same levels on the two legs.
Toe Systolic Pressure	Normally 80–90% of brachial systolic pressure.
Penile Systolic Pressure	Normally >80% of brachial systolic pressure; a value of <60% is consistent with vasculogenic impotence.
Treadmill Exercise Test	Normal walking time 5 minutes without symptoms or drop in ankle systolic pressure (2 mph, 12% grade).

CLINICAL APPLICATIONS OF NONINVASIVE TESTING

The goals of the lower extremity arterial evaluation are to confirm the diagnosis of arterial occlusive disease, indicate the location of any obstructing lesions, and quantify the resulting degree of disability. A variety of conditions produce signs and symptoms in the legs that may be confused with arterial disease (Table 14-2). Furthermore, it is not unusual for a single patient to have multiple causes for leg pain, and it may be difficult to determine which is most responsible for a patient's symptoms. The measurements of arterial pressure and flow patterns described in this chapter can be applied to both the initial evaluation and subsequent followup of patients with arterial occlusive disease.

The Initial Evaluation

In the evaluation of any patient with signs or symptoms consistent with arterial occlusive disease, two questions must be answered: (1) Is arterial occlusion present? and (2) Is arterial occlusion causing the patient's symptoms?

Table 14-2
Conditions Associated with Leg Pain

Arterial occlusive disease (claudication, rest pain)
Osteoarthritis (hip, knee)
Neurospinal disease (lumbar disc, spinal stenosis)
Nocturnal muscle cramps
Peripheral neuropathy (diabetes mellitis)
Reflex sympathetic dystrophy (causalgia)
Deep vein thrombosis (venous claudication)
Cellulitis
Trauma

Recording of ankle-pressure indexes, segmental pressure gradients, Doppler velocity waveforms and the treadmill exercise or reactive hyperemia test will answer these questions unequivocally in the majority of patients.

The finding of normal ankle pressure indexes at rest and a normal response to treadmill exercise essentially rules out any significant lower-extremity arterial occlusive disease. Some patients will have decreased ankle pressure indexes at rest and symptoms during treadmill exercise but little or no ankle pressure drop after cessation of exercise. This finding suggests that, although arterial disease is present, it is not producing the symptom in question, and another cause of leg pain should be considered. The limitations imposed by cardiac, pulmonary and musculoskeletal conditions are directly observed during exercise testing, allowing these factors to be considered in the overall management of the patient.

Followup Testing

Noninvasive testing is a convenient and practical means for serial followup of patients after their initial evaluation. Evidence of disease progression or improvement may be observed, and the results of medical or surgical therapy can be objectively documented.

In patients who have had successful arterial reconstructions for occlusive disease, ankle pressures and appropriate segmental pressure gradients should be significantly improved compared with the preoperative values.[45] If a single level of disease was present preoperatively, successful bypass grafting or endarterectomy should result in normal or near-normal ankle pressures. Failure of ankle pressures to improve immediately following surgery suggest either a problem related to surgical technique or the selection of an inappropriate reconstructive procedure.[46] Deterioration of noninvasive measurements later in the postoperative period may reflect either structural changes occurring in the reconstructed segment or progression of occlusive disease at other sites.[47,48] Serial postoperative followup is desirable, since early identification and repair of a failing arterial reconstruction results in the greatest chance of maintaining patency.

Patients whose condition is improved after surgery but still not returned to normal may have their status documented by noninvasive testing. For example, a patient may show a significant improvement in treadmill walking time after arterial reconstruction despite a persistent drop in ankle pressure. This observation is common in patients with arterial occlusive disease at multiple levels who have only one level corrected; the abnormal hemodynamic response will then reflect the remaining untreated disease. Figure 14-6 shows the ankle pressure changes recorded before and after an aortofemoral bypass graft in a patient who also has stenoses in both superficial femoral arteries. Although the treadmill walking time improved, an abnormal ankle pressure response is still present.

Specific Clinical Problems

Claudication

The term *intermittent claudication* refers to a muscular ache or cramp that occurs during exercise and is relieved by rest. It results from inadequate blood flow to muscle during exercise and is a definite, reproducible symptom. Claudica-

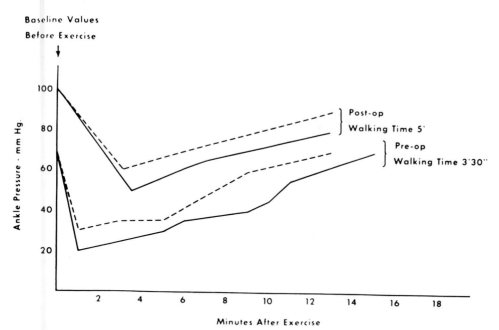

Figure 14-6. Ankle pressure response to treadmill exercise before and after an aortofemoral bypass graft in a patient with bilateral superficial femoral artery stenoses. The postoperative exercise test shows some improvement in walking time but remains abnormal. (Dashed lines) left ankle; (solid lines) right ankle. (From Strandness DE: Abnormal exercise responses after successful reconstructive arterial surgery. Surgery 59:325–333, 1966. With permission.)

tion usually involves the calf, but the thigh or buttock may also be affected when arterial occlusions reduce blood flow to these areas. Arteriosclerosis obliterans is by far the commonest cause of claudication; popliteal artery entrapment must be considered, however, when claudication occurs in young adults or children.[49,50]

When the characteristic symptoms are produced by treadmill exercise in association with a drop in ankle pressure to less than 60 mm Hg, the clinical impression of intermittent claudication is confirmed. The walking time documents the extent of disability and serves as a baseline for subsequent followup. Segmental pressure gradients indicate the location of arterial occlusive lesions.

Rest Pain

Ischemic rest pain develops in the toes or forefoot when blood flow is insufficient to maintain normal cellular function at rest. Noninvasive tests usually show multiple-level arterial occlusive disease with ankle systolic pressure less than 40 mm Hg and an ankle pressure index less than 0.35. Treadmill exercise or reactive hyperemia testing are not necessary in patients with this degree of abnormality.

Impotence

Pelvic vascular insufficiency is just one of several potential causes of impotence; hormonal, psychogenic, and neurogenic factors must also be considered. As previously discussed, a penile-to-brachial systolic pressure ratio of less than 0.6 is consistent with vasculogenic impotence; it is not, however, diagnostic.[34] A normal ratio of 0.8 or greater is helpful in excluding the problem of penile arterial insuffiency.

Healing of Ulcers and Amputations

Noninvasive pressure measurements can be used to assess the probability of achieving primary healing in the ischemic lower extremity. Ischemic foot ulcers are unlikely to heal if ankle systolic pressure is less than 55 mm Hg in nondiabetics or less than 80 mm Hg in diabetics.[51] The ankle pressures in diabetic patients may be falsely elevated because of calcific medial sclerosis that renders vessels incompressible.

Ankle pressures have not been uniformly helpful in predicting healing of BK or foot amputations.[8] A BK or calf pressure greater than 70 mm Hg correlates with primary healing of BK amputations, while the absence of detectable Doppler flow signals below the knee predicts failure of healing.[52] Primary healing may still be achieved with BK pressures less than 70 mm Hg, so the choice of amputation level should not be based on pressure measurement alone.

Predicting Results of Arterial Surgery

Noninvasive measurements of lower-extremity pressure have been used to predict the functional results of arterial reconstruction in terms of symptom relief and graft patency. In patients undergoing aortofemoral bypass procedures, a thigh pressure index of 0.85 or less is a reliable predictor of a good postoperative result; however, improvement may also occur in many patients with thigh pressure indexes greater than 0.85.[53] The presence of occlusive disease limited to the aortoiliac arteries, as demonstrated by normal segmental pressure gradients in the leg, is also predictive of a good result after aortofemoral bypass grafting. A comparison of ankle pressure indexes before and after aortofemoral bypass showed that an increase of 0.1 or more during the first 12 hours after operation correlated highly with subsequent symptomatic improvement.[53] The preoperative ankle pressure index alone also has some predictive value.[54] When the ankle pressure index is greater than 0.8, 94 percent of patients will obtain significant symptom relief after aortofemoral bypass, while only 64 percent of patients will show the same degree of improvement if the ankle pressure index is less than 0.4. These observations indicate that aortofemoral bypass grafting is most successful in those patients with significant aortoiliac occlusive disease and normal distal arteries.

The predictive value of noninvasive pressure measurements in femoropopliteal bypass procedures has not been firmly established. An early study suggested that an ankle pressure index of greater than 0.4 predicted a high graft patency rate, while an ankle pressure index of less than 0.2 was associated with early graft failure.[55] Later reports have not confirmed these observations, however, and very low ankle pressures should not be regarded as a contraindication for femoropopliteal bypass.[46]

The role of lumbar sympathectomy in the management of patients with lower-extremity arterial disease has been controversial. Sympathectomy is often considered for patients with impending limb loss due to severe, unreconstructable occlusive disease. In this situation, ankle pressure measurements have provided a means for selecting those patients most likely to benefit from the procedure.[56] An ankle pressure index greater than 0.35 predicts a favorable clinical response to sympathectomy; an index less than 0.2 correlates highly with sympathectomy failure and subsequent limb loss. The value of lumbar sympathectomy depends on the adequacy of collateral circulation in the leg, and the ankle pressure index provides an indirect assessment of the potential for increasing flow through the collateral vessels.

LOWER-EXTREMITY ARTERIAL EXAMINATION

The sequence of noninvasive tests used in the routine lower-extremity arterial examination is listed in Table 14-3. Although the basic elements of each test have been described, some additional remarks on technique and interpretation are appropriate.

The examination begins with a brief history and physical examination emphasizing the symptoms and signs of peripheral vascular disease. The status of palpable peripheral pulses, location of bruits, and the presence of ischemic skin lesions are noted. If a significant degree of cardiac or pulmonary disease is present, the patient's ability to perform treadmill exercise must be determined. When doubt exists, a physician should be consulted.

Any continuous-wave Doppler device is satisfactory for measuring ankle or segmental limb pressures. Initially, ankle systolic pressure should be measured in both DP and PT arteries (Fig. 14-7). Bilateral brachial pressures are also measured. The ankle pressure index for each leg is calculated by dividing the highest ankle pressure by the highest brachial pressure. When the ankle pressure index is normal, measurement of segmental pressure gradients is not necessary. In limbs with severe arterial disease and no detectable flow signals at the ankle, thigh pressures can often be obtained by using the popliteal artery flow signal.

Analog waveforms are usually recorded with a direction sensing continuous-wave Doppler and a strip chart recorder incorporating a zero crossing detector.

Table 14-3
The Lower Extremity Arterial Examination

---

1. Measurement of ankle pressures (DP and PT) and brachial pressures at rest.
2. Calculation of ankle pressure indexes.
3. Segmental pressure gradients if ankle pressures are abnormal.
4. Common femoral artery velocity waveforms at rest.
5. Treadmill exercise or reactive hyperemia testing with repeat common femoral artery velocity waveforms and serial ankle pressure measurements.
6. Special studies:
    Penile pressure
    Toe pressure
    Duplex scanning

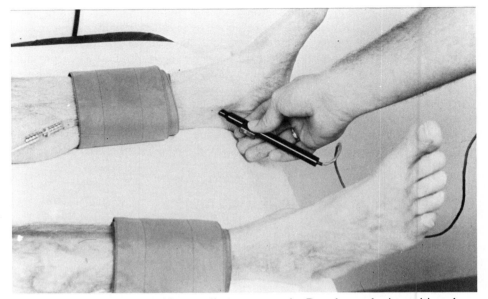

Figure 14-7. To measure ankle systolic pressures, the Doppler probe is positioned over the left posterior tibial artery.

The Doppler angle is adjusted by visual inspection to minimize noise and artifact. Although waveforms can be obtained from any site with a Doppler signal, only the common femoral artery (CFA) waveform is routinely recorded. This waveform is helpful in detecting proximal aortoiliac occlusive lesions. It is valuable to record the CFA waveforms both before and immediately after treadmill exercise or reactive hyperemia, since some less severe lesions will be apparent only at increased flow rates.

Stress testing with treadmill exercise or reactive hyperemia can be tolerated by most patients who do not have ischemic rest pain. As previously stated, the treadmill test is preferred because it is a more physiologic form of stress. The speed and grade of the electronic treadmill can be varied to suit the individual patient, but the standard test uses 2 miles/hr and a 12-percent grade. It is convenient to have the patient wear ankle cuffs and an arm cuff while walking on the treadmill (Fig. 14-8). Immediately after cessation of exercise the patient returns to the examining table where ankle and arm pressures are measured. Serial ankle pressure measurements are then made at 2–3-minute intervals for up to 10 minutes or until they return to preexercise values. An automatic cuff inflator facilitates this rapid sequence of measurements. A form for recording the noninvasive test results is shown in Fig. 14-9.

Additional studies, such as measurement of toe and penile pressures, are of value only in selected clinical circumstances. Toe pressures can be used to detect occlusive lesions between the level of the ankle and the digital arteries.

Although the duplex scanner has been developed primarily for evaluating the carotid bifurcation, this instrument can also be used to assess the arteries in the abdomen and legs.[15,16] The duplex scanner provides a B-mode image that displays

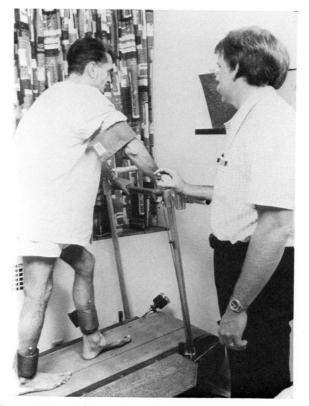

Figure 14-8.   Ankle cuffs and one arm cuff are in place to facilitate post-exercise pressure measurements in the treadmill stress test.

the artery being examined and serves as a guide for placement of the pulsed Doppler sample volume in the center of the flow stream. Thus, the B-mode and Doppler methods are combined to determine the location and extent of arterial stenoses. Center-stream pulsed Doppler signals are processed by a spectrum analyzer, and the resulting flow patterns can be used to classify the degree of disease present. A set of spectral criteria has been developed by comparing a series of flow patterns with corresponding contrast arteriograms. These criteria are based on increases in peak systolic frequency, changes in waveform contour, and increases in the width of the frequency band. In a preliminary study of 20 patients involving 230 arterial segments extending from the abdominal aorta to the popliteal bifurcation, duplex scanning had an overall accuracy of 92 percent.[16] The accuracy for each arterial segment was iliac, 97 percent; common femoral and profunda, 95 percent; proximal, mid, and distal superficial femoral, 92 percent, 94 percent, and 89 percent, respectively; and popliteal, 83 percent. Spectral analysis was most accurate for lesions in the aortoiliac segment, and the results were not affected by multiple-level occlusive disease. Duplex scanning with spectral analysis provides a direct anatomic and physiologic assessment of the leg arteries. With further refinements in technique, duplex scanning could become a powerful

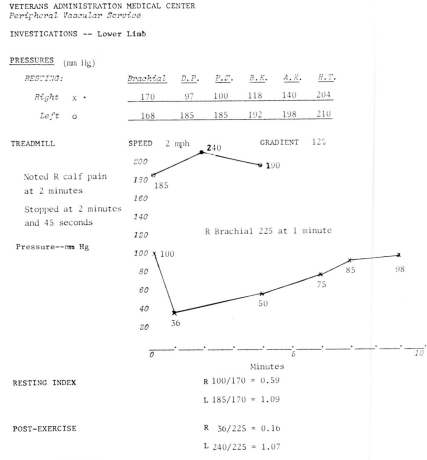

Figure 14-9. On this form for recording test results, *D.P.* and *P.T.* refer to the ankle pressures obtained by positioning the Doppler probe over the dorsalis pedis and posterior tibial arteries respectively. The results shown are for Case 14-3.

method for diagnosis of lower-extremity arterial disease. This subject is considered in greater detail in Chapter 16.

Sources of Technical Error

Variability

The variability in measurements of arterial pressure results from biologic as well as technical factors. The ankle pressure index and other ratios that relate peripheral and central arterial pressures compensate for minute-to-minute changes in central pressure, thus avoiding a major source of biologic variation. Because of variability related to technique, changes in ankle pressure index must be 0.15 or greater to be considered significant.[57]

Incompressible Vessels

Accurate measurement of arterial pressure using pneumatic cuffs requires that cuff pressure be transmitted through the arterial wall to the flow stream. The presence of medial calcification in the arterial wall results in varying degrees of incompressibility and recording of falsely high pressures.[27] Occasionally, it may be impossible to eliminate the distal flow signal, even with maximal cuff inflation pressures. When this situation is encountered, the main arteries are usually patent, since collateral vessels are easily obliterated by the cuff.

Diabetic patients are particularly prone to medial calcification, and artifactual elevation of leg pressures must always be considered in this group. In approximately 5–10 percent of diabetic patients, ankle pressures cannot be measured because of incompressible vessels.[51] In these cases, toe pressure measurement is a more reliable method for assessing the severity of arterial occlusive disease.

Cuff Artifact

As previously mentioned, cuff width should be at least 50 percent greater than limb diameter for accurate pressure measurement. The use of smaller cuffs results in falsely elevated pressure readings, particularly in obese patients. In the majority of patients, the magnitude of the cuff artifact can be anticipated, and relatively narrow thigh cuffs can be successfully used to measure segmental pressure gradients.

Other Sources of Error

In limbs with severe arterial occlusive disease and low flow rates, Doppler signals may be unobtainable even when the arteries are patent. The plethysmographic techniques may provide useful information in these cases. When very weak Doppler signals are detected, it may be difficult to distinguish between arterial and venous flow. A direction-sensing Doppler is useful in this situation. In addition, venous signals will augment with distal limb compression, while arterial signals will either remain the same or diminish.

The pressure gradients between adjacent segments may be increased in markedly hypertensive patients. On the other extreme, segmental pressure gradients may be decreased when cardiac output is low.[58] When the collateral vessels bypassing an arterial obstruction are unusually large and efficient, the corresponding segmental gradient may be normal. If this is the case, a significant gradient should become apparent after treadmill exercise.

Arterial occlusive lesions distal to the ankle will not be detected by the routine lower-extremity evaluation, since the ankle is the most distal site of pressure measurement. Lesions involving the plantar or digital arteries, such as vasculitis and microembolism, may be identified by strain-gauge plethysmography.

SUMMARY

The results of the various tests in the lower extremity arterial examination should be combined to form an overall assessment of the patient's circulatory status. Decisions are then made regarding the presence of arterial occlusive disease, its location and severity, and its contribution to the patient's symptoms. This information provides a database that can be used to plan initial therapy. If the patient is considered to be a candidate for direct arterial surgery or interventional radiologic procedures, further evaluation by arteriography is required.

CASE STUDIES

Case 14-1

A 58-year-old man complained of pain in the right calf and buttock after walking one or two blocks. There were no symptoms at rest. Fourteen years previously, he had undergone an aortoiliac endarterectomy for claudication. The results of the noninvasive evaluation are shown in Figures 14-10A and B.

DISCUSSION   The resting ankle pressure index is moderately decreased on the right and borderline normal on the left. Segmental pressures show a significant gradient on the right side between the HT and brachial levels (thigh pressure index 110/136 = 0.81), while the HT pressure on the left side is slightly below normal (thigh pressure index 158/136 = 1.16). There are no other significant gradients in either leg. The resting CFA waveform on the right side is an abnormal monophasic signal, and the left side has a normal multiphasic appearance which includes a small reverse-flow component.

Treadmill exercise reproduced the patient's symptoms after 1 minute and 40 seconds. The right PT pressure dropped to zero, and the left PT increased to 136. Left brachial artery pressure after exercise was 146. The right ankle pressure increased gradually, and at the end of 8 minutes, it had returned to the resting value of 96. The postexercise waveform on the right side is markedly abnormal with lower peak frequency and less pulsatility than the preexercise tracing. On the left side the postexercise waveform has lost the normal reverse-flow phase, suggesting a minor degree of stenosis in the left aortoiliac system.

This evaluation is consistent with symptomatic right aortoiliac stenosis. Both the resting measurements and the response to exercise suggest a single level of arterial occlusive disease. The results also suggest minimal aortoiliac disease on the left side, although this is not clinically apparent at the patient's present level of activity. Arteriography demonstrated an 80-percent stenosis of the right common iliac artery and irregularity of the left common iliac with areas of aneurysmal change. The distal runoff was satisfactory. The patient underwent placement of Dacron bifurcation aortoiliac graft.

Case 14-2

A 61-year-old man had been having right calf and thigh pain brought on by walking and relieved by a brief period of rest. This had progressed over several years until his walking was limited to less than one block at a time. The noninvasive evaluation is shown in Figures 14-11A and B.

DISCUSSION   The ankle pressure index and segmental gradients in the left leg are normal. On the right side, the ankle pressure index is markedly decreased. The right HT pressure is decreased (thigh pressure index 90/115 = 0.78), and there is a significant segmental gradient between the HT and AK levels. Resting CFA waveforms are normal on the left side and abnormal on the right side.

After just 1 minute and 5 seconds of treadmill exercise, the patient stopped with right calf and thigh pain. The postexercise right brachial pressure was 120, and the left PT pressure was 140. On the right side, the PT pressure dropped to zero where it remained until 6 minutes when it was recorded as 10. The final measurement at 10 minutes was 12.

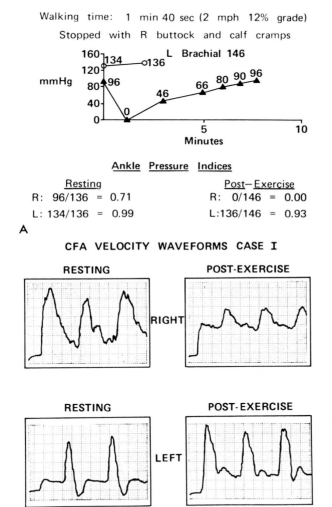

CASE I
Segmental Pressures (mmHg)

	BRACHIAL	DP	PT	BK	AK	HT
R ▲	128	88	96	96	106	110
L ○	136	132	134	142	154	158

Treadmill Exercise Test

Walking time: 1 min 40 sec (2 mph 12% grade)

Stopped with R buttock and calf cramps

L Brachial 146

mmHg

Minutes

Ankle Pressure Indices

Resting
R: 96/136 = 0.71
L: 134/136 = 0.99

Post–Exercise
R: 0/146 = 0.00
L: 136/146 = 0.93

A

CFA VELOCITY WAVEFORMS CASE I

RESTING   POST-EXERCISE

RIGHT

RESTING   POST-EXERCISE

LEFT

B

Figure 14-10A and B. Results of noninvasive evaluation for Case 14-1. (CFA) common femoral artery

CASE II
Segmental Pressures (mmHg)

	BRACHIAL	DP	PT	BK	AK	HT
R ▲	115	35	48	50	62	90
L ○	115	115	122	130	134	145

Treadmill Exercise Test

Walking time: 1 min 5 sec (2 mph 12% grade)

Stopped with R calf and thigh pain

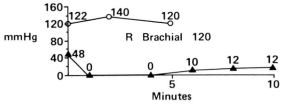

R Brachial 120

Ankle Pressure Indices

Resting	Post-Exercise
R: 48/115 = 0.42	R: 0/120 = 0.00
L: 122/115 = 1.06	L: 140/120 = 1.17

A

CFA VELOCITY WAVEFORMS CASE II

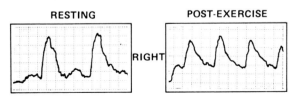

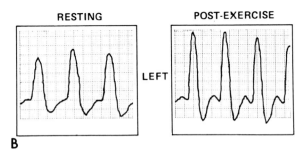

B

Figure 14-11A and B. Results of noninvasive evaluation for Case 14-2.

The right postexercise waveform shows an increased degree of abnormality, while the left side retains its normal, multiphasic pattern.

In this patient, the resting pressure measurements indicate multiple-level arterial occlusive disease affecting the right aortoiliac and femoropopliteal segments. The right-ankle pressure response to exercise is also consistent with multiple levels of occlusion. The CFA waveforms suggest right aortoiliac disease. Arteriography showed a 60-percent stenosis of the right external iliac artery and right superficial femoral artery occlusion. The profunda femoris artery was widely patent. There were no significant lesions involving the arteries to the left leg.

Case 14-3

A 68-year-old man complained of right calf pain after walking approximately one block, which had not improved on an exercise program. A noninvasive evaluation was performed (see Fig. 14-9).

DISCUSSION   The resting ankle pressure index and all segmental gradients in the left leg are normal. On the right side, the ankle pressure index is decreased, and there are significant gradients at the HT to AK and AK to BK levels. The thigh pressure indexes are normal, as are the CFA waveforms (not shown).

The patient became symptomatic after 2 minutes of treadmill exercise but was able to continue walking for an additional 45 seconds. The left PT pressure increased to 240 after exercise, with a right brachial pressure of 225. The right PT pressure fell to 36 and then increased slowly, reaching the resting value at 9 minutes. Postexercise waveforms remained normal.

This evaluation indicates arterial occlusive disease involving the right femoropopliteal segment. There is no evidence of significant aortoiliac disease. Arteriography showed occlusion of the right superficial femoral artery with moderate narrowing of the popliteal artery. The patient underwent a common femoral-to-distal popliteal bypass graft using autogenous saphenous vein. After surgery, the right ankle pressure index was 0.93, and all segmental gradients were within normal limits.

R. Eugene Zierler, M.D.
Assistant Professor of Surgery
University of Washington
School of Medicine, and
Chief, Vascular Surgery Section
Seattle Veterans Administration Medical Center
1660 South Columbian Way
Seattle, Washington 98108

D. Eugene Strandness, Jr., M.D.
Professor of Surgery
University of Washington
School of Medicine
RF 25
Seattle, Washington 98195

REFERENCES

1. Marinelli MR, Beach KW, Glass MJ, et al.: Noninvasive testing vs. clinical evaluation of arterial disease. JAMA 241:2031–2034, 1979

2. Beales JSM, Adcock FA, Frawley, JE, et al.: The radiological assessment of disease at the profunda femoris artery. Br J Radiol 44:854–857, 1971

3. Crummy AB, Rankin RS, Turnipseed WD, et al.: Biplane arteriography in ischemia of the lower extremity. Radiology 126:111–115, 1978

4. Sethi GR, Scott SM, Takaro T: Multiple-plane agiography for more precise evaluation of aortoiliac disease. Surgery 78:154–159, 1975

5. Thomas M, Andrews MR: Value of oblique projections in translumbar aortography. Am J Roentgenol 116:187–193, 1973

6. Castenada-Zuniga W, Knight L, Formanek A, et al.: Hemodynamic assessment of obstructive aortoiliac disease. Am J Roentgenol 127:559–561, 1976

7. Karayannacus PE, Talukder N, Nerem RM, et al.: The role of multiple noncritical arterial stenoses in the pathogenesis of ischemia. J Thorac Cardiovasc Surg 73:458–469, 1977

8. Kempczinski RF, Rutheford RB: Current status of the vascular diagnostic laboratory. Advances in Surgery 12:1–52, 1978

9. Nippa JH, Hokanson DE, Lee DR, et al.: Phase rotation for separating forward and reverse blood velocity signals. IEEE Trans Sonics Ultrasonics 22:340–346, 1975

10. Blackshear WM: Surgical indications for lower extremity arterial occlusive disease. Part I. Curr Probs Cardiology 6:22–32, 1981

11. Baker DW: Pulsed ultrasonic Doppler blood flow sensing. IEEE Trans Sonics Ultrasonics 17:170–185, 1970

12. Mozersky DJ, Hokanson DE, Sumner DS, et al.: Ultrasonic visualization of the arterial lumen. Surgery 72:253–259, 1972

13. Fell G, Phillips DJ, Chikos PM, et al.: Ultrasonic Duplex scanning for disease of the carotid artery. Circulation 64:1191–1195, 1981

14. Zierler RC, Bodily KC, Blackshear WM, et al.: Current status of ultrasonic Duplex scanning of the carotid bifurcation, in Diethrich EG (ed): Noninvasive Cardiovascular Diagnosis (ed 2). Littleton, MA, PSG Publishing, 1981, pp 33–51

15. Blackshear WM, Phillips DJ, Strandness DE: Pulsed Doppler assessment of normal human femoral artery velocity patterns. J Surg Res 27:73–83, 1979

16. Jager KA, Langlois Y, Roederer GO, et al.: Noninvasive assessment of lower extremity ischemia, in Bergan JJ, Yao JST (eds): Evaluation and Treatment of Upper and Lower Extremity Circulatory Disorders. Orlando, Fl, Grune & Stratton, 1984, pp 97–121

17. Berstein EF, Dilley RB, Goldberger LE, et al.: Growth rates of small abdominal aortic aneurysms. Surgery 80:765–773, 1976

18. Leopold GR, Goldberger LE, Bernstein EF: Ultrasonic detection and evaluation of abdominal aortic aneurysms. Surgery 72:939–945, 1972

19. Marcus R, Edell SL: Sonographic evaluation of iliac artery aneurysms. Am J Surg 140:666–670, 1980

20. Johnston KW, Marozzo BC, Cobbold RSC: Errors and artifacts of Doppler flowmeters and their solution. Arch Surg 112:1335–1342, 1977

21. Strandness DE, Sumner DS: Hemodynamics for Surgeons. New York, Grune & Stratton, 1975, p 29

22. Knox RA, Strandness DE: Ultrasound techniques for evaluation of lower extremity arterial occlusion. Semin Ultrasound 2:264–275, 1981

23. Strandness DE, Sumner DS: Hemodynamics for Surgeons. New York, Grune & Stratton, 1975, p 21

24. Carter SA: Clinical measurements of systolic pressures in limbs with arterial occlusive disease. JAMA 207:1869–1874, 1969

25. May AG, Van de Berg L, De Weese JA, et al.: Critical arterial stenosis. Surgery 54:250–259, 1963

26. Strandness DE, Sumner DS: Hemodynamics for Surgeons. New York, Grune & Stratton, 1975, p 233

27. Strandness DE, Bell JW: Peripheral vascular disease: Diagnosis and objective evaluation using a mercury strain-gauge. Ann Surg (Suppl) 161:1–35, 1965

28. Yao JST, Hobbs JT, Irvine WT: Ankle systolic pressure measurements in arterial diseases affecting the lower extremities. Br J Surg 56:676–679, 1969

29. Sumner DS, Strandness DE: The relationship between calf blood flow and ankle blood pressure in patients with intermittent claudication. Surgery 65:763–771, 1969

30. Yao JST: Hemodynamic studies in peripheral arterial disease. Br J Surg 57:761–766, 1970

31. Pascarelli EF, Bertrand CA: Comparison of blood pressures in the arms and legs. N Engl J Med 270:693–698, 1964

32. Cutajar CL, Marston A, Newcombe JF: Value of cuff occlusion pressures in assessment of peripheral vascular disease. Br J Med 2:392–395, 1973

33. Carter SA, Lezack JD: Digital systolic pres-

sures in the lower limbs in arterial disease. Circulation 43:905–914, 1971

34. Kempczinski RF: Role of the vascular diagnostic laboratory in the evaluation of male impotence. Am J Surg 138:278–282, 1979

35. Lane RJ, Appleberg M, Williams W: A comparison of two techniques for the detection of the vasculogenic component of impotence. Surg Gynecol Obstet 155:230–234, 1982

36. Fronek A, Johanson K, Dilley RB, et al.: Ultrasonically monitored postocclusive reactive hyperemia in the diagnosis of peripheral arterial occlusive disease. Circulation 48:149–152, 1973

37. Hummell BW, Hummel BA, Mowbry A, et al.: Reactive hyperemia vs treadmill exercise testing in arterial disease. Arch Surg 113:95–98, 1978

38. Keagy BA, Pharr WF, Thomas D, et al.: Comparison of reactive hyperemia and treadmill tests in the evaluation of peripheral vascular disease. Am J Surg 142:158–161, 1981

39. Strandness DE, Schultz RD, Sumner DS, et al.: Ultrasonic flow detection: A useful technique in the evaluation of peripheral vascular disease. Am J Surg 113:311–320, 1967

40. Johnston KW, Taraschuk I: Validation of the role of pulsatility index in quantitation of the severity of peripheral arterial occlusive disease. Am J Surg 131:295–297, 1976

41. Gosling RG, Dunbar G, King DH, et al.: The quantitative analysis of occlusive peripheral arterial disease by a noninvasive ultrasonic technique. Angiology 22:52–55, 1971

42. Thiele BL, Bandyk DF, Zierler RE, et al.: A systematic approach to the assessment of aortoiliac disease. Arch Surg 118:477–481, 1983

43. Baird RN, Bird DR, Clifford PC, et al.: Upstream stenosis—its diagnosis by Doppler signals from the femoral artery. Arch Surg 115:1316–1322, 1980

44. Campbell WB, Baird RN, Cole SEA, et al.: Physiological interpretation of Doppler shift waveforms—the femorodistal segment in combined disease. Ult Med Bio 9:265–269, 1983

45. Strandness DE, Bell JW: Ankle pressure

responses after reconstructive arterial surgery. Surgery 59:514–516, 1966

46. Corson JD, Johnson WC, LoGerfo RS, et al.: Doppler ankle systolic blood pressure: Prognositic value in vein bypass grafts of the lower extremity. Arch Surg 113:932–935, 1976

47. Blackshear WM, Thiele BL, Strandness DE: Natural history of above- and below-knee femoropopliteal grafts. Am J Surg 140:234–241, 1980

48. Strandness DE: Abnormal exercise responses after successful reconstructive arterial surgery. Surgery 59:325–333, 1966

49. Insua JA, Young JR, Humphries AW: Popliteal artery entrapment syndrome. Arch Surg 101:771–775, 1970

50. Rich NM, Collins GJ, McDonald PT, et al.: Popliteal vascular entrapment: Its increasing interest. Arch Surg 114:1377–1384, 1979

51. Raines JK, Darling RC, Both K, et al.: Vascular laboratory criteria for the management of peripheral vascular disease of the lower extremities. Surgery 79:21–29, 1976

52. Barnes RW, Shanik GD, Slaymaker EE: An index of healing in below-knee amputation: Leg blood pressure by Doppler ultrasound. Surgery 79:13–20, 1976

53. Bone GE, Hayes AC, Slaymaker EE, et al.: Value of segmental limb blood pressures in predicting results of aortofemoral bypass. Am J Surg 132:733–738, 1976

54. Bernstein EF, Stuart SH, Fronek A: The predictive value of noninvasive testing in peripheral vascular disease, in Bernstein EF (ed): Noninvasive Diagnostic Techniques in Vascular Disease. St. Louis, MO, The C.V. Mosby Co., 1982, pp 396–403

55. Dean RH, Yao JST, Stanton PE, et al.: Prognostic indicators in femoropopliteal reconstruction. Arch Surg 110:1287–1293, 1975

56. Yao JST, Bergan JJ: Predictability of vascular reactivity relative to sympathetic ablation. Arch Surg 107:676–680, 1973

57. Baker JD, Dix D: Variability of Doppler ankle pressures with arterial occlusive disease: An evaluation of ankle index and brachial-ankle pressure gradient. Surgery 89:134–137, 1981

58. Winsor T: Influence of arterial disease on the systolic blood pressure gradients of the extremity. Am J Med Sci 220:117–126, 1950

Robert W. Barnes, M.D.

15

Doppler Techniques for Evaluation of Lower-Extremity Venous Disease

The clinical symptoms and signs of leg-vein thrombosis require the clinician to establish a diagnosis objectively, but the fallibility of the clinical diagnosis[1] precludes complete treatment of the patient based solely on clinical findings. Contrast phlebography is the "gold standard" for the diagnosis of venous thrombosis of the lower extremity. However, the time, expense, discomfort, and slight risk of inducing venous thrombosis or allergic reaction prevents the routine use of this invasive procedure for screening and followup studies of patients with lower-extremity venous disease. Several noninvasive diagnostic techniques have been developed in the past 15 years to evaluate patients for both acute and chronic venous disease. Of the various noninvasive methods, Doppler ultrasound in experienced hands provides the most versatile, accurate, and inexpensive technique for evaluating the superficial, communicating, and deep veins of the lower extremity.[2] In addition, veins of the upper extremity as well as the major veins of the abdomen and thorax may be examined by this technique. The objective of this chapter is to review the instrumentation, pertinent anatomy, diagnostic method, interpretation, and applications of Doppler ultrasound in venous thromboembolic disease.

Instrumentation

The most useful diagnostic instrument for evaluating the venous system is a portable, continuous-wave, nondirectional Doppler ultrasonic velocity detector operating at a nominal frequency of 5 MHz.* For examination of the superficial (saphenous) veins of the lower extremity, the use of the pencil probe of a directional Doppler detector operating at a transmission frequency of 8–10 MHz is preferable. The examination may be conveniently carried out by an experienced

This work was supported in part by NIH grant #5 ROL HL 22852-03.
* e.g., MedaSonics ultrasonic stethoscope. Model BF 4A. Mountain View, CA.

vascular technologist using the audible output of the Doppler instrument. The audio output may be presented by means of a stethoscope earpiece, a loud-speaker, or a recordable analog waveform. Although the latter technique provides hard-copy output, the recording of Doppler signals does not provide any greater accuracy than that obtained by auditory interpretation of the Doppler velocity signals.

RELEVANT ANATOMY

The venous system may be conveniently divided into deep, communicating (perforating), and superficial veins (Fig. 15-1). In the lower extremity, the deep veins accessible to Doppler venous examination include the posterior tibial vein behind the medial malleolus, the popliteal vein, the superficial femoral vein in the mid-thigh, and the common femoral vein at the groin. The communicating veins, which are most prominent in the medial aspect of the lower leg, connect the posterior arch branch of the greater saphenous vein with the deep (posterior tibial) vein of the calf. The superficial veins in the lower extremity include the greater

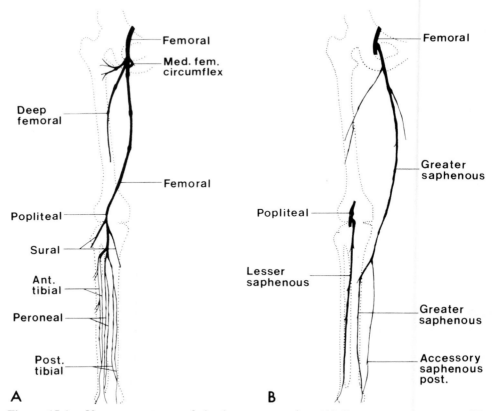

Figure 15-1. Venous anatomy of the lower extremity. (A) Deep venous system. (B) Superficial venous system.

saphenous, which runs from the anterior border of the medial malleolus, up the medial aspect of the lower leg and thigh to the saphenofemoral junction near the groin crease.

DIAGNOSTIC TECHNIQUE

The patient is examined in the supine position with the head of the bed elevated 20–30° to permit pooling of blood in the lower extremity. Footwear and stockings should be removed. The patient should be informed about the purpose and method of the procedure and should be encouraged to relax so that muscle tension does not inhibit the examination. The leg should be slightly flexed at the knee and hip, with the hip externally rotated. The examination is initiated by placing acoustic gel over the posterior tibial vein just posterior to the medial malleolus. The Doppler instrument is then gently positioned over the site of the posterior tibial vein and the venous signal located adjacent to the pulsatile posterior tibial artery signal (Fig. 15-2). If the signal cannot be elicited because of peripheral vasoconstriction, the foot is compressed to augment venous flow in the posterior tibial vein. Next, the calf is compressed to establish the competence of the posterior tibial venous valves. Finally, the calf is released to determine the presence of augmentation of flow from the posterior tibial vein into the deep calf veins.

The Doppler probe is then positioned over the saphenous vein just anterior to the medial malleolus (Fig. 15-3). Care should be taken not to exert any pressure on the skin with the Doppler probe. The spontaneous signal is elicited, and, if necessary, the foot is compressed to augment venous flow in the saphenous vein. Next, the saphenous vein is compressed in the calf to establish the competence of the superficial venous valves.

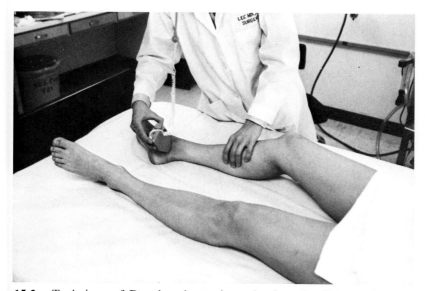

Figure 15-2. Technique of Doppler ultrasonic evaluation of calf (posterior tibial) vein during calf compression.

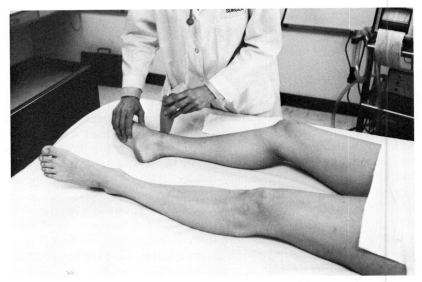

Figure 15-3. Technique of Doppler examination of superficial (greater) saphenous vein.

The Doppler probe is then positioned over the common femoral vein in the groin (Fig. 15-4). The exact location of the femoral vein is determined by detecting the velocity signal in the common femoral artery at the site of the palpable femoralartery pulse. By angling the Doppler probe slightly medially, the femoral venous velocity signal should be heard. After spontaneous femoral vein signals have been observed the calf and thigh are compressed to augment flow in the

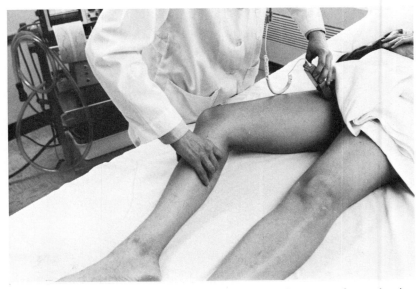

Figure 15-4. Technique of Doppler examination of common femoral vein.

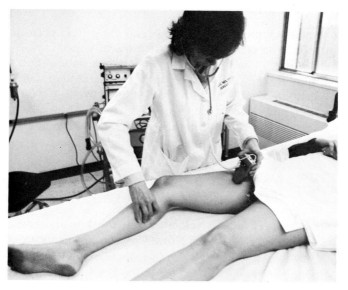

Figure 15-5. Technique of Doppler evaluation of superficial femoral vein during calf compression.

common femoral vein. Finally, a Valsalva maneuver or passive compression of the abdomen may be carried out to establish the competence of the femoral venous valves.

Next, the Doppler probe is moved over the superficial femoral vein on the anteromedial aspect of the proximal third of the thigh (Fig. 15-5). The venous signal is usually heard along with the superficial femoral artery signal, inasmuch

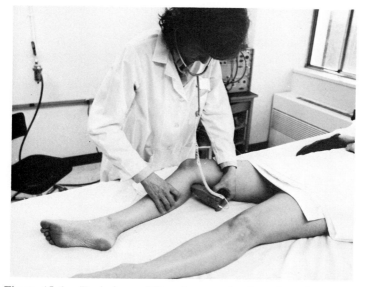

Figure 15-6. Technique of Doppler examination of popliteal vein.

as the two vessels are superimposed at this location in the thigh. The calf is compressed to augment femoral venous flow, and the patient performs a Valsalva maneuver to establish the competence of the femoral vein.

The popliteal vein can be evaluated by having the patient flex the knee and externally rotate the hip (Fig. 15-6). Alternatively, the patient can be positioned prone with the feet on a pillow. With the Doppler probe positioned over the popliteal fossa, the popliteal venous signal is usually heard adjacent to the popliteal artery signal. The calf is compressed to augment venous flow, and the thigh is compressed to establish competence of the popliteal venous valves.

INTERPRETATION

The Doppler ultrasonic venous velocity signal must be distinguished from the arterial velocity waveform (Fig. 15-7). Normally arterial signals are pulsatile with each heartbeat. Venous flow signals have five qualities that should be elicited at each location of Doppler examination (Fig. 15-8). The first quality is *spontaneity;* that is, the venous flow signal normally is heard spontaneously at its expected location. An exception to this is the posterior tibial signal, which may not be heard spontaneously if venous flow is reduced because of cool, vasoconstricted feet. In such instances, flow velocity may be accelerated by compression of the foot to elicit an audible Doppler venous signal. Absence of a spontaneous venous flow signal in major deep veins suggests venous obstruction due either to thrombosis or to extrinsic compression.

The second quality of normal venous flow is *phasicity,* which refers to the cyclic increase and decrease in flow velocity which varies with respiration. In the lower extremity, venous flow decreases or ceases during inspiration as a result of increased intra-abdominal pressure during descent of the diaphragm. Venous flow

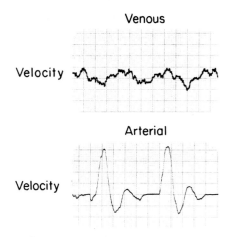

Figure 15-7. Comparison of phasic velocity alterations in the venous system and arterial pulsations.

DOPPLER VENOUS VELOCITY SIGNALS

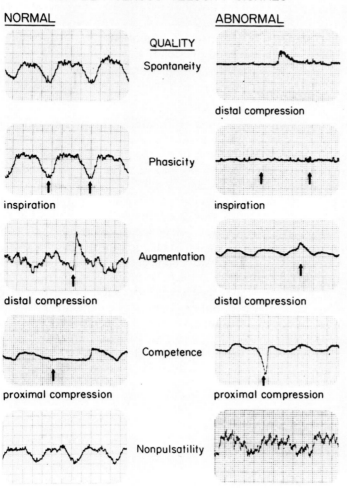

Figure 15-8. Normal and abnormal findings in lower-extremity veins.

increases during expiration. A more *continuous* venous flow signal, without respiratory variation, suggests proximal venous obstruction.

The third characteristic of the normal venous signal is *augmentation* in pitch and amplitude in response to distal limb compression or release of proximal limb compression. Such maneuvers should accelerate venous flow velocity if the intervening venous system is patent. Thrombosis or extrinsic venous compression may result in attenuation or absence of flow augmentation during limb-compression maneuvers.

The fourth characteristic of the venous Doppler signal reflects *competence* of the venous valves, manifested by obliteration of flow during proximal limb compression or a valsalva maneuver. Venous flow during such maneuvers suggests *incompetence* of venous valves due to prior (post-thrombotic) venous thrombosis or varicose veins.

The fifth quality of the normal venous-flow signal is its *nonpulsatility*. This term refers to the fact that venous flow is normally cyclic with respiration but not with each heartbeat. *Pulsatile* venous flow signals with each cardiac contraction suggest systemic venous hypertension, as may occur with congestive heart failure, tricuspid insufficiency, fluid overload, and so on.

DIAGNOSTIC ACCURACY

In experienced hands, the Doppler ultrasonic velocity detector is one of the most sensitive and versatile methods to evaluate the deep, communicating, and superficial veins. Several reports have suggested that the sensitivity of the venous Doppler examination may exceed 95 percent in detecting major calf vein thrombosis and deep vein thrombosis at or above the level of the knee.[3-6] Partial venous thrombosis or small clots behind venous valves might not be detected by this technique, however. Venous Doppler examination is somewhat nonspecific, inasmuch as any condition that may extrinsically compress the venous system may result in a false-positive diagnosis. Such conditions as subfascial hematoma, ruptured Baker's cyst, or extrinsic compression of the venous system by malignancy or other masses may result in false-positive diagnoses. In situations of trauma, arthritis, malignancy, or other conditions that may extrinsically compress the venous system, a contrast phlebogram is recommended to establish the diagnosis. Duplex ultrasound examination may enhance the accuracy of diagnosis of partial venous thrombosis and conditions resulting in extrinsic venous compression. Further study of this technique is needed, however. B-mode and duplex ultrasound methods for venous diagnosis are described in Chapter 16.

CLINICAL APPLICATIONS

Acute Deep Vein Thrombosis

The Doppler venous examination is our preferred technique to screen patients for acute deep vein thrombosis. The patient may be rapidly screened at the bedside. The method permits fairly accurate assessment of calf vein thrombosis[7,8] as well as major iliofemoral venous thrombosis. The technique may be performed in patients who are in traction or in plaster casts; however, modifications of the examination around the orthopedic appliances may be required for assessment of major venous thrombosis. Other techniques, such as plethysmography, may not be used in these conditions. Patients who have a normal venous Doppler examination may be considered to have some condition other than venous thrombosis, because the sensitivity of the Doppler examination in our hands exceeds 95 percent. In patients who have suffered trauma or have some other illness that may cause venous compression, contrast phlebography is neccesary to rule out false-positive results when the Doppler study is abnormal (Fig. 15-9). We treat patients for acute deep vein thrombosis based on an abnormal venous examination. If a patient has a normal venous Doppler examination, we pursue other studies to attempt to establish the cause of the leg complaints. In our experience, withholding anticoagulation in patients with

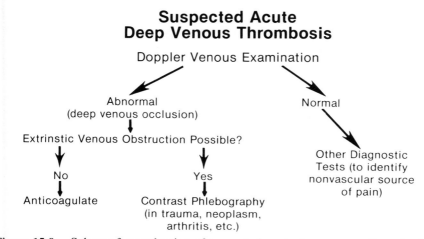

Figure 15-9. Schema for evaluation of suspected acute deep venous thrombosis.

normal venous Doppler examination has never resulted in a serious or fatal pulmonary embolus.

Recurrent Venous Thrombosis

A Doppler venous examination is useful to screen patients with complaints compatible with recurrent leg vein thrombosis (Fig. 15-10). Many patients suffer recurrent symptoms but have never been adequately studied to establish the diagnosis of venous disease. If the venous Doppler examination is normal, we assume that the patient has never had significant leg vein thrombosis. We do, however, obtain a contrast phlebogram following normal Doppler studies to establish the diagnosis once and for all. If a patient has an abnormal venous Doppler examination, this test does not prove that the recurrent symptoms are due to active recurrent venous thrombosis. Such patients should be evaluated by a test that is specific for activity of venous disease, such as the ^{125}I-fibrinogen uptake test. In our experience, 70 percent of patients with recurrent leg symptoms have a normal ^{125}I-fibrinogen test and thus do not have true recurrent venous thrombosis.[9] These patients are considered to have the postthrombotic syndrome and are treated with bed rest, leg elevation, and elastic support. Anticoagulants are not required in these patients, and no patient has suffered a recurrent pulmonary embolus in the face of a negative fibrinogen uptake test. Similarly, no patient with symptoms of recurrent venous thrombosis and a normal venous Doppler examination has been treated with prolonged anticoagulation, and no patient has developed a recurrent pulmonary embolus.

Postthrombotic Syndrome

Patients with postthrombotic venous insufficiency may be evaluated by Doppler ultrasound to establish the presence or absence of venous outflow obstruction and venous valvular incompetence.[10] In our experience, most patients

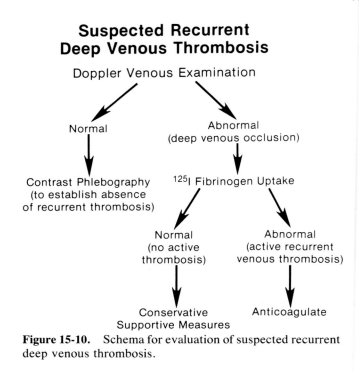

Figure 15-10.   Schema for evaluation of suspected recurrent
deep venous thrombosis.

do not have venous obstruction as a major pathophysiologic sequela of prior deep
vein thrombosis. Such patients will reveal venous reflux by Doppler examination
during proximal calf or thigh compression maneuvers. In addition, abnormal communicating venous incompetence may be established by Doppler ultrasound, as
reported by Folse and Alexander.[11] Most patients may be treated with bed rest,
leg elevation, and elastic support. Patients with active venous stasis ulcers may be
treated with medicated bandage (Unna boot) therapy and may be healed on an
ambulatory basis. Subsequently, these patients require an elastic support stocking
for life. These patients do not require chronic anticoagulation unless true recurrent active venous thrombosis is established by the ^{125}I-fibrinogen uptake test.

Varicose Veins

Patients with varicose veins must be evaluated for the presence or absence of
concomitant deep vein disease (secondary varicose veins).[12] The Doppler examination is useful to determine the presence or absence of associated deep vein
abnormality. If the deep veins are normal, the varicose veins are considered to be
primary (inherited). Patients with primary varicose veins usually have a more
favorable outcome, and the varicosities are only a cosmetic problem. Occasionally, recurrent superficial thrombophlebitis may develop in primary varicose veins
or the varicosities may rupture and bleed, but the complications of postthrombotic
syndrome and pulmonary embolus are rare in these patients. Conversely, patients
with secondary varicose veins due to underlying deep venous disease have a less
satisfactory course with more significant edema, venous stasis dermatitis or ul-

ceration, and possible recurrent pulmonary embolism. Such patients may demonstrate deep venous obstruction but more commonly reveal deep venous valvular incompetence by Doppler examination. These patients do not usually benefit from stripping of varicose veins. More appropriate therapy involves elastic support stockings or treatment of the venous stasis ulceration by medicated bandage.

Superficial Thrombophlebitis

Patients with inflammation along the course of the greater or lesser saphenous veins are usually considered to have superficial thrombophlebitis. In the presence of predisposing varicose veins, the diagnosis of superficial thrombophlebitis may be evident at the bedside. In the absence of obvious varicosities, however, superficial inflammation may be due to lymphangitis or cellulitis, since lymphatic vessels parallel the saphenous veins. To establish the diagnosis, Doppler ultrasound is very useful and much less painful than a contrast phlebogram[13] (Fig. 15-11). In the presence of superficial thrombophlebitis, the venous velocity signals will be obliterated at the site of inflammation, although there may be numerous prominent arterial signals associated with the inflammatory condition. In the presence of lymphangitis or cellulitis, venous flow velocity will be markedly increased in the saphenous vein, which drains the inflamed area. The Doppler examination is also useful to establish the patency of the deep venous system in the presence of superficial thrombophlebitis. If the deep veins are patent, and the superficial veins are thrombosed, anti-inflammatory therapy is indicated. If the deep veins are also thrombosed, anticoagulants are indicated. If the superficial veins are patent, lymphangitis or cellulitis should be treated by antibiotic therapy.

Pulmonary Embolism

Doppler ultrasound is useful to screen patients with suspected pulmonary embolus for a source of venous thrombosis in the lower extremities.[14] In our experience, 70 percent of patients with suspected pulmonary embolus have

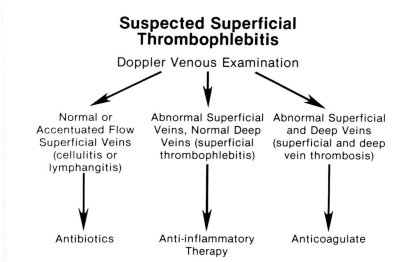

Figure 15-11.   Schema for evaluation of suspected superficial thrombophlebitis.

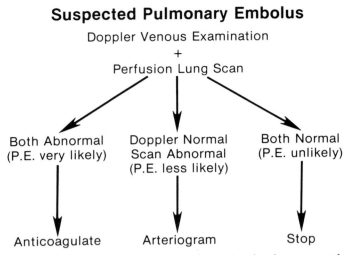

Suspected Pulmonary Embolus

Doppler Venous Examination
+
Perfusion Lung Scan

| Both Abnormal (P.E. very likely) | Doppler Normal Scan Abnormal (P.E. less likely) | Both Normal (P.E. unlikely) |

Anticoagulate   Arteriogram   Stop

Figure 15-12. Schema for evaluation of suspected pulmonary embolus.

normal deep veins. A pulmonary embolus is difficult to diagnose on a clinical basis. A perfusion lung scan is notoriously nonspecific. The use of a Doppler venous examination may increase the specificity of lung scans; that is, an abnormal perfusion lung scan and an abnormal venous Doppler examination should be considered strongly suggestive of pulmonary embolus (Fig. 15-12). If the perfusion lung scan is associated with a normal venous Doppler examination, however, the probability of a pulmonary embolus is markedly reduced. In the latter situation, we would consider a pulmonary arteriogram indicated unless the combined perfusion/ventilation lung scan demonstrates a high probability of pulmonary embolism.

TRAINING OPPORTUNITIES

New opportunities for training technologists have become available with the institution of teaching seminars and the establishment of a Society for Noninvasive Vascular Technology. Although physicians may become skilled in the use of Doppler ultrasound in venous disease, the performance of venous Doppler examinations by an experienced technologist is the most cost-effective method of carrying out this procedure. The Society for Noninvasive Vascular Technology conducts educational seminars and provides a useful forum for regular meetings of individuals experienced in this discipline. Although many vascular laboratories initially use a more objective technique, such as venous plethysmography, to evaluate patients for venous disease, with increasing experience such centers gradually appreciate the rapidity, versatility, and cost-effectiveness of venous Doppler examination. With proper attention to technical details, Doppler ultrasonic evaluation of the venous system can prove to be the most accurate and versatile method to evaluate patients for acute and chronic venous disease. The acquisition of skill in use of this technique may be accelerated by the use of a programmed audiovisual instructional series, including tape recordings of normal and abnormal venous flow velocity signals.[4]

SUMMARY

Doppler ultrasound is a very versatile technique to evaluate the venous system. Not only may the major deep veins of the lower extremities be examined, but the communicating and superficial veins may be separately interrograted, a situation which is not possible with other noninvasive techniques such as plethysmography of ^{125}I-fribrinogen uptake testing. In addition, the Doppler detector provides useful information about upper-extremity venous disease, and the technique may be used in patients who are in orthopedic traction or a plaster cast. In experienced hands, the Doppler examination may be rapidly performed on a portable basis in about 5–10 minutes.

The greatest limitation of the Doppler ultrasonic venous evaluation is the subjectivity of the test. Considerable experience is required before maximal accuracy is achieved by this technique. A vascular technologist must use the method on a daily basis for several months before becoming sufficiently familiar with the technique to permit a reliable diagnosis.

CASE STUDIES

Case 15-1

A 67-year-old man had swelling and pain in the right thigh and leg 6 days after resection of the colon for carcinoma. Physical examination revealed obvious swelling of the entire right lower extremity, which was slightly cyanotic. The superficial veins were prominent. The right groin, the medial thigh, and the calf were tender. Representation of the Doppler venous evaluation of both lower extremities is depicted in Figure 15-13. What is your diagnosis?

DISCUSSION   The venous flow signals in the left common femoral, superficial femoral and posterior tibial veins were normal. They revealed the normal qualities of spontaneity, phasicity, augmentation, and competence and were slightly pulsatile.

The venous flow signals in the right lower extremity were abnormal. At the location of the common femoral vein there was a spontaneous signal, which was continuous, i.e., not influenced by respiration. It probably represented a collateral vein in the groin. This flow signal did not augment with calf compression. No flow signal was elicited in the superficial femoral vein. The posterior tibial venous flow was not spontaneous, and there was decreased augmentation upon release of calf compression.

These findings are compatible with right iliofemoral venous thrombosis.

Case 15-2

A 28-year-old woman had left calf pain of 3 days' duration. The pain was not related to exercise. There was no history of trauma, and the patient was not taking oral contraceptives. Physical examination revealed mild edema of the left ankle and tenderness of the left calf. The representative tracings from the venous Doppler examination are shown in Figure 15-14. What is your conclusion in this case?

DISCUSSION   The venous flow signals in the right lower extremity were normal. Lack of spontaneous flow in the right greater saphenous vein was associated with cool extremities. In the left lower extremity, the common and superficial femoral venous flow signals were normal except for decreased augmentation in response to calf compression. The posterior tibial flow signal was continuous and was augmented by calf compression and

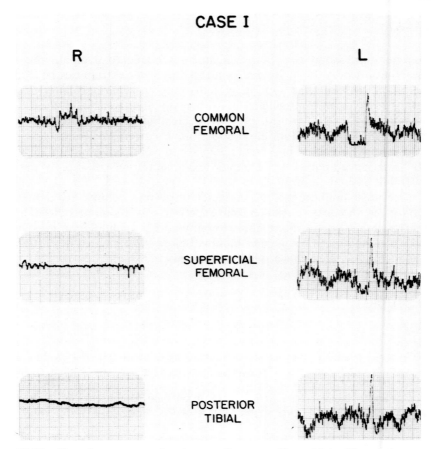

Figure 15-13. Doppler venous signal recordings on Case 15-1: The patient was a 67-year-old man.

interrupted by compression of the saphenous vein. Augmentation of posterior tibial flow in response to release of calf compression was demonstrated. The flow signal in the left greater saphenous vein was spontaneous and continuous.

These findings are compatible with calf vein thrombosis with collateral circulation through the saphenous vein.

Case 15-3

A 47-year-old man suffered from a chronic, nonhealing ulcer on the medial aspect of the left leg for 8 months. The ulcer developed after minor trauma. He also noted chronic swelling and hyperpigmentation of the left ankle for 5 years since an ankle fracture associated with a skiing accident. Examination revealed chronic venous stasis dermatitis with hyperpigmentation and scaling of the left ankle, particularly on the medial aspect. Proximal to the medial malleolus there was a 2-cm ulcer with a granulating base and a moderate amount of yellow exudate. The tracings from the venous Doppler examination are shown in Figure 15-15. Your impression?

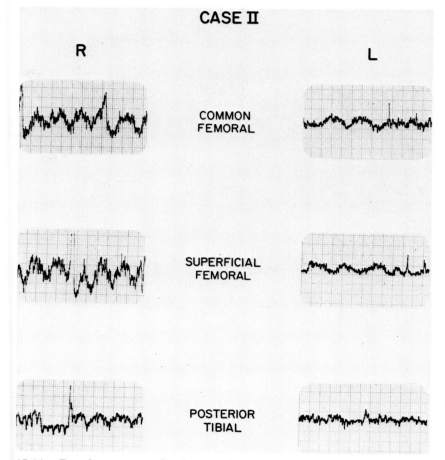

Figure 15-14. Doppler venous signal recordings on Case 15-2: The patient was a 28-year-old woman.

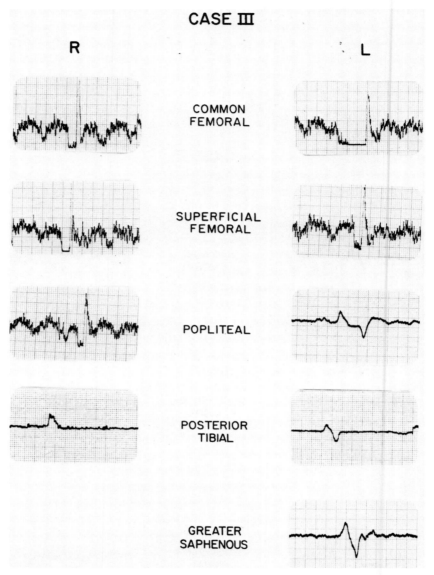

Figure 15-15. Doppler venous signal recordings on Case 15-3: The patient was a 47-year-old man.

DISCUSSION   The venous signals in the right lower extremity were normal. The left common and superficial femoral venous signals were normal. The left popliteal, posterior tibial, and saphenous venous signals demonstrated incompetent venous valves. There was reduced augmentation of the left posterior tibial venous flow in response to release of calf compression.

These findings are compatible with chronic venous insufficiency associated with old left calf vein thrombosis. The incompetence of the left saphenous vein is probably the result of secondary varicosity due to the underlying deep venous disease.

Professor and Chairman
Department of Surgery-520
University of Arkansas for Health Sciences
and McClellan Memorial VA Hospital
4301 West Markham
Little Rock, Arkansas 72205

REFERENCES

1. Barnes RW, Wu KK, Hoak JC: The fallibilty of the clinical diagnosis of venous thrombosis. JAMA 234:605–607, 1975
2. Barnes RW, Russell HE, Wilson MR: Doppler Ultrasound Evaluation of Venous Disease: A Programmed Audiovisual Instruction (ed 2). Iowa City, University of Iowa Press, 1975, p 200
3. Sigel B, Popky GL, Wagner DK, et al: Comparison of clinical and Doppler ultrasound evaluation of confirmed lower extremity venous disease. Surgery 64:332–338, 1968
4. Strandness DE Jr, Sumner DS: Ultrasonic velocity detector in the diagnosis of thrombophlebitis. Arch Surg 104:180–183, 1972
5. Sumner DS, Baker DW, Strandness DE Jr: The ultrasonic velocity detector in a clinical study of venous disease. Arch Surg 97:75–80, 1968
6. Yao JST, Courmos C, Hobbs JR: Detection of proximal vein thrombosis by the Doppler ultrasound flow detection method. Lancet 1:4, 1972
7. Barnes RW, Russell HE, Wu KK, et al.: Accuracy of Doppler ultrasound in clinically suspected venous thrombosis of the calf. Surg Gynecol Obstet 143:425–428, 1976
8. Sumner DS, Lambeth A: Reliability of Doppler ultrasound in the diagnosis of acute venous thrombosis both above and below the knee. Am J Surg 138:205–209, 1979
9. Barnes RW, Turley DG, Qureshi GD, et al.: Objective diagnosis of recurrent deep vein thrombosis. Thromb Haemostas 46:168, 1981
10. Barnes RW, Collicott PE, Sumner DS, et al.: Noninvasive quantitation of venous hemodynamics in the postphlebitic syndrome. Arch Surg 107:807–814, 1973
11. Folse R, Alexander RH: Directional flow detection for localizing venous valvular incompetency. Surgery 67:114–121, 1970
12. Barnes RW, Ross EA, Strandness DE Jr: Differentiation of primary from secondary varicose veins by Doppler ultrasound and strain gauge plethysmography. Surg Gynecol Obstet 141:207–211, 1975
13. Barnes RW, Wu KK, Hoak JC: Differentiation of superficial thrombophlebitis from lymphangitis by Doppler ultrasound. Surg Gynecol Obstet 143:23–25, 1976
14. Barnes RW, Kinkead LR, Wu KK, et al.: Venous thrombosis in suspected pulmonary embolism: Incidence detectable by Doppler ultrasound. Thromb Haemostas 36:150–156, 1976

Steven R. Talbot, R.V.T.

16

B-Mode Evaluation of Peripheral Arteries and Veins

Our experience at LDS Hospital with B-mode sonography of peripheral veins and arteries began in 1981 when we discovered, in the course of carotid examination, that the jugular vein was very well visualized. This observation led to highly successful attempts at imaging arm and leg veins. We quickly realized that B-mode imaging of extremity vessels uniquely complemented Doppler examination through (1) precise localization of thrombus, (2) identification of nonobstructive thrombus that could not be detected with Doppler methods or phleborheography, (3) characterization of thrombus (''spongy'', solid, attached, loose), (4) direct observation of clot dissolution in response to thrombolytic therapy, and (5) direct assessment of valve function and blood flow.

Our experience with venous and arterial imaging has led us to develop detailed examination protocols. The objective of this chapter is to instruct others in the examination technique that we have found to be of considerable benefit in the management of patients with extremity venous and arterial disease.

INSTRUMENTATION

Venous and arterial imaging in the extremities requires high-resolution, real-time ultrasound equipment, preferably with pulsed, range-gated Doppler. Since thrombus is, in most cases, poorly echogenic, the ultrasound instrument should be capable of resolving low-level echoes. It should also have excellent resolution for imaging small vessels and small thrombi. General-purpose ultrasound instruments are usualy not acceptable for peripheral vascular work. The scanner used in our laboratory is a commercially available real-time unit with 8 and 4 MHz scanheads. The 4-MHz scanhead is helpful in following deeper vessels and is a must with obese patients. The scanheads feature phased focusing that allows selection of focus in the near, mid, and far fields. This variable focus capability is helpful, since the depth of the vessels being imaged may vary. The instrument also is equipped with pulsed, range-gated Doppler.

INTRODUCTION TO VASCULAR ULTRASONOGRAPHY, SECOND EDITION

The instrumentation availability in a given laboratory may influence the clinician's ability to image some vessels. Most instruments operating at frequencies of 8–10 MHz are limited to a depth of only 4 cm. Deeper vessels, such as the distal femoral artery and vein and the popliteal vessels, may be out of the range of higher frequency probes. The availability of a lower frequency probe that allows greater scanning depth is desirable, even though these probes do not have resolving capabilities equivalent to the higher frequency transducers.

VENOUS IMAGING TECHNIQUES AND ANATOMY, LOWER EXTREMITY

Lower-extremity venous imaging is performed with the patient in the supine position. The entire bed is tilted 10–20° (head elevated) (Fig. 16-1). The patient should be well informed about the examination and encouraged to relax. We stress that there will be no injections or x-ray exposure during the examination. First, the continuous-wave Doppler examination is completed, as described in Chapter 15. The Doppler examination may also be performed using the pulsed Doppler of the duplex probe, if desired. The leg is next positioned for the B-mode study with the knee extended and the hip in slight external rotation. A large amount of gel is applied from the groin crease to the lower thigh, approximating the course of the superficial femoral vein. Imaging is begun as high in the groin as possible. Transverse scanning is performed first, rather than longitudinal imaging, to ensure proper identification of the thigh vessels. Immediately below the inguinal ligament only the common femoral artery and vein are seen (Fig. 16-2). The common femoral vein will usually be located behind and slightly lateral to the common femoral artery. If duplex equipment is available, the Doppler component may be used to differentiate between the artery and vein. When the artery and vein have been correctly identified, light probe pressure is applied over the vessels. The vein should collapse until the walls touch, which confirms that no thrombus is present at this point. The artery will not collapse unless much greater pressure is used. Even when the artery collapses partially, it will snap back quickly when pressure is decreased. The vein will stay closed as long as light probe pressure is maintained, and this finding is crucial for verifying that the vein is thrombus-free. Venous compression should be performed every inch or so as the examiner moves down the leg.

As the examination is slowly continued down the medial thigh, the common femoral artery starts its division, just below the groin crease, to form the superficial femoral artery and the profunda femoris artery. At about the same point, the saphenous vein joins the lateral border of the common femoral vein (the saphenofemoral junction) (Fig. 16-3). Inferior to this point, four distinct vessels will be visible, the superficial femoral artery and vein, the profunda femoris artery, and the saphenous vein (Fig. 16-4). As the examiner proceeds down the leg, the saphenous vein will quickly move toward the skin line while the profunda femoris artery dives deeply into the musculature and usually is lost from view. In some patients, the deep femoral vein may be seen adjacent to the profunda femoris artery. After the saphenous vein and profunda femoris artery have disappeared from the screen, only the superficial femoral artery and vein will be

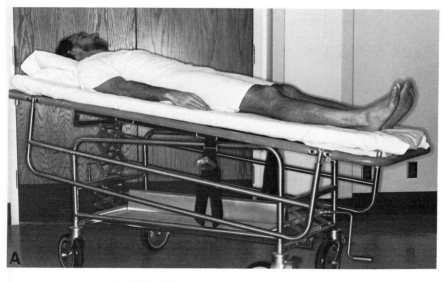

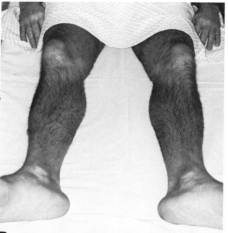

Figure 16-1. Patient position for lower-extremity venous examination. (A) The bed is tilted 10–20° to enhance venous filling. (B) The legs are positioned with knees slightly extended and hips in slight external rotation.

seen lying side by side. The artery is usually more superficial, with the vein behind, as seen in Figure 16-5. The examiner next follows these two vessels into the lower third of the thigh (Fig. 16-6), where they penetrate deeply into the adductor canal and are lost from view.

The patient is then rolled on to the side opposite that being examined, into the lateral decubitus position. The leg being examined should be placed in front of the other leg and should be rested comfortably on the bed, slightly flexed at the hip and knee. Venous imaging is continued in a transverse plane as high in the popliteal space as possible. The popliteal vein will usually be seen superficial to

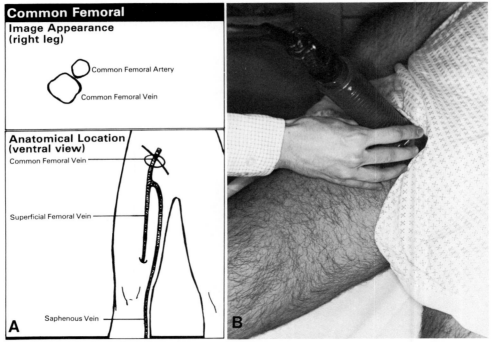

Figure 16-2. Common femoral level. Venous imaging in the lower extremity is begun at the inguinal ligament in the transverse plane. The common femoral vein and artery are seen at this level.

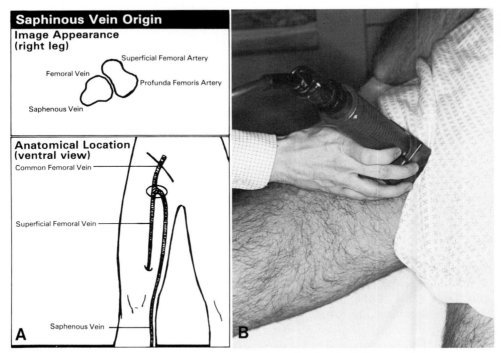

Figure 16-3. Saphenous vein origin. Just below the inguinal ligament, the common femoral artery divides to form the superficial femoral and profunda femorus arteries. At the same level, the greater saphenous vein joins the lateral border of the common femoral vein.

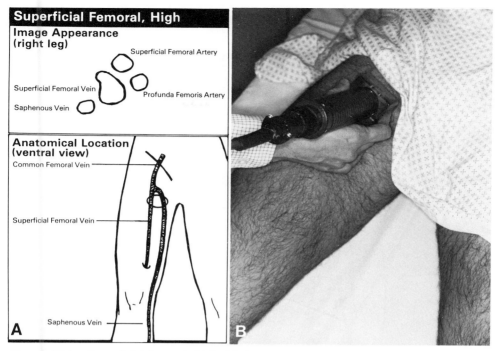

Figure 16-4. Superficial femoral, high. Slightly below the level shown in Figure 16-3, the saphenous vein moves medially toward the skin line, while the profunda femorus artery dives deeply into the musculature.

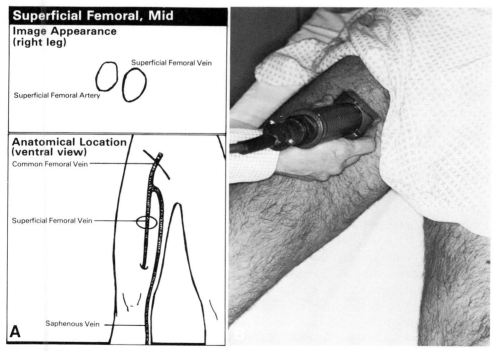

Figure 16-5. Superficial femoral, mid-thigh. At this level, only the superficial femoral artery and vein are seen.

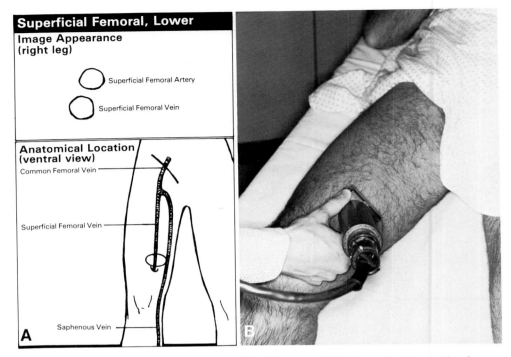

Figure 16-6. Superficial femoral, low thigh. The superficial femoral artery and vein are followed until they dive deeply into the musculature at the level of the adductor canal.

the artery (Fig. 16-7). As the examination is continued down to the mid-portion of the popliteal space, the popliteal vein will come to lie directly lateral to the popliteal artery but the vein will remain closer to the skin line than the artery (Fig. 16-8). As scanning is continued farther down toward the calf, several veins will branch off of the main popliteal trunk (Fig. 16-9). One of the branches, the lesser saphenous vein, may be followed, in some patients, from the popliteal vein down the posterolateral surface of the calf to the lateral malleolus. The posterior tibial vein also may be followed, in some cases, from its junction with the popliteal vein all the way down to the medial malleolus. Below the popliteal vein all deep veins are paired and follow the main arterial trunks (see Fig. 15-1, page 334). If the examiner loses track of the posterior tibial vein in the upper calf, the vein is easily found at the level of the medial malleolus (Fig. 16-10), from which point it may be followed back up toward the popliteal vein. Many parts of the deep calf veins may not be clearly imaged, but the examiner should always investigate as many veins as can be seen. After all the veins that can be followed in the calf have been studied, the patient is returned to the supine position and the saphenous vein is followed starting at the saphenofemoral junction (Fig. 16-11A) and ending just above the medial malleolus (Fig. 16-11B). A very light touch with the transducer head is required when the examiner is trying to locate superficial veins such as the saphenous vein. The probe should glide along the gel-coated surface of the skin with minimal pressure or the vein will be compressed and will not be visualized.

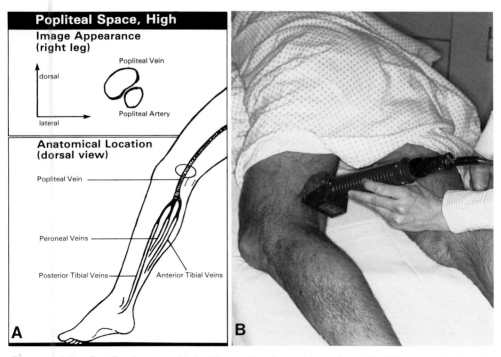

Figure 16-7. Popliteal space, high. The patient is on his or her side. The examination is continued high in the popliteal space, where the popliteal and vein are seen.

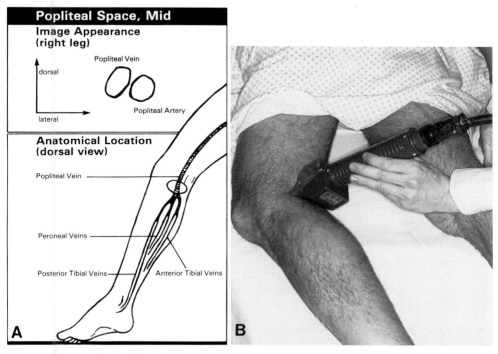

Figure 16-8. Mid-popliteal space. The popliteal vein lies superficial to the popliteal artery.

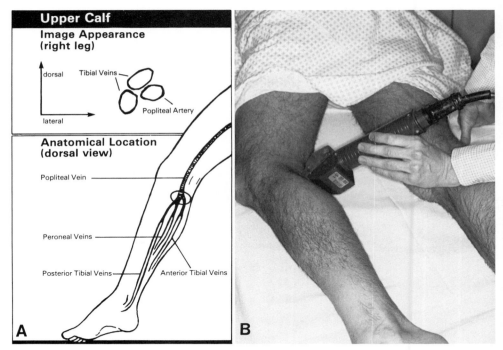

Figure 16-9. Upper calf level. In the upper calf, several venous bifurcations occur. All venous branches are scanned as far as possible into the calf.

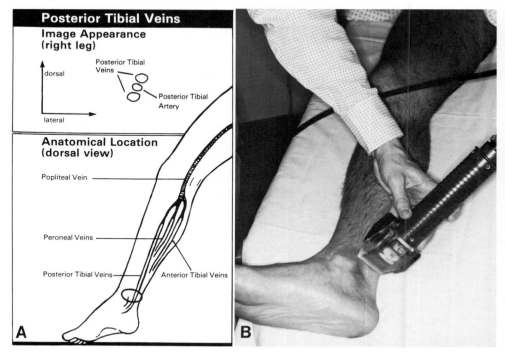

Figure 16-10. Posterior tibial venous examination. With the patient in the supine position, the posterior tibial veins can be located at the level of the medial malleolus. The posterior tibial veins are paired.

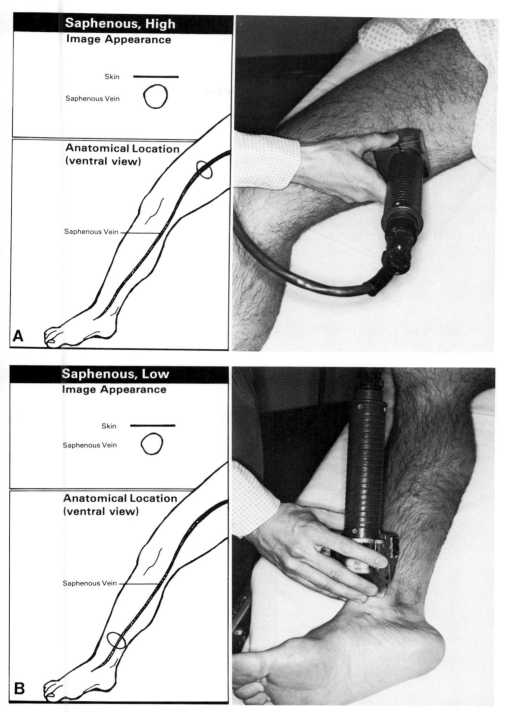

Figure 16-11. Greater saphenous examination. (A) With the patient supine, the greater saphenous vein is traced from the saphenofemoral junction to the level of the ankle. For saphenous vein examination, the transducer should be focused in the near field (if possible) and minimal probe pressure applied to avoid compressing the vein. (B) The greater saphenous vein may be followed down to the medial malleolus.

359

VENOUS EXAMINATION TECHNIQUES AND ANATOMY, UPPER EXTREMITY

Upper-extremity examination takes place with the patient in the supine position with the arm raised to permit access to the axilla. The transverse scan plane is usually prefered for upper-extremity examination because it simplifies the correct identification of vascular anatomy. Starting high in the axilla, the axillary artery and vein are first identified. The vein is superficial to the artery, as shown in Figure 16-12. As the examiner moves down the arm, the basilic vein will branch off medially. The major venous trunk visible below this point is called the brachial vein. In many individuals, the brachial vein will split into two separate trunks that follow the brachial artery down the medial aspect of the arm (Fig. 16-13). The brachial artery and vein(s) cross the elbow medially and can be followed into the forearm, where they divide into the radial and ulnar vessels (Fig. 16-14). The forearm veins are paired and are very small. With a good-quality instrument, the radial and ulnar veins may be followed all the way down to the wrist (Fig. 16-15 and Fig. 16-16). To examine the basilic vein, the examiner returns to its junction with the axillary vein and follows it in transverse section down the medial aspect of the arm. The basilic vein is located nearer to the skin than the brachial veins (Fig. 16-17) and may be followed past the elbow into the forearm. The cephalic vein is also superficially located and may be identified along the anterior border of the biceps muscle (Fig. 16-18). It joins with the basilic vein near the elbow,

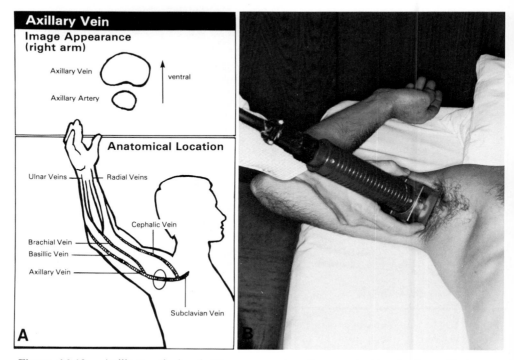

Figure 16-12. Axillary vein level. The upper-extremity examination begins with transverse views of the axilla that demonstrate the axillary artery and vein.

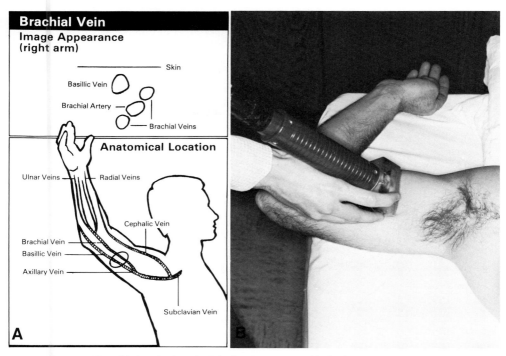

Figure 16-13. Brachial vein level. Within the upper third of the arm, the basilic vein branches off medially. The major venous trunk accompanying the brachial artery below this point is the brachial vein, which frequently is paired.

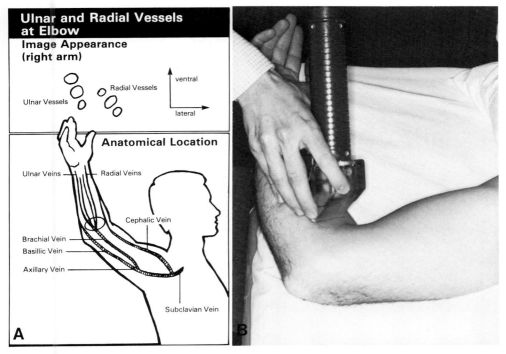

Figure 16-14. Ulnar and radial vessels. In the medial portion of the forearm, just below the elbow, the brachial artery and vein divide into the radial and ulnar arteries and veins.

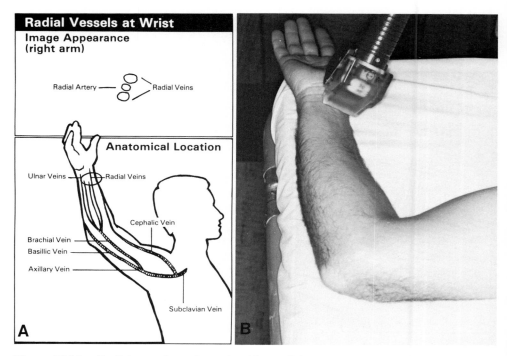

Figure 16-15. Radial vessels at the wrist. The radial artery and veins may be followed down the forearm to the wrist.

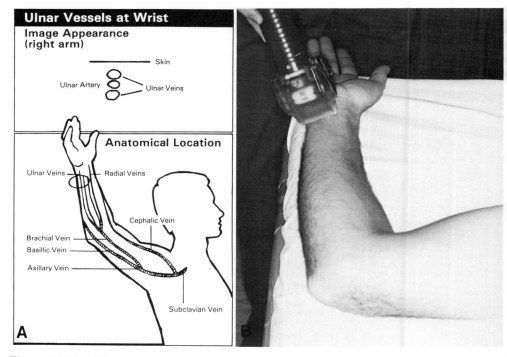

Figure 16-16. Ulnar vessels at the wrist. The ulnar artery and veins may be followed down the forearm to the wrist.

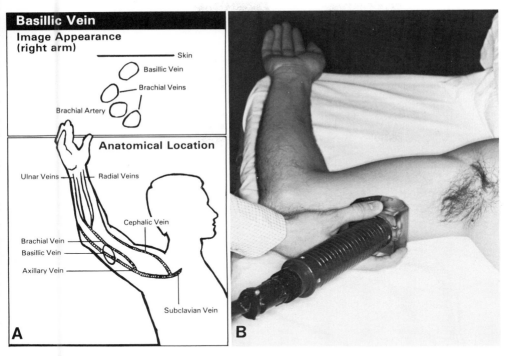

Figure 16-17. Basilic vein. The basilic vein is located on the posteromedial aspect of the arm. (See also Fig. 16-16.)

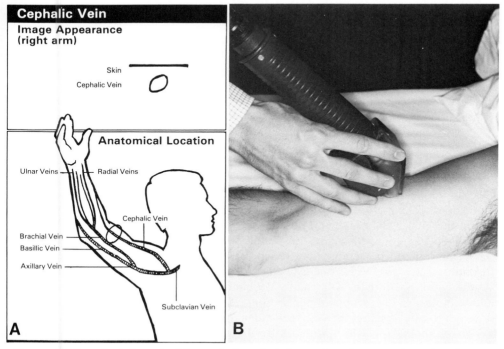

Figure 16-18. Cephalic vein. The cephalic vein is located on the anterolateral surface of the arm.

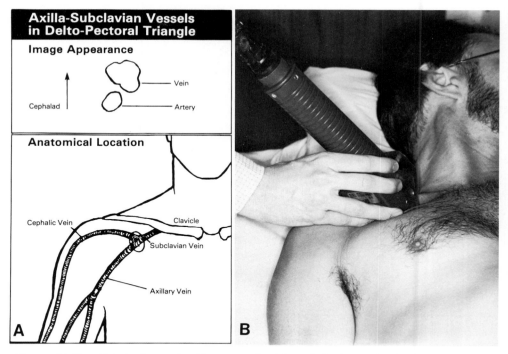

Figure 16-19. Subclavian and axillary vessels. The subclavian and axillary vessels may be imaged in the deltopectoral triangle.

the elbow, through the medial cubital vein, which crosses the anticubital fossa. The cephalic vein may also be followed into the forearm as well as up over the shoudler to its junction with the subclavian vein. A small section of the subclavian and axillary vein may also be imaged below the clavicle in the area of the deltopectoral triangle (Fig. 16-19). With a deeply focused scanhead of small dimensions, the subclavian vein may also be imaged in the supraclavicular fossa.

NORMAL AND ABNORMAL APPEARANCE OF VEINS

All venous imaging should first be conducted in a transverse plane, with the clinician checking closely to make sure the vein is compressable at every level. When the vein walls touch and no echogenic material is seen, the vein is free of thrombus (Fig. 16-20). If echogenic material is clearly seen within the lumen and the vein walls do not completely touch, or if the vein does not collapse at all, thrombus is present. Veins that are totally obstructed will have echogenic material visible within the lumen, will usually be dilated, will not respond to compression, and will not produce Doppler signals (Fig. 16-21). When thrombus is present but does not totally obstruct the vein, echogenic material will be seen in the lumen and venous compression will be limited by the contained thrombus (Fig. 16-22). In such cases flow may very well be detected in the vein even though thrombus is present. New, nonobstructive thrombus may be difficult to visualize because such

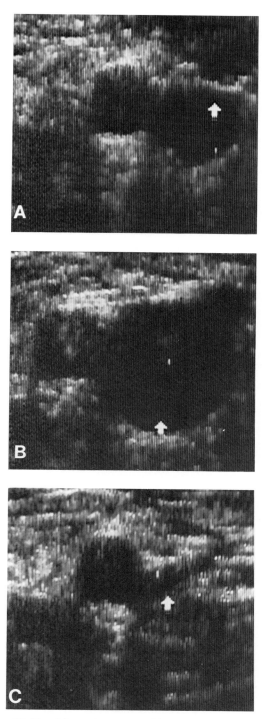

Figure 16-20. Normal sonographic appearance of an extremity vein. (A) A transverse view demonstrates the common femoral artery and vein (arrow within lumen) at the level of the inguinal ligament. (B) During the Valsalva maneuver, the common femoral vein dilates (arrow). (C) Light probe pressure causes the normal common femoral vein to collapse (arrow), indicating absence of intraluminal thrombus.

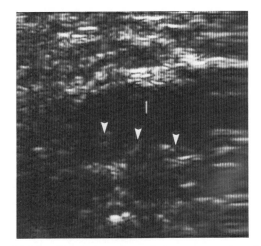

Figure 16-23. Fresh thrombus. A transverse view demonstrates a focal, low echogenicity thrombus (arrowheads) that
occupies a portion of the vein lumen. Artifacts (vertical line)
are present in the superficial portion of the lumen.

indication that the vein is not clear. On further inspection, a fine echo pattern will
be seen centrally in the lumen, but the periphery of the lumen will frequently be
clear (Fig. 16-23). These findings must hold up in both transverse and longitudinal
planes. The "texture" of fresh thrombus will usually be spongy, as demonstrated
by slight deformation of the thrombus when gentle pressure is applied. In many
cases acute thrombus can actually be seen floating freely from a small point of
attachment. The free-floating "tail" may be short or extremely long. The long tails
are quite dramatic, and visualization of a long, loosely attached thrombus tail will
impress even the most skeptical individual with the value of venous imaging.
Wherever a thrombus tail is seen freely moving within a vein, extra care should be
taken to prevent breaking the thrombus loose. When we image a loose thrombus
tail, we return the patient to his or her room on a stretcher and make sure the
physician and the nurse in charge are aware of our observation.

Other characteristics associated with fresh thrombus are smooth borders and
homogeneous echogenicity. Although the identification of fresh thrombus usually
means the patient is at greater risk of pulmonary embolism, the finding also
suggests greater possibility of resolution with thrombolytic therapy. Venous
imaging should be used to follow the response of a loose thrombus tail to therapy
until the thrombus dissolves or adheres to the vein wall.

Chronic Thrombosis

As a venous clot ages and becomes more organized, it also becomes more
rigid, as witnessed by sonographic findings that fresh thrombus evolves from
spongy to firm until it becomes difficult or impossible to compress the thrombus
with light or even moderate probe pressure. With older thrombus, the vein wall
will not oppose even when enough pressure is applied to cause an adjacent artery
to collapse. As thrombus ages, it also becomes more echogenic. In our experience, "the older the clot, the more echogenic its appearance", has been a fairly
reliable rule (Figs. 16-24 to 16-26), and very old thrombus may become highly

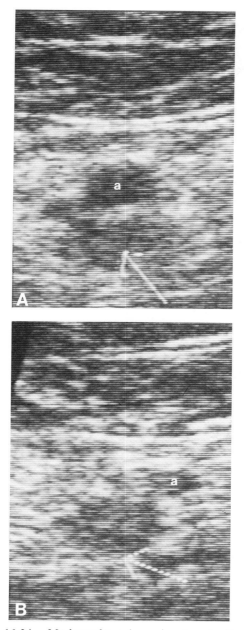

Figure 16-24. Moderately echogenic chronic thrombus. (A) A transverse section at the superficial femoral vein demonstrates complete opacification of the common femoral vein (arrows) with medium echogenicity, chronic thrombus (a, superficial femoral artery). (B) Compression with the transducer demonstrates the rigidity of the thrombosed femoral vein (arrow). Note that the superficial femoral artery (a) is flattened by the pressure, yet the shape of the vein changes little if at all.

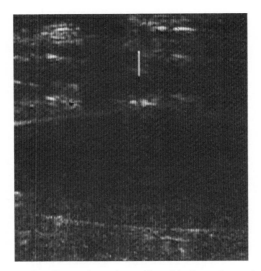

Figure 16-25. Strongly echogenic old thrombus. A partially calcified old venous thrombus is seen attached to the near wall of the superficial femoral vein. Note the acoustic shadow distal to the thrombus.

echogenic. One would expect markedly echogenic, chronic thrombus to be easily identified; however, as years go by, the thrombus becomes so echogenic that it begins to blend in with surrounding tissue and becomes difficult to spot. It is not unusual to image a patient with a history of deep venous thrombosis several years ago and find, at first glance, an artery but no visible structure where the vein should be. Then, with close inspection, the examiner may make out the echo-filled vein that blends so well with surrounding tissue that it is almost invisible. Those experienced with carotid imaging often encounter this appearance in chronically occluded carotid arteries. Not all chronic thrombi are totally obstructive; some thrombi do not totally obstruct the vessel in the first place and simply adhere to the vein wall. Other veins that have been totally obstructed at one time have recanalized. In either case, there is irregular, residual thrombus resembling arterial plaque along one or both surfaces of the vein wall (Fig. 16-26). The vein will compress until the thrombus prevents complete opposition of both surfaces of the vein wall, and pulsed Doppler examination may demonstrate flow in the residual lumen.

In some cases of chronic thrombosis we have encountered an intraluminal object that resembles a thrombus tail, except that it is very echogenic and does not "wave" in the flow stream (Fig. 16-26A). On transverse images this appearance is seen to result from nearly complete recanalization of the vein, with only a residual stringlike area of thrombus that is firmly attached to one wall surface (Fig. 16-26B).

A final observation that may be made in a chronic thrombosis is the presence of collateral veins. Collateral venous channels are usually seen in cases of very chronic thrombosis; however, collateral veins may also be seen in some cases just a few days after clot forms.

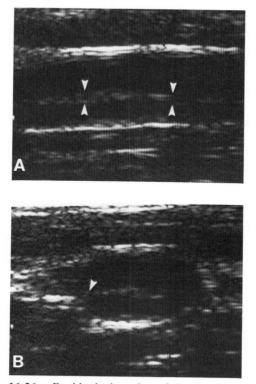

Figure 16-26. Residual thrombus following recannalization. (A) A rigid, string-like thrombus (arrowheads) is seen in a patient with chronic venous thrombosis. Recannalized thrombus such as this may have an appearance similar to a loose thrombus tail, except that this type of thrombus is attached to the wall and does not move freely within the lumen. (B) A transverse view demonstrates the point of attachment (arrowhead) of the thrombus remnant shown in A.

Superficial Thrombosis

Superficial veins are well visualized with B-mode ultrasound imaging. Although thrombosis of superficial veins is common, most of the medical literature plays down the importance of this condition. Hence, in many cases the physician may palpate a thrombus in a superficial vein and decide that no other diagnostic test is needed. Usually the clot is palpated in the saphenous vein, and if the "cord" is palpable in the calf but not above the knee, the patient most likely will be treated conservatively based on the assumption that the thrombus ends where the cord ends. On many occasions, when we have imaged the superficial vein in such cases, we have found older-looking, solid thrombus in the calf, but a loose, compressable thrombus tail that trails all the way into the saphenofemoral junction. The compressible portion of the thrombus, of course, cannot be detected by palpation. The thrombus tail is not attached to the vein wall and is not associated with inflammatory signs or symptoms. Because we have frequently identified extensive thrombosis in cases where clinical findings suggested only limited superficial vein thrombosis, we now recommend B-mode imaging of patients with superficial phlebitis to make sure the clot is attached to the vein wall and terminates well away from the deep system.

VALVE ABNORMALITIES

Valves are visible sonographically in most patients, but their identification may be difficult with poorer-quality instruments. Valves appear as bright, string-like projections that dip into the lumen of the vein. Healthy valves exhibit movement as flow advances and ebbs. The valve leaves remain partially open most of the time in resting patients but close promptly with proximal compression. Diseased valves may continue to exhibit motion at rest, but if the vein is dilated, the cusps may not touch and thus may allow reverse flow. If thrombus is present, or has previously been present, the valve cusps may be attached to the vein wall or frozen in place. Clot may also been seen behind the valve cusps. If the ultrasound instrument is equipped with a pulsed Doppler, flow information may be of great help in identifying the competency of the valve. Duplex examination has great advantage over reliance on continuous-wave Doppler because the examiner can be sure that the flow signals arise from the vessel of interest rather than from another vein in the vicinity.

VISUALIZATION OF VENOUS BLOOD FLOW

With some high-resolution scanners, blood flow in veins may be imaged directly. In our experience with venous imaging, we quickly learned that flow visualization is enhanced by a variety of conditions that slowed blood flow and that the ability to image flow is not neccessarily the result of venous obstruction. For instance, we often see slowed blood flow in pregnant women who are in the supine position (Fig. 16-27). The pressure of the uterus on the vena cava is usually responsible, and when the patient rolls on her side the flow will increase as the pressure is released. Extremely slow or stagnated venous blood flow, however, is usually the result of either proximal venous compression or obstruction, and in many cases of proximal obstruction, blood flow will be stopped. This stationary column of blood has the appearance of fresh thrombus but will evacuate with probe pressure. It has been our experience that stagnant blood within the vein will soon become clot if flow is not restored. In any situation in which slow flow results from the patient's position, appreciable increase in flow should be seen when that position is altered. When proximal obstruction causes stagnant flow, changes in position will have little, if any, effect on speeding up the flow.

CLINICAL APPLICATION FOR VENOUS EVALUATION

Before the use of B-mode imaging, noninvasive examination for suspected venous thrombosis was limited to determining whether the deep veins were patent or obstructed. The extent of thrombosis was only vaguely indicated, and more

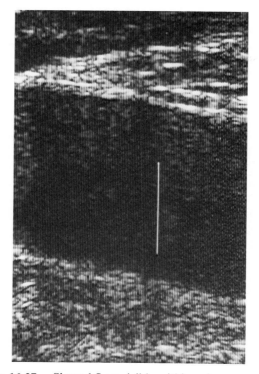

Figure 16-27. Slowed flow visible within vein as a result of pressure on vena cava when pregnant patient is in supine position.

definitive assessment of the status of the venous system required contrast venography. The recent addition of real-time imaging to traditional tests such as plethysmography and Doppler flow assessment provides numerous advantages, including the following: (1) small, nonobstructive thrombi may be detected that would not be identified on Doppler examination, (2) the exact location and extent of thrombosis may be determined, and (3) thrombus may be characterized as acute, subacute, or chronic. The B-mode and Doppler studies may be performed at bedside, which is a particular advantage for orthopedic and intensive care patients. Furthermore, B-mode imaging may be used more freely than venography, since it is less expensive, involves no radiation exposure, is painless, and carries no significant risk. The safety and comfort of B-mode venous evaluation makes possible the serial study of patients with venous thrombosis to ensure maximal resolution of thrombus in response to lytic therapy. The opportunity to monitor clot disollusion may be of great value in determining when medication may be safely discontinued. Our experience has shown that as clot is disolved with lytic agents, loose thrombus tails may form. Patient ambulation is not advisable when loose thrombus is present, and with serial followup examination, the point at which ambulation is safe may be determined.

Improved management of superficial thrombosis is also possible with venous imaging. Our experience suggests that it is advisable to image all thrombosed superficial veins because thrombi may extend far beyond the level detectable on physical examination. With B-mode imaging, the point at which the thrombus terminates may be identified, and the clinician may determine whether clot is present in or near the deep venous system.

The effectiveness of venous imaging may be limited in muscular, obese, or severely edematous patients in whom portions of the vascular system may be too deep for clear visualization. When the results of venous imaging are equivocal because vessels are poorly seen, venography may be indicated, but referral for venography should be required only rarely. As indicated by our experience at LDS Hospital, clinical reliance on B-mode venous imaging markedly decreased the need for venography. In 1980, before B-mode venous imaging was available, approximately 120 extremity venograms were performed, as compared with fewer than 50 extremity venograms in 1984, when over 600 noninvasive venous studies were performed. The reduction in the use of venography has broad implications in terms of patient risk and comfort.

ACCURACY OF B-MODE VENOUS DIAGNOSIS

In our opinion, ultrasonic venous imaging in the hands of experienced examiners can be extremely accurate. Unfortunately, only one study[3] has been published that addresses the accuracy of ultrasonic venous imaging, and this study includes only a small number of patients in whom ultrasound findings were confirmed with venography. Nonetheless, the report is encouraging. In 23 cases of lower-extremity venous thrombosis, both the sensitivity and positive predictive value of B-mode diagnosis were 92 percent, and both specificity and negative predictive value were 100 percent. Furthermore, this study suggests that venous imaging is highly accurate for differentiating among acute thrombus, chronic thrombus, and combinations of acute and chronic thrombus. The technologist employed to learn venous imaging for the Sullivan study was trained at our laboratory at LDS Hospital. He and his colleagues subsequently accumulated several years of experience, and the results reported by Sullivan and associates reflect this level of experience. Experience is the key to accuracy with this modality. The "learning curve" for B-mode venous examination is lengthy, and the technologist must be willing to spend several months developing expertise in the art of venous imaging before accuracy such as that reported by Dr. Sullivan and associates may be expected. Physician interpretation training is also extremely important, as is the quality of the imaging equipment used. Attempts at venous imaging with a poor-quality instrument may be extremely discouraging, if not dangerous. The point must also be made that venous imaging should be used in conjunction with a modality that is sensitive to venous obstruction, such as continuous-wave Doppler, phleborheography, or impedance plethysmography. We have found continuous-wave Doppler examination with a nonimaging instrument, as described in Chapter 15, to be the best companion study for B-mode venous imaging,[4] but others may prefer duplex flow evaluation performed simultaneously with the imaging procedure.

PERIPHERAL ARTERY IMAGING

If one can image peripheral veins in the extremities with ultrasound, then it follows that peripheral arteries may also be imaged. In the course of examining patients for venous obstruction, we often observed plaque in arteries as well as arterial thrombus or aneurysm. These observations led us to investigate the clinical value of B-mode arterial imaging. We have found ultrasound arterial imaging helpful for localization of peripheral arterial thrombus in the lower extremities. In some cases, B-mode thrombus localization may be sufficiently definitive to allow for surgical removal of the thrombus without arteriography.

Many of the skills used for venous imaging are applicable to peripheral arterial examination. For arterial imaging, however, correlative Doppler examination is much more important than in venous studies. Because arteries do not compress as readily as veins, it is more difficult to identify soft, poorly echogenic thrombus. In some cases, the artery may appear free of thrombus yet may contain plaque or thrombus that will only be identified with Doppler evaluation. An additional problem encountered in arterial imaging is acoustic shadowing from plaque calcification. Acoustic shadows may obscure the arterial lumen as well as plaque or thrombus within the lumen. Because of these technical difficulties, arterial imaging should always be performed in conjunction with other functional tests, such as pulse-volume recording or Doppler flow assessment.

TECHNIQUE FOR LOWER-EXTREMITY ARTERIAL EXAMINATION

Imaging of peripheral arteries, in our laboratory, is done selectively following pulse volume recording, continuous-wave Doppler, and photoplethysmography. The examination is conducted with the patient in the supine position with the bed or table flat. We have found that a transverse scanning plane is most useful. Imaging is begun at the groin crease with localization of the common femoral artery. Doppler signals are used frequently so that patency of the artery can be confirmed. The vessel is closely interrogated for atherosclerotic plaque or thrombus using the same techniques that are applied during carotid artery ultrasound examination, as described in Chapter 7. In the thigh, the common femoral, superficial femoral, and a short segment of the profunda femorus arteries may be imaged in most cases. The examination is continued into the leg by having the patient roll onto his or her side, as described previously, to allow examination of the popliteal artery. Although the anterior and posterior tibial arteries occasionally may be identified below the popliteal fossa, these branches are small and difficult to see clearly in most cases. It is also difficult to obtain Doppler signals in these branch arteries; therefore, the value of duplex examination is limited below the popliteal space.

Peripheral arterial imaging is most useful for identification of arterial thrombus that may be surgically removed. If the location and extent of thrombus can be determined, arteriography may not be necessary before surgery. Thrombus is identified through visualization of echogenic material in the lumen (Fig. 16-28) and through the absence of Doppler signals or the detection of a "thumping" Doppler

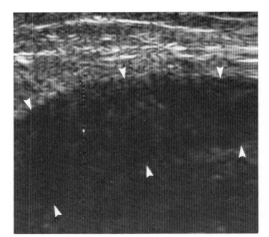

Figure 16-28.   Arterial thrombosis. Fresh thrombus is identified by diffuse, fine echogenicity that fills the lumen (arrowheads) of the superficial femoral artery. (Longitudinal view.)

signal. Fresh, poorly organized thrombus may be seen to move within the lumen
with each arterial pulse.

Plaque depositions may also be seen within peripheral arteries (Fig. 16-29).
The efficacy of B-mode plaque assessment is questionable, however. Plaque
deposition in lower-extremity vessels is often very extensive, but B-mode or
duplex imaging is restricted to relatively localized areas. Hence, the full extent of
arteriosclerotic involvement is difficult to assess with duplex technique. Furthermore, existing Doppler and plethysmographic techniques that are commonly used
in peripheral vascular laboratories have a recognized high level of accuracy for
assessment of obstructive lesions in the lower extremities. It is not clear that

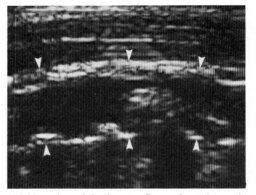

Figure 16-29.   Arterial plaque. Strongly echogenic plaque
deposits are seen in this longitudinal view of a peripheral
artery (arrowheads).

direct examination of arteries with duplex techniques offers a diagnostic advantage over older methods.

It is also possible to identify atherosclerotic aneurysms (Fig. 16-30) with B-mode or duplex methods. This function of B-mode imaging may be of considerable clinical value in patients with embolic symptoms in whom the source of embolization is uncertain. B-mode imaging is also useful for determining the nature of postoperative or arteriographic complications. Hematoma or abscess formation adjacent to a graft anastomosis or arterial puncture site may transmit pulsations and give the appearance of an aneurysm, and B-mode or duplex techniques may be used to evaluate such collections. It is quite simple in most cases to determine whether the pulsations are intrinsic to the collections, as is the case with an aneurysm (Fig. 16-31), or whether the pulsations are transmitted through a collection lying adjacent to the vessel. The Doppler component of the duplex instrument may also be used to confirm directly the presence of blood flow in an aneurysm.

SUMMARY

The addition of venous and arterial imaging to other traditional examinations in use in the vascular laboratory can greatly enhance diagnostic accuracy. The potential benefits from the use of venous imaging are only now being realized. Those who fully explore the many applications of these new techniques will enjoy the satisfaction of providing referring physicians with much more accurate and complete information than ever before possible from the noninvasive laboratory.

CASE STUDIES

Case 16-1

We were called into the intensive care unit to examine a 79-year-old male receiving ventilator therapy following a suspected pulmonary embolus. The patient was in distress, and augmented respiratory effects of the volume ventilator made Doppler venous examination difficult. As a result, the Doppler examination results were equivocal. Real-time venous imaging was performed, with findings shown in Figure 16-32.

DISCUSSION The B-mode scans shown in Figure 16-32 reveal a large, loose thrombus tail high in the common femoral vein, with attachment much lower within the vein. The thrombus would move from side-to-side within the vein with each sigh breath given by the ventilator. Following the scan, placement of an inferior vena cava umbrella was discussed, but this form of therapy was rejected because of the patient's advanced age and bleak prognosis. The patient died 5 days later.

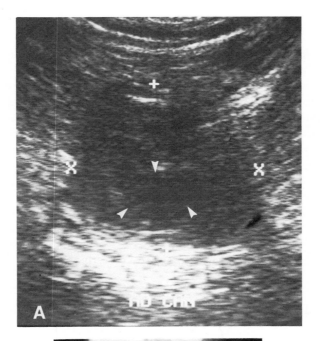

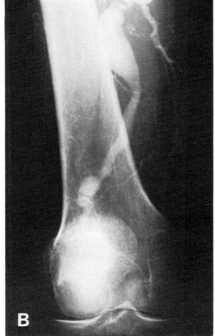

Figure 16-30. Atherosclerotic aneurysm. (A) This transverse section of the superficial femoral artery (cursors) demonstrates aneurysmal dilatation measuring 4 cm. Most of the lumen of the aneurysm is filled with organized thrombus. The patent portion of the lumen is indicated by arrowheads. (B) An arteriogram in the same patient demonstrates arterial dilatation, but the true size and extent of the aneurysm was evident only with ultrasound examination.

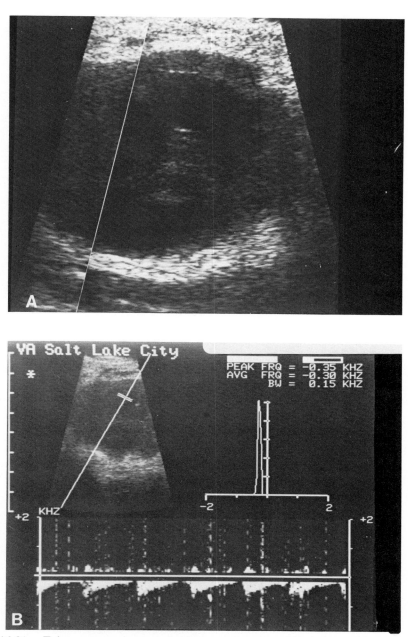

Figure 16-31. False aneurysm, superficial femoral artery. (A) A large false aneurysm (composite, longitudinal view) is seen adjacent to the superficial femoral artery (not shown) at the site of previous arterial catheterization. Echoes recorded in the aneurysm resulted from slowly swirling blood. (B) The aneurysm was clearly pulsatile and blood flow was also detected within the lumen of the aneurysm with the duplex device.

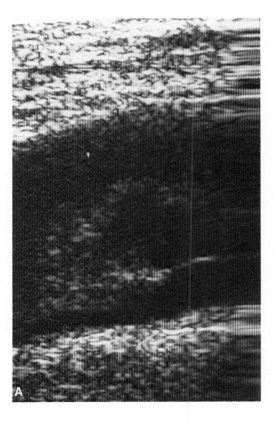

Figure 16-32. Case 16-1. Longitudinal (A) and transverse (B) images of the common femoral vein.

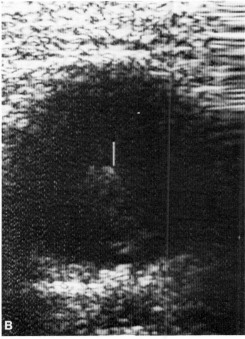

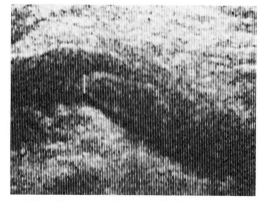

Figure 16-33. Case 16-2. Longitudinal image of the popliteal vein.

Case 16-2

This 70-year-old woman, who complained of 4 days of right calf pain, was seen in our vascular laboratory as an outpatient. Phleborheography and Doppler examination were normal. Venous imaging revealed absence of thrombus in the common femoral, superficial femoral, and saphenous veins. B-mode findings low in the right popliteal vein are shown in Figure 16-33.

DISCUSSION   The popliteal vein seen in Figure 16-33 contains a loose, nonobstructive thrombus that was not detected with Doppler examination (continuous wave or duplex). The patient was treated in the hospital for 5 days and released with a regimen of warfarin therapy.

Case 16-3

This 78-year-old male was initially seen because of left leg swelling of 24-hours duration. Phleborheography and Doppler studies of the left leg were abnormal, and B-mode images demonstrated obstruction of the common femoral vein. The patient was treated with streptokinase and strict bed rest. After 72 hours, significant clinical improvement was evident, and the physician intended to allow the patient to ambulate if repeat ultrasound examination demonstrated resolution of the thrombus. Findings from B-mode examinations at 72, 96, and 120 hours are shown in Figure 16-34.

DISCUSSION   The scan performed at 72 hours (Fig. 16-34A) demonstrated a long, loose thrombus tail in the superficial femoral vein. The referring physician, who was present during the scan, decided to continue streptokinase therapy for an additional 24-hour period, based on demonstration of the loose thrombus tail. The second followup scan, performed at 96 hours (Fig. 16-34B), showed that the tail was thinner but even more loosely attached. Based on these findings, an additional 24 hours of streptokinase therapy was elected. A third followup scan after 120 hours of therapy (Fig. 16-34C) demonstrated resolution of the thrombus. Ambulation was permitted thereafter, and the patient was released from the hospital 5 days later. The value of B-mode examination in following the course of therapy for venous thrombosis is illustrated in this case.

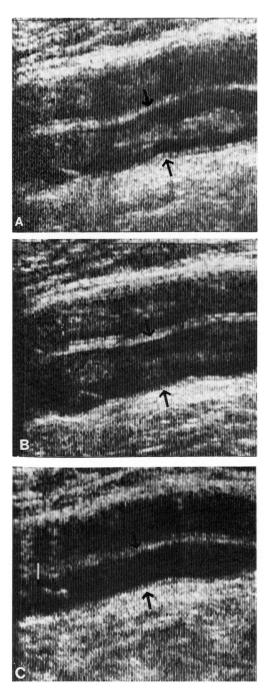

Figure 16-34. Case 16-3. Longitudinal images of the left common femoral vein (arrows) obtained at (A) 72 hours, (B) 96 hours, and (C) 120 hours after inauguration of streptokinase therapy.

ACKNOWLEDGMENTS

Special thanks to Clynn R. Ford, M.D., Medical Director at LDS Hospital Peripheral Vascular Laboratory and to technologists Sally Barraclough, and Gary Rohde.

Steven R. Talbot, R.V.T.
Technical Director
Peripheral Vascular Laboratory
LDS Hospital
8th Avenue and C Streets
Salt Lake City, Utah 84143

REFERENCES

1. Barnes RW: Doppler ultrasound evaluation of venous disease: a programmed audiovisual instruction (ed 2). Iowa City, University of Iowa Press, 1975

2. Cranley JL. Vascular Surgery Volume II, Peripheral Venous diseases. Harper and Row 1975; 11

David S. Sumner, M.D.

17

Plethysmography in Arterial and Venous Diagnosis

Before the advent of ultrasonic techniques, plethysmography was the principal method employed by the clinician who wished to document objectively the physiologic impact of arterial and venous disease. For more than a century, plethysmography has been used extensively by physiologists in their investigation of circulatory mechanisms. Indeed, most of our basic concepts of peripheral vascular physiology have been derived from studies undertaken with these instruments. Even today, the plethysmograph remains a powerful and clinically valuable tool for the diagnosis and assessment of arterial and venous disorders, complementing and supplementing results obtained with ultrasound.

This chapter will describe the instruments that are available, explain their mode of action, list their advantages and disadvantages, summarize their clinical applications, and discuss how they may be used in conjunction with ultrasonic methods.

INSTRUMENTATION

All plethysmographs are designed to measure changes in the volume of selected parts of the body.[1] Because transient changes in the volume of the extremities are largely attributable to changes in blood content, plethysmographic techniques can be adapted to measure arterial and venous dilation or constriction, mean blood flow, arterial pulsations, and peripheral blood pressure. Volume changes are either measured directly or are inferred from changes in circumference, electrical impedance, or reflectivity of infrared light. Thus, all plethysmographs perform basically the same function, and the preference for one or another variety is dictated by the precision required, the answers being sought, and convenience, cost, and personal prejudice. At times, it is expedient to sacrifice sensitivity for stability or accuracy for ease of use.

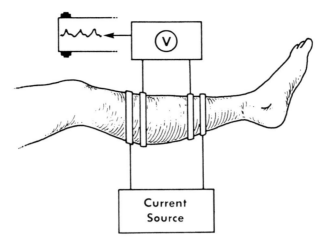

Figure 17-4. In impedance plethysmography, a high-frequency current is applied to the outer two electrodes, and the inner two electrodes record the voltage drop. A collecting cuff placed around the thigh is necessary when venous outflow and venous expansion are being measured. (From Sumner DS: Volume plethysmography in vascular disease: An overview, in Berstein EF (ed): Noninvasive Diagnostic Techniques in Vascular Disease (ed 3). St. Louis, CV Mosby, 1985, pp 97–118. With permission.)

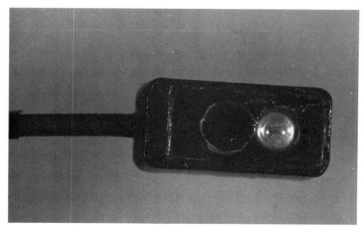

Figure 17-5. A light-emitting diode and photoelectric sensor are mounted side by side on the photoplethysmograph.

In a strict sense, photoelectric plethysmographs are not true plethysmographs, since they do not actually measure volume change and the information that they provide pertains only to the cutaneous circulation. The pulse contours that are obtained, however, closely resemble those recorded by the strain-gauge method, and although they cannot be calibrated, relative changes in blood content can be inferred from DC tracings. Photoplethysmographs are finding an ever-increasing role in vascular laboratories because they are simple to use and can be applied to areas that are not easily studied with other plethysmographs.

EXAMINATION TECHNIQUES

In the clinical laboratory, plethysmographs are used in four ways: (1) to measure arterial inflow or venous outflow (venous occlusion plethysmography), (2) to record periodic fluctuation in limb volume related to the arrival of arterial pulses (pulse plethysmography), (3) to document transient changes in venous volume due to exercise or venous incompetence (volumetry) and (4) to estimate systolic arterial pressure (segmental pressure measurement).

Venous Occlusion Plethysmography

Venous-occlusion plethysmography is one of the oldest yet one of the most reliable methods for measuring mean blood flow.[1,13,14] The technique can be applied to the forearm, calf, hand, foot, fingers, or toes. A volume sensor, such as a water, air, or strain-gauge plethysmograph, is placed around the part in which blood flow is to be measured. A pneumatic cuff with a bladder that is at least 20 percent wider than the diameter of the part is wrapped around the extremity above the plethysmograph (see Figures 17-2 and 17-3). This cuff, which is referred to as the "collecting cuff," is rapidly inflated to a pressure exceeding that in the underlying veins but less than the diastolic pressure. In most cases, a pressure of 50 mm Hg will suffice. Arterial inflow is not impeded by the pressure, but the veins are temporarily occluded, causing total cessation of blood flow from the extremity. Since no blood escapes, the rate at which the volume of the extremity increases is equal to the rate of arterial inflow. As the venous pressure rises, the pressure gradient across the capillaries is reduced, blood flow decreases, and the slope of the volume change becomes progressively less steep. When the venous pressure rises to the level of the pressure in the collecting cuff, the veins underlying the cuff reopen, once again permitting blood to flow out of the extremity. A new equilibrium is established with the venous outflow equaling the arterial inflow; the extremity no longer expands and the volume tracing levels off. When the cuff is deflated, the entrapped blood escapes and the volume tracing falls rapidly to baseline levels.[1,15]

If blood flow is being measured in a terminal organ (such as the hand, foot, finger, or toe), a distal cuff is not required, but if flow is being measured in a more proximal organ (such as the calf or forearm), it is necessary to apply an "exclusion cuff" around the ankle or wrist (Figs. 17-2 and 17-3). This cuff is inflated to a pressure that exceeds arterial pressure in order to prevent blood flow into the foot or hand. Allowing blood flow to continue into these areas—which have a much greater flow rate than the arm or calf—would yield erroneously high values.

Calculations

Arterial inflow in $cm^3/min/100cm^3$ of tissue volume may be calculated by drawing a straight line connecting the systolic peaks or diastolic valleys of the pulsations that constitute the initial upward slope of the volume tracing (Fig. 17-6). The slope of this line can be expressed in terms of the number of divisions on the recording paper that the line rises in 1 minute. The number of divisions are converted into volume change by using the appropriate calibration factor. Details of the formulas that must be applied are given in references 1 and 7.

Maximum venous outflow, the initial rate at which entrapped blood leaves the extremity when the collecting cuff is suddenly deflated, is calculated in the same way as mean arterial inflow.[16] The line depicting the slope is drawn connecting the peaks or valleys of any visible pulses, starting at the point where the volume curve begins to fall. In these determinations, the slope is negative and therefore is defined as the number of divisions that the line falls in 1 minute.

The volume change that occurs when the collecting cuff is inflated is almost entirely due to the accumulation of blood in the veins, and the magnitude of the change is a function of the increase in venous pressure. When the curve levels off, the pressure in the veins distal to the cuff is equivalent to the pressure in the cuff.[17] Thus, venous compliance may be determined at any given pressure by dividing the volume change by the cuff pressure ($\Delta V/P$).

Pulse Plethysmography

Limbs, digits, and all organs composed of soft tissue expand and contract coincidentally with each cardiac cycle, producing a volume pulse that can be detected with any sensitive plethysmograph (Fig. 17-7). During the initial (sys-

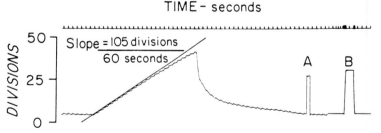

Figure 17-6. Plethysmographic measurement of calf blood flow with the mercury strain gauge: (A) electrical calibration corresponds to a 1-percent volume change (22 divisions). (B) Mechanical calibration indicates a 0.2-cm stretch of the gauge (26 divisions). Calf circumference is 34.6 cm.

Flow (electrical calibration)   = 105 div/min ÷ 22 div/1% vol. change
                                  = 4.8 $cm^3/100cm^3/min.$

$$\text{Flow (mechanical calibration)} = 2 \times \frac{105 \text{ div/min } (0.2cm/26 \text{ div})}{34.6 \text{ cm}} \times 100$$

                                     = 4.7 $cm^3/100cm^3/min.$

See equations 17-2 and 17-3.

PLETHYSMOGRAPHIC PULSE FORMS

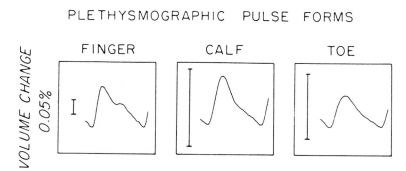

Figure 17-7. Normal plethysmographic pulses: Note that the finger pulse is larger than the toe or calf pulse. Vertical bars indicate a volume change of 0.05 percent. (From Strandness DE Jr, Sumner DS: Hemodynamics for Surgeons. New York, Grune & Stratton, 1975. With permission.)

tolic) phase of the cycle, arterial inflow exceeds venous outflow, and the volume of the part increases. During the more prolonged, second (diastolic) phase of the cycle, outflow exceeds inflow, and the volume of the part decreases. Although most of the blood flows out through the veins, there is often some retrograde flow in the arteries in early diastole. This retrograde flow is responsible for the dicrotic wave that appears on the downslope of the pulse.

The question whether the volume change responsible for the pulse occurs in the veins or in the arteries has been the subject of some debate.[17] Peripheral venous flow and pressure pulses are similar to those observed in the central veins and reflect the pressure and flow changes that occur on the right side of the heart. On the other hand, the contour of the plethysmographic pulse closely resembles that of the arterial pressure pulse, and the differentiated plethysmographic pulse resembles the arterial flow wave (Fig. 17-8). Therefore, the weight of the evidence appears to support the arterial theory.[18]

In the digits, the pulses that coincide with the cardiac cycle are superimposed on larger but less frequent cyclical changed in volume—the so-called alpha, beta, and gamma waves (Fig. 17-9).[19,20] Marked decreases in digital volume and in the excursion of the digital pulse occur in response to a deep breath, mental arithmetic, painful stimuli, and exposure of a remote part of the body to cold.[21,22,23] Warming one hand or a large part of the body can cause an increase in the volume of the pulse in the other hand or toes. All these effects have been attributed to sympathetic activity and are absent in the sympathectomized extremity.[17] They represent reflex vasodilation or vasoconstriction of the terminal arterioles and veins.

Other volume changes occur as a direct effect of quiet respiration. In the supine subject, inspiration causes a slight rise in lower-limb volume that is followed by a decrease in volume with expiration.[24,25] These volume changes, which are due to the effect of varying abdominal pressure on venous outflow, are analogous to the phasic changes in venous flow that are detected with the Doppler flow meter. As the diaphragm descends during inspiration, the intra-abdominal pressure rises, venous outflow from the legs is impeded, and the volume in the

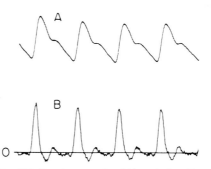

Figure 17-8. Digit volume pulse (A) and simultaneous electrically differentiated pulse (B): Note that the differentiated pulse closely resembles an arterial velocity flow recording. From Strandness DE Jr, Sumner DS: Hemodynamics for Surgeons. New York, Grune & Stratton. 1975. With permission.

legs rises. Sympathetic outflow may also be partially responsible for the volume changes that occur with respirations, particularly in the digits (Fig. 17-9).

Plethysmographic pulses are best recorded with an AC amplifier, which serves to stabilize the baseline and to eliminate the larger but slower changes in limb volume due to sympathetic activity or respiration. If one wishes to observe the larger fluctuations in limb or digit volume, it is necessary to employ a DC

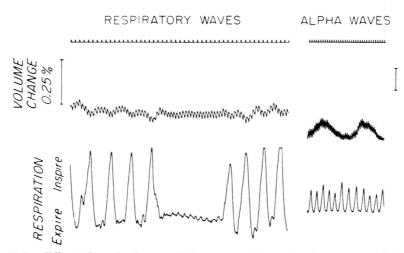

Figure 17-9. Effect of respiration on plethysmographic tracing from a normal finger tip. Alpha waves are less frequent but of greater magnitude. Time in seconds is indicated at the top. (From Strandness DE Jr, Sumner DS: Hemodynamics for Surgeons. New York, Grune & Stratton. 1975. With permission.)

amplifier. For most clinical purposes calibration is unnecessary. If required, calibration can be accomplished as described in the previous section.

Volumetry

Volume changes many times the magnitude of those associated with the arterial pulse are caused by the movement of blood into or out of the veins of the limbs. Because of the effect of gravity, postural changes evoke large shifts of blood; veins distend in the dependent positions of the body and collapse in elevated parts. Exercise, by compressing intramuscular or intermuscular veins, rapidly depletes venous volume. Extrinsic mechanical compression has a similar effect. Because venous volume is closely correlated with venous pressure, the measurement of limb volume changes produced by gravity, muscular exercise, or mechanical compression affords a convenient method for assessing venous function.

Any of the plethysmographs can be used for volumetry, but most investigators have employed strain-gauge plethysmographs, photoplethysmographs, or the water foot-volumeter. DC amplification is required, since volume changes are relatively large and occur over many seconds. Most of the volumetric studies are concerned with the rate at which the changes occur rather than their actual volume; therefore, calibration is usually unnecessary.

Pressure Measurement

Systolic blood pressure can be measured at almost any location along a limb or digit with a pneumatic cuff, a sensitive plethysmograph, and a DC amplifier.[6,26,27] The anatomic level at which pressure is to be measured determines the placement of the cuff, but the plethysmograph, which merely serves as a flow sensor, can be positioned at any convenient point on the limb or digit distal to the cuff. After the cuff has been inflated well above systolic pressure, the plethysmographic pulses disappear and the tracing begins to fall slowly, indicating a gradual loss in volume of the part. The tracing continues to fall as the cuff is slowly deflated. When systolic pressure is reached, blood again flows into the distal part of the extremity, causing the tracing to rise sharply and pulsations to reappear. The pressure in the cuff at the point at which the tracing rises is equivalent to the systolic blood pressure in the arteries at the level of the cuff (Fig. 17-10).

Measurement of blood pressure is one of the most valuable clinical applications of the plethysmograph. Although the manipulations are somewhat more difficult than those required for similar measurements conducted with the Doppler flowmeter, the plethysmograph can be used when no Doppler signals are available and can be used on the fingers and toes—sites where it is often impossible to employ the Doppler method.[28,29]

Any of the various plethysmographs will serve adequately, but because of their small size and easy application, the photoplethysmograph has proved to be exceedingly helpful, particularly for measuring pressures in the digits. Calibration of the volume tracing is not required. Errors are similar to those made with the Doppler technique and are related to cuff size, placement of the cuff, and calcification of the underlying arteries. For accurate pressure measurements, it is imperative that the width of the cuff exceed the circumference of the limb by at

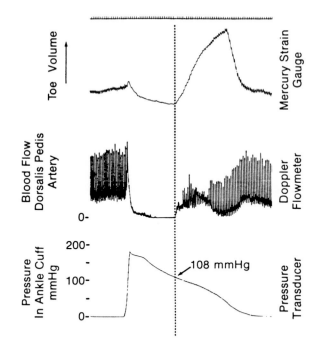

Figure 17-10. Systolic blood pressure is recorded simultaneously at the ankle with a mercury strain gauge on the second toe and a Doppler probe positioned over the posterior tibial artery. (From Sumner DS: Measurement of segmental arterial pressure, in Rutherford RB (ed): Vascular Surgery. (Ed. 2) Philadelphia, WB Saunders, 1984. pp 109–135. With permission.)

least 20 percent. Occasionally, it is necessary, for logistic reasons, to use a cuff that is too narrow. Under these circumstances, the person interpreting the data must realize that the pressure recorded will be spuriously high.[26]

EVALUATION OF OBSTRUCTIVE ARTERIAL DISEASE

Plethysmography can be used to detect the presence of arterial disease, localize the site or sites of obstruction, evaluate its functional severity, follow its natural course, assess the effects of treatment, and determine the presence or absence of sympathetic activity.

Segmental Pressure

Measurement of the systolic blood pressure at the ankle is the single most valuable noninvasive test for detecting hemodynamically significant arterial obstructions in the legs. An ankle-pressure index (systolic blood pressure at the ankle/brachial systolic blood pressure) less than 1 is highly suggestive of arterial disease, and an index that is less than 0.92 almost certainly implies disease.[26] By applying pneumatic cuffs at various levels along the leg, one can often determine the principal site of arterial obstruction. In our laboratory, we use four cuffs, placed around the upper thigh, lower thigh just above the knee, upper calf, and ankle. Between any two levels, the pressure gradient should not exceed 30 mm Hg; and at all levels the index should exceed 1. The detailed interpretation of pressure measurements is discussed more completely in preceding chapters and need not be elaborated on here.

Use of the Doppler flow meter is by far the easiest and most practical method for measuring systolic blood pressure in the leg. On rare occasions, however, no Doppler signal can be obtained distal to the cuff. In such situations, a plethysmograph can be used to detect the return of flow as the cuff is deflated. A mercury strain-gauge plethysmograph or a photoplethysmograph applied to the big toe or one of the adjacent toes serves admirably for this purpose. As an alternative, an air plethysmograph can be placed at any convenient site along the limb distal to the pressure cuff.[30] The location of the flow sensor is not particularly important as long as there is enough blood flow to provide a detectable volume change when the systolic pressure is reached.

Techniques for measuring arm pressure are analogous to those used in the lower extremity. Again, the Doppler flowmeter is preferred, and plethysmography is seldom required. Cuffs are placed around the arm, forearm, and wrist. The brachial pressure is the most reliable measurement and should not differ from arm to arm by more than 10 percent or 15 mm Hg. Pressures at all levels should be roughly equal, and a difference of more than 15 mm Hg between levels may be significant.[31] For measuring arm pressures, the mercury strain-gauge plethysmograph or photoplethysmograph is placed on one of the fingers.

Digit Pressure

Although Doppler techniques can be used to measure blood pressure in the digits, it is frequently difficult to obtain a consistently good digital arterial signal by those means. This is especially true in the toes, which, because of their short length, do not afford ready access to a digital artery when a pneumatic cuff is in place. Either the mercury strain-gauge plethysmograph or the photoplethysmograph can be used as a flow sensor, but the latter is preferred because it is easier to apply, occupies less space, and is less subject to motion artifacts than the strain gauge.

To measure finger pressures, a pneumatic cuff is placed around the proximal or middle phalanx, and the plethysmograph is attached to fingertip (Fig. 17-11). The mercury strain gauge is wrapped around the terminal phalanx at the base of the nail, and the photoplethysmograph is placed over the fleshy pad on the volar surface. Toe-pressure measurements are slightly more cumbersome, because the cuff (whose width must be greater than 1.2 times the diameter of the toe) frequently impinges on the terminal phalanx, leaving little room for the plethysmographic flow sensor. This is especially true for the third, fourth, and fifth toes.

Carter and Lezack[32] report that the toe index (toe pressure/brachial pressure) averaged 0.86 ± 0.12 in young subjects and 0.91 ± 0.13 in old subjects. We found

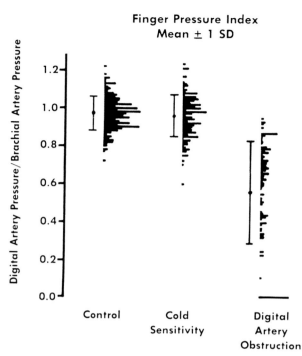

Figure 17-13. Finger pressure indices in control subjects, patients with primary Raynaud's disease, and in patients with digital or palmar arterial obstructions are compared. Vertical bars indicate mean ± one standard deviation. From Sumner DS, Lambeth A, Russel JB: Diagnosis of upper extremity obstructive and vasospastic syndromes by Doppler ultrasound, plethysmography, and temperature profiles, in Puel P, Boccalon H, Enjalbert A (eds): Hemodynamics of the Limbs I, Toulouse, G.E.P.E.S.C., 1979, With permission.

tion, the earliest change is the loss of the "reflected" wave on the downslope. With more severe disease, the slope of the anacrotic limb decreases, the peak is delayed and becomes more rounded, and the downslope bows away from the baseline. The volume of the pulse progressively decreases so that, in very severe obstructions, it may not be possible to record a pulse wave. By combining criteria of volume and contour, Raines has categorized the segmental pulses into five groups, which correlate with the degree of arterial obstruction.[30]

Because segmental pulses supplement the more easily obtained pressure data, they are not usually required in the routine diagnostic evaluation. However, segmental pulses can be useful when accurate pressure measurements cannot be made because of incompressible underlying arteries. Although air-filled cuffs are most commonly used to obtain segmental pulses, mercury strain gauges serve just as well.

Digital Plethysmographic Pulses

The contour of the digital pulse resembles those recorded from other areas of the upper and lower extremity (see Fig. 17-7). Obstruction in any artery proximal to the tip of the finger or toe produces a rounded pulse with no dicrotic wave, a slow upslope, and a downslope bowed away from the baseline (Fig. 17-14). In the fingers, a peculiar pulse having a contour intermediate between the normal and obstructive contours has been recognized. This so-called "peaked pulse" has a fairly rapid upswing, an anacrotic notch or bend, and a dicrotic wave located high on the downslope. In our experience, such pulses are commonly observed in patients with collagen diseases, Buerger's disease, frostbite, and traumatic arteritis.[39]

The volume and contour of the digital pulse bears a reasonably close relationship to the digital pressure (Fig. 17-15).[30,40] However, terminal arterial disease or vasoconstriction may produce an abnormal digital pulse even when digital pressures are normal. Thus, a "peaked" or obstructive digital pulse may be the only objective manifestation of arterial disease in some individuals. For this reason, plethysmographic studies are a valuable diagnostic adjunct to Doppler examinations—especially when the Doppler studies are negative and ischemic disease of the terminal portion of the limb is suspected.

The ability of the peripheral arterioles to vasodilate can be assessed by performing a reactive hyperemia test.[6] A pneumatic cuff placed around the limb at some convenient point proximal to the digits is inflated to a pressure well in excess of that in the underlying arteries. After a 5-minute period of ischemia, the cuff is suddenly deflated and the pulses are continuously recorded until maximal hyperemia is reached. In normal extremities, the volume of the pulse will at least double, and maximum pulse excursion will be attained within a few seconds after restoration of flow (Fig. 17-16). In the presence of obstruction proximal to the digits, peak pulse volume will be delayed—sometimes for more than 1 minute. Failure of the pulse volume to increase either indicates that the peripheral arterioles are too stiff to expand, as might occur in collagen diseases, or that they are already maximally dilated in an effort to compensate for the high resistance imposed by a proximal obstruction. In either case, surgical sympathectomy or vasodilators would not be efficacious as a method of treatment.[41]

Occasionally, the pulse volume will decrease after a reactive hyperemia test, a finding that is indicative of proximal arterial obstruction (Fig. 17-17). Vasodilatation in the more voluminous proximal muscles that lie distal to the arterial obstruction diverts blood from the digits, causing decreased digital flow. Flow increases in the digits only after the metabolic requirements of these muscles have been satisfied.

Because vasodilatation following a period of ischemia also occurs in sympathectomized extremities, a positive response to a reactive hyperemia test does not necessarily indicate that the patient would benefit from a surgical sympathectomy. Sympathetic activity is best demonstrated plethysmographically by having the patient take a deep breath (Fig. 17-18). If there is little or no reduction in pulse volume or in the volume of the digit, the limb is already effectively sympathectomized, and no response to surgical sympathectomy would be expected. Ice placed on the forehead or mental arithmetic can also be used to

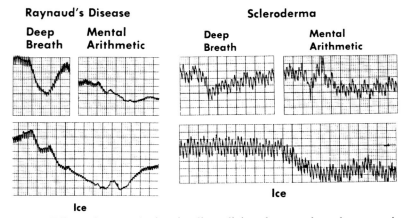

Figure 17-18. Effect of sympathetic stimuli on digit volume and on the excursion of the digit-volume pulse: normal response in a patient with primary Raynaud's disease is compared with abnormal response in a patient with scleroderma. Tracings on the patient with scleroderma were recorded at a higher sensitivity than those on the patient with Raynaud's disease. (From Sumner DS, Lambeth A, Russell JB: Diagnosis of upper extremity obstructive and vasospastic syndromes by Doppler ultrasound, plethysmography, and temperature profiles, in Puel P, Boccalon H, Enjalbert A (eds): Hemodynamics of the Limbs I, Toulouse, G.E.P.E.S.C., 1979. With permission.)

detect sympathetic activity, but these tests are less reliable than the deep-breath test (Fig. 17-18). If the pulses are already reduced, sympathetic activity can be demonstrated by warming the patient's body with an electric blanket, leaving the digits exposed. If the reduction in pulse volume is due to an increased sympathetic tone, this maneuver will result in vasodilatation.

Volume Flow Measurements

One of the first methods for investigating peripheral arterial disease made use of venous-occlusion plethysmography to quantitate blood flow to the tissues.[42] These measurements were usually made in the calf or forearm. Because the peripheral arterioles dilate to maintain blood flow at a nearly normal rate, even in the presence of significant proximal arterial obstruction, measurement of resting blood flow proved to be far less sensitive than measurement of peripheral pressure.[43] Reductions in resting blood flow occur only when arterial disease is far advanced.

Under conditions of maximal vasodilatation, however, blood flow to the calf or forearm will be reduced in comparison to that occurring under similar conditions in a normal extremity.[42,43] For example, after exercise, flows in excess of 40 ml/100 ml/min are commonly recorded in normal calves. The maximum flow rate is attained almost instanteously, following which the flow rapidly decreases, returning to preexercise levels within a few minutes (Fig. 17-19).[17] In the presence of proximal arterial obstruction, calf blood flow usually increases somewhat, reaching values of 5 to 30 ml/100 ml/min, but the peak flow rate is often delayed for 1 to 20 minutes, and the flow may not return to preexercise levels by 30

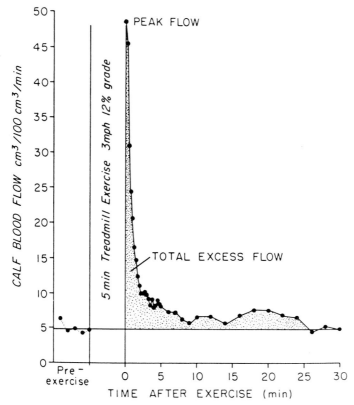

Figure 17-19. Postexercise hyperemia in a normal human calf, measured by venous occlusion plethysmography. (From Strandness DE Jr, Sumner DS: Hemodynamics for Surgeons. New York, Grune & Stratton, 1975. With permission.)

minutes (Fig. 17-20). Responses are similar after a reactive hyperemia test, but peak values are reached more rapidly and the hyperemia is less prolonged.[17]

Although these tests have contributed greatly to our understanding of the physiology of arterial obstructive disease, they are far too cumbersome to be used in routine laboratory practice. Because changes in pressure reflect alterations in flow, and because pressure is much easier to record, pressure measurements (usually obtained with the Doppler flowmeter) have now largely replaced quantitative flow determinations. Venous occlusion plethysmography is now largely restricted to physiologic investigations.[43,44]

EVALUATION OF VASOSPASTIC DISEASE

In patients with episodic digital ischemia, the major diagnostic responsibility of the vascular laboratory is to determine whether the process is purely vasospastic (primary Raynaud's disease) or whether the cold sensitivity represents normal vasoconstriction acting on a substrate of macrovascular or micro-

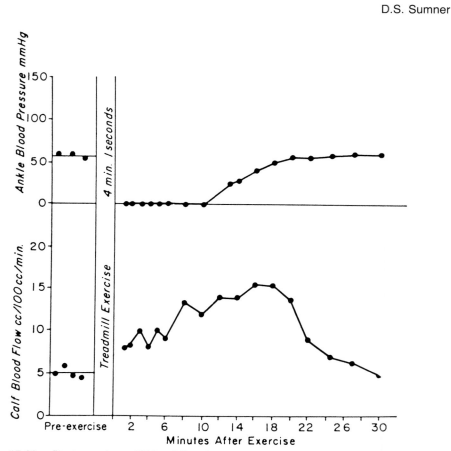

Figure 17-20. Postexercise calf blood flow is compared with ankle systolic pressure in a limb with stenosis of the iliac artery and occlusion of the superficial femoral artery. Note the reduction in peak hyperemia, the delay in reaching peak hyperemia response, and the persistence of hyperemia for more than 20 minutes. (From Sumner DS, Strandness DE Jr: The relationship between calf blood flow and ankle blood pressure in patients with intermittent claudication. Surgery 65:763–771, 1969. With permission.)

vascular arterial disease (secondary Raynaud's phenomenon).[17] The disease entities responsible for "secondary" Raynaud's phenomenon are legion, but all cause reductions in digital pressure or changes in the contour of the digital pulse. As mentioned above, the only abnormality in some patients with collagen disease (such as scleroderma or lupus) may be a peaked or obstructive finger pulse. The diagnosis of "primary" Raynaud's disease is one of exclusion. In my experience, if a patient complaining of cold sensitivity is found to have normal digital pressures, normal digital pulse contours, normal reactive hyperemia responses, and normal sympathetic activity, it is extremely rare to identify any biochemical abnormality signifying an underlying disease process.[31] Such patients have a benign prognosis. A few patients whose digital studies are otherwise normal appear to have a hyperactive sympathetic response (deep-breath test), but this finding has been difficult to quantify.

Patients who demonstrate an active reactive hyperemia response, reflex vasodilatation, and an active vasoconstriction to a deep breath or other sympathetic stimulus may benefit from vasodilator drugs or a surgical sympathectomy (though this procedure is rarely necessary). Patients with "fixed" microvasculature, or those in whom the peripheral arteriolar bed is already maximally vasodilated to compensate for severe proximal arterial obstruction, will not benefit from vasodilator therapy or sympathectomy (see Fig. 17-18).

Inciting an attack of Raynaud's phenomenon in the office or vascular laboratory is often difficult. We have found the simple cold-tolerance test proposed by Porter[45] to be quite useful for documenting cold-induced vasospasm. Nielsen and Lassen[46] have devised a more quantitative plethysmographic test that demonstrates critical closure of the digital arteries in response to cold exposure. Briefly, the technique employs a mercury strain-gauge plethysmograph to measure the digital pressure in fingers that have been precooled to a well-defined temperature by fluid circulating in a digital cuff. In normal fingers, the systolic blood pressure decreases as the skin temperature falls, but even at 10°C, the average pressure is only 16 ± 3 percent less than it is when the fingers are warm. In contrast, the digital artery pressure in patients with primary Raynaud's disease falls rapidly as finger temperatures are reduced. Complete closure of the digital arteries (recognized by a zero digital-artery pressure) occurs at different temperatures (ranging from <10°C to 22°C), depending on the severity of the cold sensitivity. Because the temperature associated with critical closure is reproducible in the same patient, this test can be used to assess the efficacy of vasodilator therapy and to determine the duration of its effect.

DIAGNOSIS OF ACUTE VENOUS OBSTRUCTION

Plethysmographic methods for detecting deep-venous thrombosis have developed pari passu with ultrasonic techniques used for the same purpose. Currently, plethysmography enjoys a great deal of popularity, not only because it has proved to be reasonably accurate, but also because it requires less technician input than the Doppler methods.

Venous Outflow and Venous Volume Measurements

Two of the most widely used tests, measurement of venous incremental capacity and the rate of venous outflow, are often combined into one procedure. Equipment consists of a pneumatic cuff wrapped around the thigh and a plethysmograph placed around the calf. An ankle cuff is not required. Although impedance plethysmographs are most often used, mercury strain gauges and air-filled devices work equally well.[16,25,47] As described earlier in this chapter, the pneumatic cuff is rapidly inflated to a specific pressure (usually 50 mm Hg) and allowed to remain inflated until the volume of the calf expands to a stable level. A plateau is reached when the pressure in the veins in the calf equals that within the cuff. Ordinarily, this requires about 45 seconds (range 15 to 180 seconds). Calf volume expansion may be calculated in terms of ml/100 ml of calf or may simply

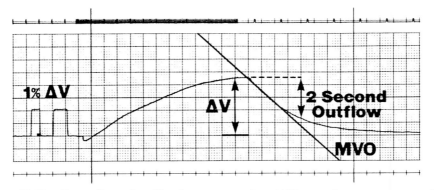

Figure 17-21. Recording of calf volume expansion (ΔV), maximum venous outflow (MVO), and 2-second outflow. (From Sumner DS: Strain-gauge plethysmography, in Bernstein EF (ed): Noninvasive Diagnostic Techniques in Vascular Disease (ed 3), St. Louis, CV Mosby, 1985, pp 742–754. With permission.)

be noted in terms of the number of divisions that the tracing rises on the recording paper (Fig. 17-21).

After full expansion has been achieved, the cuff is suddenly deflated, allowing the blood backed up in the calf to rapidly escape into the thigh veins. The initial rate at which the tracing falls, the so-called maximum venous outflow (MVO), is calculated in ml/100 ml/min. A more commonly used method is to record the volume decrease that occurs within 2 or 3 seconds after release of cuff pressure (Fig. 17-21).[25,48]

At low transmural pressures, veins are quite complaint because of their semicollapsed state. A rise in venous pressure of only a few mm Hg produces a great increase in venous volume. At high transmural pressures, veins assume a circular cross-section, their walls become quite stiff, and even a large increase in venous pressure will result in only a small increase in venous volume.[17] Because obstruction of the deep veins of the legs causes the venous pressure to rise, venous compliance is reduced. Therefore, the extent to which the calf expands in response to inflation of a thigh cuff is reduced in limbs with venous obstruction.

In normal limbs at a congesting pressure of 50 mm Hg, calf-volume expansion approximates 2–3 percent.[49] Expansion is usually less than 2 percent in limbs with acute venous obstruction.[50] There is, however, a great deal of overlap between individual values in normal and abnormal limbs. Postphlebitic legs may or may not have normal values, depending on the extent of the obstructive process and the extent of collateral development (Fig. 17-22). Owing to the increased capacity of varicose veins, limbs with prominent varicosities often show increased venous expansion. Because of these factors, measurement of calf volume expansion, as an isolated test, has not proved to be a sufficiently reliable method for identifying the presence of deep-venous thrombosis.

The rationale for using the rate of venous outflow to detect deep venous thrombosis is quite straightforward.[17] The rate of venous outflow (Q) is directly proportional to the pressure gradient propelling blood from the calf veins (Pcv) to

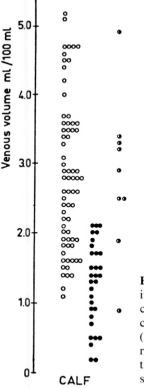

Figure 17-22. Calf volume expansion with the collecting cuff inflated to 50 mm Hg. Open circles represent normal legs; closed circles, acute deep-venous thrombosis; and half-closed circles, postphlebitic limbs. Note extensive overlap of values. (Adapted from Hallböök T, Göthlin J: Strain-gauge plethysmography and phlebography in diagnosis of deep venous thrombosis. Acta Chir Scand 137:37–52, 1971. With permission.)

the inferior vena cava (P_{ivc}), and inversely proportional to the resistance of the interposed venous channels (R).

$$Q = \frac{Pcv - P_{ivc}}{R} \tag{17-6}$$

Because cuff inflation provides a consistent elevation of venous pressure within the calf (e.g., 50 mm Hg) and because central venous pressure is quite low, the rate of venous outflow is decreased in the presence of acute venous obstruction. As shown in Figure 17-23, there is a fairly good separation between the MVO of normal limbs and limbs with acute venous thrombosis. When an MVO of 20 ml/100 ml/min was selected as the dividing line between normal and abnormal values, Barnes and colleagues[16] found the test to be 91-percent sensitive and 88-percent specific.

Venous outflow, especially when measured 2 or 3 seconds after cuff release, is not merely a function of the factors included in equation 17-6, but, among other things, also depends on the extent of volume expansion.[17] In general, venous outflow increases as the extent of volume expansion increases.[25,51,52] It has been

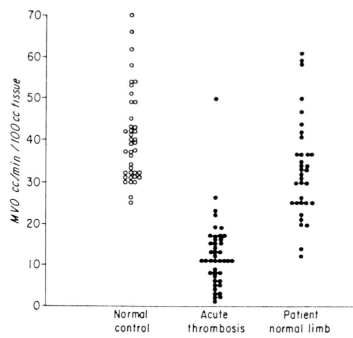

Figure 17-23. Maximum venous outflow (MVO) in normal limbs and in lims with acute deep venous thrombosis (From Barnes RW, Collicott PE, Mozersky DJ, et al.: Noninvasive quantitative of maximum venous outflow in acute thrombophlebitis. Surgery 72:971–9079, 1972.With permission.)

found that the overall accuracy of these tests is increased by plotting venous outflow versus venous volume expansion on a graph.[25,53] A discriminate line that slopes upward from left to right on a graph, with venous outflow on the ordinate and calf volume expansion on the abscissa, provides excellent separation between normal values, lying above the line, and abnormal values, lying below the line (Fig. 17-24). A composite analysis of reported data in which this method has been compared with 1930 phlebograms reveals an overall sensitivity of 95 percent and specificity of 93 percent.[54]

False-positive studies occur when there is residual obstruction in postphlebitic extremities and when there is extrinsic compression from tumors, hematomas, and Baker's cysts. Nonocclusive thrombi and venous thrombi confined to the calf are responsible for most of the false-negative results. With time, collateral development also returns the values to normal. Cramer and associates found that only 17 percent of limbs remained abnormal more than 1 month after an episode of deep venous thrombosis.[47]

Combined venous-outflow and venous-expansion plethysmography have proved to be an excellent method for diagnosing acute venous thrombosis proximal to the popliteal segment. Overall accuracy can be improved by combining this test with the Doppler venous survey[55] or with the ^{125}I-fibrinogen uptake test,[56] both of which are more sensitive to calf-vein thrombosis.

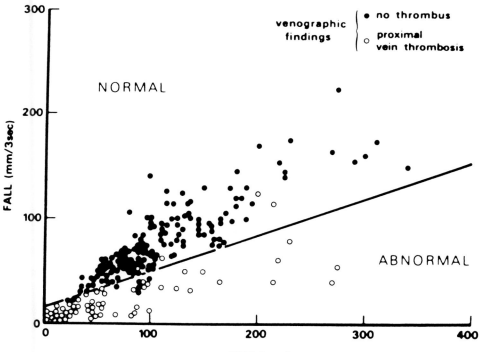

Figure 17-24. Three-second venous outflow (fall) plotted against calf volume expansion (rise) in normal limbs and limbs with thrombosis in the popliteal or more proximal veins. Dimensions are divisions on the recording paper. (From Hull R, Van Aken WG, Hirsh J, et al.: Impedance plethysmography using the occlusive cuff technique in the diagnosis of venous thrombosis. Circulation 53:696–700, 1976. With permission.)

Phleborheography

Phleborheography is an entirely different plethysmographic test for detecting deep-venous thrombosis.[24] Its rationale is similar to that of the Doppler method. Volume-sensing pneumatic cuffs are placed around the thorax, midthigh, upper calf, lower calf, and foot. The two lower cuffs also serve as compression devices. Normally, respiration causes phasic variations in the venous-flow pattern and in the transmural pressure within the leg veins (Fig. 17-25). In turn, this causes phasic changes in limb volume. Reduction or absence of these respiratory waves indicates the presence of venous obstruction. In the initial part of the test, the foot cuff is inflated rapidly three times to a pressure of 50 mm Hg. Normally, no increase in limb volume is detected by the cuffs on the thigh and calf. When venous outflow is impeded by proximal venous obstruction, however, foot pumping causes the limb to swell perceptibly below the site of obstruction. The second portion of the test consists of rapid inflation and deflation of the lower calf cuff to 30 mm Hg. In normal limbs, this maneuver tends to empty the foot veins, causing a decrease in foot volume and no increase in calf volume. In the presence

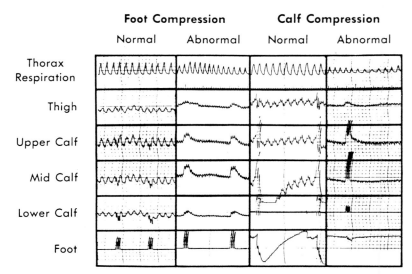

	Foot Compression		Calf Compression	
	Normal	Abnormal	Normal	Abnormal
Thorax Respiration				
Thigh				
Upper Calf				
Mid Calf				
Lower Calf				
Foot				

Figure 17-25. Phleborheographic tracings from normal limbs and limbs with deep venous obstruction. (From Sumner DS: The approach to diagnosis and monitoring of venous disease, in Rutherford RB (ed): Vascular Surgery. Philadelphia, WB Saunders, 1977. With permisssion.)

of venous obstruction, calf pumping causes little or no decrease in foot volume but an increase in the volume of the proximal calf and thigh.

Cumulative figures from four reports of 798 extremities indicate that phleborheography has a sensitivity of 92 percent and a specificity of 95 percent.[57] Most of the false-negative results were due to small clots below the knee.

EVALUATION OF CHRONIC VENOUS INSUFFICIENCY

Although chronic venous insufficiency is more easily diagnosed clinically than acute venous thrombosis, noninvasive tests can help by documenting the presence of venous obstruction and venous valvular incompetence. Some degree of quantitation of the physiologic abnormality is also possible. These tests can distinguish between deep- and superficial-vein incompetence, thereby permitting a more accurate differentiation of primary from secondary varicose veins.

Venous Reflux Flow

Barnes and colleagues[58] have devised a method for measuring the volume and rate at which blood is forced retrograde down the leg in response to thigh compression (Fig. 17-26). The apparatus is identical to that employed for measuring maximum venous outflow, except that a narrow arterial occlusion cuff is placed around the upper thigh just cephalad to the wider venous occlusion cuff. A mercury strain gauge is used to measure volume changes in the calf. With the upper-thigh cuff inflated well above systemic arterial pressure, the distal (venous

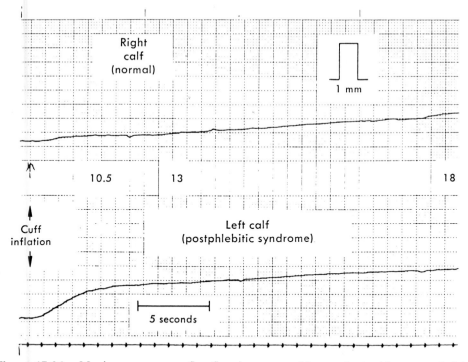

Figure 17-26. Maximum venous reflux flow is compared in a patient with a normal right leg and incompetence of the deep veins of the left leg. (From Barnes RW, Collicott PE, Mozersky DJ, et al.: Noninvasive quantitation of venous reflux in the postphlebitic syndrome. Surg Gynecol Obstet 136:769–773, 1973. With permission.)

occlusion) thigh cuff is suddenly inflated to 50 mm Hg. Since the arterial cuff precludes the egress of blood through the proximal venous channels, blood is displaced distally toward the calf.

In normal subjects, the maximum rate of venous reflux flow is quite low, averaging 3 ± 1 ml/100 ml/min, with an upper limit of 6 ml/100 ml/min. In postphlebitic limbs, the reflux flow rate averages 13 ± 7 ml/100 ml/min.[4] To distinguish between primary and secondary varicose veins, a Penrose drain tourniquet is applied to the calf just below the knee but above the strain gauge. This serves to compress the superficial veins, but has little effect on the deep veins. When venous incompetence is restricted to the superficial veins—as in limbs with primary varicose veins—the tourniquet tends to normalize the venous reflux flow.[59] Little or no effect is observed in normal legs or in those with deep-vein insufficiency.

Foot Volumetry

Norgren, Thulesius, and their colleagues[4,60] have introduced a new technique, called "foot volumetry," for measuring the volume of blood displaced from the foot during exercise. Because venous-volume changes reflect venous-pressure changes, this method can be substituted for the more tedious and invasive pressure measurements that have held a time-honored place in the physiologic evaluation of chronic venous insufficiency.

The patient stands with each foot in a water plethysmograph and is then requested to perform 20 deep-knee bends. In limbs with chronic venous insufficiency, less blood is pumped from the foot, and the foot refills more rapidly than in normal limbs. Whereas in normal limbs, refilling occurs exclusively from the arterial side, in abnormal limbs, blood refluxes down the incompetent veins, thereby accelerating the refilling process. Tourniquets can be applied to the thigh, calf, and ankle to differentiate between superficial- and deep-vein incompetence.

More recently, Schanzer and colleagues have proposed using the mercury strain gauge in a similar fashion.[61] Because both chronic deep-venous obstruction and deep-venous valvular incompetence interfere with foot emptying during exercise, it is difficult to distinguish between these two causes of venous insufficiency. Use of the mercury strain gauge permits the evacuation of blood from the foot by elevation of the leg to 45°. When the legs are returned to a dependent position, venous refilling occurs rapidly in limbs with venous incompetence but slowly in limbs with deep-venous obstruction and functioning valves.

Photoplethysmography and Calf Volumetry

The volume of blood in the calf (Fig. 17-27) responds to exercise in much the same way as the foot volume. In most recent reports, a mercury strain gauge has been used as the volume sensor. Patients are examined in either the standing or the sitting position and are asked to raise themselves on their toes, or plantar-flex

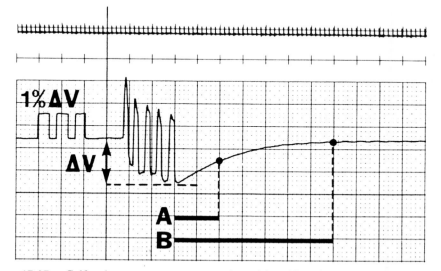

Figure 17-27. Calf volume response to exercise with subject in a sitting position: After five plantar flexions, volume was reduced (ΔV) by 2 percent. Recovery half-time ($T_{1/2}$) was 10 seconds (A), and total recovery time was 35 seconds (B). (From Sumner DS: Strain gauge plethysmography, in Bernstein EF (ed): Noninvasive Diagnostic Techniques in Vascular Disease (ed 3), St. Louis, CV Mosby, 1985, pp 742–754. With permission.)

their feet a standard number of times (usually 5 or 20). With the patients standing, Fernandes e Fernandes and colleagues[62] found that the calf volume decreased 2.2 ± 0.5 percent in normal limbs, 1.3 ± 0.3 percent in limbs with superficial venous insufficiency and 0.06 ± 0.5 percent in limbs with chronic venous insufficiency. These differences seem to be less evident when the patient exercises in the sitting position.

Reported average venous refilling times in the standing position range from 14 to 22 seconds in normal limbs, 5 to 7 seconds in limbs with superficial venous incompetence and 3 to 7 seconds in limbs with chronic venous insufficiency.[62,63] Because it is sometimes difficult to recognize the precise point at which the calf volume returns to preexercise levels or establishes a new baseline, the recovery half-time ($T_{1/2}$) may be used. This is defined as the time after cessation of exercise required for the calf to regain half the volume it lost during exercise. With the patients in the sitting position, Barnes reports recovery half-times of 3.4 ± 1.4 seconds in normal limbs and 1.3 ± 1 seconds in postphlebitic limbs.[64] Application of a tourniquet to compress the superficial veins will have no effect on the decrease in calf volume or recovery time in normal limbs or in limbs with chronic venous insufficiency but will tend to normalize these values in limbs with primary varicose veins.

Hyperemia developing as a result of exercise may accelerate venous refilling even in normal limbs. This tends to mimic rapid refilling caused by venous reflux and could lead to false-positive studies. In order to avoid the problem of hyperemia, manual compression of the calf has been substituted for exercise as a method for emptying the underlying veins.[65] Because there is relatively much less muscle mass in the foot, foot volumetry is less affected by the hyperemia induced by exercise.[61]

Photoplethysmography has also been used to follow changes produced by exercise in the amount of blood contained within the cutaneous veins.[12,66,67] Studies are performed with the patient sitting. A photoplethysmograph is affixed to the skin above the medial malleolus, and the patient is instructed to plantar-flex the feet five times. Recordings are made with a DC amplifier. Three different patterns have been observed. In the "decompressive" pattern, the tracing falls, indicating a transient decrease in skin blood content; in the "static" pattern, no change is observed; and in the "congestive" pattern the tracing actually rises.[12] The latter two patterns are associated with severe venous disease and stasis ulceration. The decompressive pattern occurs in normal limbs and in limbs with stasis dermatitis. It is less commonly seen in association with ulcers.

The total time required for the tracing to rise to preexercise levels usually exceeds 20 seconds in normal legs. When the decompressive pattern is observed in limbs with chronic venous insufficiency, recovery times are usually much less than 20 seconds.[66] Recovery half-times ($T_{1/2}$) average 9.7 ± 4.3 seconds in normal extremities, 3.7 ± 2 seconds in legs with varicose veins, and 3.6 ± 3.1 seconds in legs with chronic venous insufficiency.[12] Again, the recovery time is unaffected by a calf tourniquet in normal limbs or in limbs with chronic venous insufficiency, but is prolonged toward normal values in limbs with primary varicose veins. Norris and associates have recently demonstrated that it is possible to calibrate the PPG to accurately predict changes in ambulatory venous pressure, both during and after exercise.[68] Such quantitation may prove to be of value in clinical research.

On theoretic grounds, it has been proposed that photoplethysmographic studies may have certain advantages over similar studies conducted with the strain gauge. Because the photoplethysmograph is sensitive only to venous volume changes occurring in the skin, the abnormalities that are detected with this instrument bear a closer relationship to the physiologic derangements responsible for postphlebitic dermatitis and stasis ulceration than do similar abnormalities detected with the mercury strain gauge. A normal photoplethysmographic study may be obtained in patients with deep-vein incompetence (as demonstrated by Doppler ultrasound or strain-gauge plethysmography), but these patients have no stasis dermatitis, pigmentation, or ulceration.[12]

Although venous Doppler surveys provide an accurate and convenient way of documenting the presence or absence of chronic venous insufficiency, plethysmographic studies offer the dual advantage of quantitating the reflux and of distinguishing between disease affecting only the deep tissues and that which also produces derangements of the cutaneous circulation.

SUMMARY

Plethysmographs are devices that measure changes in the volume of selected body parts. A variety of plethysmographs have been developed for medical applications as described herein. Plethysmographs may be used for extremity vascular diagnosis in four ways: (1) to measure arterial inflow or venous outflow (venous occlusion plethysmography), (2) to record periodic fluctuation in limb volume related to the arrival of arterial pulses (pulse plethysmography), (3) to document transient changes in venous volume due to exercise or venous incompetence (volumetry), and (4) to estimate systolic arterial pressure (segmental pressure measurement).

Despite advancements in Doppler techniques, plethysmography may remain a commonly used and valuable technique for extremity vascular diagnosis.

David S. Sumner, M.D.
Professor of Surgery
Chief, Section of Peripheral Vascular Surgery
Southern Illinois University
School of Medicine
PO Box 3926
Springfield, IL 62708

REFERENCES

1. Sumner DS: Volume plethysmography in vascular disease: An overview, in Bernstein EF (ed): Noninvasive Diagnostic Techniques in Vascular Disease (ed 3). St. Louis, CV Mosby, 1985, pp 97–118
2. Dahn I: On the calibration and accuracy of segmental calf plethysmography with a de-scription of a new expansion chamber and a new sleeve. Scand J Clin Lab Invest 16:347–356, 1964
3. Greenfield ADM, Whitney RJ, Mowbray JF: Methods for the investigation of peripheral blood flow. Br Med Bull 19:101–109, 1963
4. Thulesius O, Norgren L, Gjöres JE: Foot

volumetry: A new method for objective assessment of edema and venous function. Vasa 2:325–329, 1973

5. Darling RC, Raines JK, Brener BJ, et al.: Quantitative segmental pulse volume recorder: a clinical tool. Surgery 72:873–887, 1973

6. Strandness DE Jr, Bell JW: Peripheral vascular disease: diagnosis and objective evaluation using a mercury strain gauge. Ann Surg 161(suppl):1–35, 1965

7. Sumner DS: Mercury strain-gauge plethysmography, in Bernstein EF (ed): Noninvasive Diagnostic Techniques in Vascular Disease (ed 3). St. Louis, CV Mosby, 1985, pp 133–150

8. Whitney RJ: The measurement of volume changes in human limbs. J Physiol (Lond) 121:1–27, 1953

9. Hokanson DE, Sumner DS, Strandness DE Jr: An electrically calibrated plethysmograph for direct measurement of limb blood flow. IEEE Trans Biomed Eng 22(1):25–29, 1975

10. Nyboer J: Electrical impedance plethysmography (ed 2). Springfield, Charles C Thomas, 1970

11. Wheeler HB, Penny BC: Impedance plethysmography: Theoretical and experimental basis, in Bernstein EF (ed): Noninvasive Diagnostic Techniques in Vascular Disease. St. Louis, CV Mosby, 1982, pp 104–116

12. Barnes RW, Yao JST: Photoplethysmography in chronic venous insufficiency, in Bernstein EF (ed): Noninvasive Diagnostic Techniques in Vascular Disease (ed 2), St. Louis, CV Mosby, 1982, pp 514–521

13. Conrad MC, Green HD: Evaluation of venous occlusion plethysmography. J Appl Physiol 16:289–292, 1961

14. Raman ER, Vanhuyse VJ, Jageneau AH: Comparison of plethysmographic and electromagnetic flow measurements. Phys Med Biol 18:704–711, 1973

15. Greenfield ADM, Patterson GC: The effect of small degrees of venous distention on the apparent rate of blood inflow to the forearm. J Physiol (Lond) 125:525–533, 1954

16. Barnes RW, Collicott PE, Mozersky DJ, et al.: Noninvasive quantitation of maximum venous outflow in acute thrombophlebitis. Surgery 72:971–979, 1972

17. Strandness DE Jr, Sumner DS: Hemodynamics for Surgeons. New York, Grune & Stratton, 1975

18. Noordergraaf A, Horman HW: Numerical evaluation of volume pulsations in man, II: Calculated volume pulsations of forearm and calf. Phys Med Biol 3:59–70, 1958

19. Burch GE: Digital Plethysmography. New York, Grune & Stratton, 1954

20. Honda N: The periodicity in volume fluctuations and blood flow in the human finger. Angiology 21:442–446, 1970

21. Browse NL, Hardwick PJ: The deep breath-venoconstriction reflex. Clin Sci 37:125–135, 1969

22. Delius W, Kellerova E: Reactions of arterial and venous vessels in the human forearm and hand to deep breath or mental strain. Clin Sci 40:271–282, 1971

23. Jamieson GG, Ludbrook J, Wilson A: Cold hypersensitivity in Raynaud's phenomenon. Circulation 44:254–264, 1971

24. Cranley JJ, Canos AJ, Sull WJ, et al.: Phleborheographic technique for diagnosis of deep venous thrombosis of the lower extremities. Surg Gynecol Obstet 141:331–339, 1975

25. Wheeler HB, Anderson FA Jr.: Impedance phlebography: The diagnosis of venous thrombosis by occlusive impedance plethysmography, in Bernstein EF (ed): Noninvasive Diagnostic Techniques in Vascular Disease (ed 2), St. Louis, CV Mosby, 1982, pp 482–496

26. Sumner DS: Measurement of segmental arterial pressure, in Rutherford RB (ed); Vascular Surgery (ed 2). Philadelphia, WB Saunders, 1984, pp 109–135

27. Winsor T: Influence of arterial disease on the systolic blood pressure gradient of the extremity. Am J Med Sci 220:117–126, 1950

28. Gundersen, J: Segmental measurements of systolic blood pressure in the extremities including the thumb and great toe. Acta Chir Scand (suppl) 426:1–90, 1972

29. Nielsen PE, Bell G, Lassen NA: The measurement of digital systolic blood pressure by strain-gauge technique. Scand J Clin Lab Invest 29:371–379, 1972

30. Raines JK, Darling RG, Buth J, et al.: Vascular laboratory criteria for the management of peripheral vascular disease of the lower extremities. Surgery 79:21–29, 1976

31. Sumner DS, Lambeth A, Russell JB: Diagnosis of upper extremity obstructive and vasospastic syndromes by Doppler ultrasound, plethysmography, and temperature profiles, in Puel P, Boccalon H, Enjalbert A (eds): Hemodynamics of the Limbs I. Toulouse, France, G.E.P.E.S.C., 1979, pp 365–373

32. Carter SA, Lezack JD: Digital systolic pres-

sures in the lower limb in arterial diseases. Circulation 43:905–914, 1971

33. Ramsey DE, Manke DA, Sumner DS: Toe blood pressure—a valuable adjunct to ankle pressure measurement for assessing peripheral arterial disease. J Cardiovasc Surg 24:43–48, 1983

34. Barnes RW, Thornhill B, Nix L, et al.: Prediction of amputation wound healing. Arch Surg 116:80–83, 1981

35. Bone GE, Pomajzl MJ: Toe blood pressure by photoplethysmography: An index of healing in forefoot amputations. Surgery 89: 569–574, 1981

36. Noer I, Tønnesen KH, Sager PH: Minimal distal pressure rise after reconstructive arterial surgery in patients with multiple obstructive arteriosclerosis. Acta Chir Scand 146: 105–107, 1980

37. Holstein P, Noer I, Tønnesen KH, et al.: Distal blood pressure in severe arterial ischemia, in Bergan JJ, Yao JST (eds): Gangrene and Severe Ischemia of the Lower Extremities. New York, Grune & Stratton, 1978, pp 95–114

38. Hirai M: Arterial insufficiency of the hand evaluated by digital blood pressure and arteriographic findings. Circulation 58:902–908, 1978

39. Sumner DS, Strandness DE Jr: An abnormal finger pulse associated with cold sensitivity. Ann Surg 175:294–298, 1972

40. Sumner DS: Rational use of noninvasive tests in designing a therapeutic approach to severe arterial disease of the legs, in Puel P, Boccalon H, Enjalbert A (eds): Hemodynamics of the Limbs II. Toulouse, France, G.E.P.E.S.C., 1981, pp 369–376

41. Strandness DE Jr: Long-term value of lumbar sympathectomy. Geriatrics 21:144–155, 1966

42. Shepherd JT: Physiology of the Circulation in Human Limbs in Health and Disease. Philadelphia, WB Saunders, 1963

43. Sumner DS, Strandness DE Jr: The relationship between calf blood flow and ankle blood pressure in patients with intermittent claudication. Surgery 65:763–771, 1969

44. Manke DA, Sumner DS, Van Beek AL, et al.: Hemodynamic studies of digital and extremity replants or revascularizations. Surgery 88:445–452, 1980

45. Porter JM, Snider RL, Bardana EJ, et al.: The diagnosis and treatment of Raynaud's phenomenon. Surgery 77:11–23, 1975

46. Nielsen SL, Lassen NA: Measurement of

digital blood pressure after local cooling. J Appl Physiol 43:907–910, 1977

47. Cramer M, Beach KW, Strandness DE Jr: The detection of proximal deep vein thrombosis by strain gauge plethysmography through the use of an outflow/capacitance discriminant line. Bruit 7:17–21, December 1983

48. Barnes RW, Hokanson DE, Wu KK, et al.: Detection of deep vein thrombosis with an automatically calibrated strain gauge plethysmograph. Surgery 82:219–223, 1977

49. Barnes RW, Collicott PE, Sumner DS, et al.: Noninvasive quantitation of venous hemodynamics in postphlebitic syndrome. Arch Surg 107:807–814, 1973

50. Halböök T, Göthlin J: Strain-gauge plethysmography and phlebography in diagnosis of deep venous thrombosis. Acta Chir Scand 137:37–52, 1971

51. Cramer M, Langlois Y, Beach K, et al.: Standardization of venous flow measurements by strain gauge plethysmography in normal subjects. Bruit 7:33–40, March 1983

52. Hull R, Taylor W, Hirsh J, et al.: Impedance plethysmography: The relationship between venous filling and sensitivity and specificity for proximal vein thrombosis. Circulation 58:898–902, 1978

53. Hull R, van Aken WG, Hirsh J, et al.: Impedance plethysmography using the occlusive cuff technique in the diagnosis of venous thrombosis. Circulation 53:696–700, 1976

54. Wheeler HB, Anderson FA Jr: Can noninvasive tests be used as the basis for treatment of deep vein thrombosis?, in Bernstein EF (ed): Noninvasive Diagnostic Techniques in Vascular Disease (ed 2). St. Louis, CV Mosby, 1982, pp 545–559

55. Richards KL, Armstrong JD, Tikoff G, et al.: Noninvasive diagnosis of deep venous thrombosis. Arch Intern Med 136:1091–1096, 1976

56. Hull R, Hirsh J, Sackett DL, et al.: Combined use of leg scanning and impedance plethysmography in suspected venous thrombosis. New Engl J Med 296:1497–1500, 1977

57. Cranley JJ, Hyland LJ, Comerota AJ: Diagnosis of deep venous thrombosis of the lower extremity by phleborheography, in Bernstein EF (ed): Noninvasive Diagnostic Techniques in Vascular Disease (ed 2). St. Louis, CV Mosby, 1982, pp 459–467

58. Barnes RW, Collicott PE, Mozersky DJ, et al.: Noninvasive quantitation of venous

reflux in the postphlebitic syndrome. Surg Gynecol Obstet 136:769–773, 1973

59. Barnes RW, Ross EA, Strandness DE Jr: Differentiation of primary from secondary varicose veins by Doppler ultrasound and strain gauge plethysmography. Surg Gynecol Obstet 141:207–211, 1975

60. Norgren L, Thulesius O, Gjöres JE, et al.: Foot-volumetry and simultaneous venous pressure measurements for evaluation of venous insufficiency. Vasa 3:140–147, 1974

61. Schanzer H, Lande L, Premus G, Peirce EC II: Noninvasive evaluation of chronic venous insufficiency. Use of foot mercury strain-gauge plethysmography. Arch Surg 119:1013–1017, 1984

62. Fernandes e Fernandes J, Horner J, Needham T, et al.: Ambulatory calf volume plethysmography in the assessment of venous insufficiency. Br J Surg 66:327–330, 1979

63. Holm JS: A simple plethysmographic method for differentiating primary from secondary varicose veins. Surg Gynecol Obstet 143:609–612, 1976

64. Barnes RW: Strain gauge plethysmography (abstract). Symposium on Noninvasive Diagnostic Techniques in Vascular Disease. San Diego, CA, 1979, p 51

65. Sakaguchi S, Tomita T, Endo I, et al.: Functional segmental plethysmography: A new venous function test. J Cardiovasc Surg 9:87–98, 1968

66. Abramowitz HB, Queral LA, Flinn WR, et al.: The use of photoplethysmography in the assessment of venous insufficiency: A comparison to venous pressure measurements. Surgery 86:434–441, 1979

67. Gorsuch G, Kempczinski R: Role of photoplethysmography in the evaluation of venous insufficiency. Bruit 5:23–26, 1981

68. Norris CS, Beyrau A, Barnes RW: Quantitative photoplethysmography in chronic venous insufficiency: A new method of noninvasive estimation of ambulatory venous pressure. Surgery 94:758–764, 1983

SECTION IV

ABDOMINAL VASCULAR DIAGNOSIS

**Chapter 18. B-Mode and Duplex Examination of the Aorta, Iliac Arteries
and the Portal Vein**

In this section, Dr. Gooding presents techniques and concepts of B-mode and duplex evaluation of the aorta, iliac arteries, and portal veins. The reader is directed, in particular, to the discussion of techniques for assessment of aortic and iliac aneurysms. Diagnosis and followup of an abdominal aneurysm appears to be a straightforward matter, but accurate evaluation requires both technical expertise and diligence. Methods for obtaining good technical results are described by Dr. Gooding. Diligence must be supplied by the sonographer.

Gretchen A.W. Gooding, M.D.

18

B-Mode and Duplex Examination of the Aorta, Iliac Arteries, and Portal Vein

AORTIC SONOGRAPHY

Equipment and Technique

The ideal ultrasound examination of the aorta encompasses both static and real-time B-mode examinations. The static examination provides a "global" view of the aorta and its surroundings that is especially useful for documenting the location of an aneurysm and for measuring its length. The real-time examination indicates the intrinsic pulsatility of the vessel (but not the actual blood flow) and serves as an effective way to determine its course, particularly if the vessel is markedly tortuous, as is frequently the case with a diseased aorta.

The standard technique for static examination of the aorta consists of parasagittal and transverse scans to define aortic anatomy. Parasagittal scans typically are obtained at 1-cm intervals and transverse scans at 2-cm intervals. A 3.5-MHz transducer is typically used for static imaging, but in very obese patients a 2.25-MHz transducer may provide better penetration.

The patient is examined in the supine position with respiration suspended. The transducer is initially angled in a cephalic direction, and a sweep is made along the length of the aorta in a sagittal or parasagittal plane. Localizing marks are made on the image to indicate the xiphoid and the umbilicus. In general, the aorta tends to bifurcate at about the level of the umbilicus. Transverse scans at 2-cm intervals from the xiphoid to the aortic bifurcation are used to examine the aorta in cross-section. Real-time imaging may be substituted for the transverse scans. If the aorta is markedly tortuous and real-time instrumentation is not available, cross-sectional images may be used to define the course of the aorta for subsequent static scanning along its primary axis.

All types of real-time equipment can effectively image the aorta, but individual units have advantages and limitations determined by their design.[1]

Sector scanners produce a pie-shaped image narrowest at the skin. In thin patients, the aorta lies very near the anterior abdominal wall and within the narrowest portion of the sector image. Thus, only a very small segment of the aorta may be included in the image when such devices are used. Because the scanning head of the sector units is fairly small, however, angulation of the transducer cephalad in the region of the proximal aorta produces excellent images of the celiac and superior mesenteric artery origins. Linear array units are ideal for aortic examination because a rectangular image is produced that encompasses a large segment of the vessel. Because of the bulk of the transducer, however, they are less helpful in the high epigastrium.

The difference between static and real-time scanning of the aorta can be compared with radiography and fluoroscopy as used in gastrointestinal studies. The static scans are analogous to the radiographic sequence and the real-time study to fluoroscopy. Real-time study adds another dimension to the morphologic information, since motion can be evaluated. The examiner can actually appreciate the pulsatility of the vessels. Furthermore, the course of a tortuous aorta can be quickly identified, a factor that greatly facilitates examination and ensures accurate measurement of aneurysmal segments. Real-time examination is sometimes more effective than static scanning in difficult cases because a multitude of angulated planes may be used to bypass the effects of overlying bowel gas.

If real-time sonography is the primary medium for aortic evaluation, it is important to establish a standard examination protocol. Transverse real-time aortic images should be obtained at the level of the diaphragm, near the area of the superior mesenteric artery–renal arteries, and in the distal aorta as well as at any points of dilatation. When longitudinal scans of the aorta are obtained with a real-time device, it is important to document the entire length of an aneurysm if present, and it is also important to document the position of the aneurysm relative to the great vessels such as the renal, superior mesenteric or celiac arteries. Often, the renal arteries cannot be identified sonographically, but the celiac axis or superior mesenteric artery is easy to find and indicates the approximate location of the renal arteries.

The Normal Aorta

The aorta extends in the abdomen from the diaphragmatic hiatus to the region of the umbilicus, where is bifurcates into the iliac arteries (Fig. 18-1). The normal abdominal aorta lies immediately adjacent to the spine, and there should be no tissue between it and the vertebral column. Since the aorta follows the thoracic and lumbar curvatures, it lies far posterior in its cephalic portion and distally becomes more anterior in location. The aorta tapers during its course in the abdomen and should measure less than 3 cm in diameter at any point. Real-time examination reveals prominent aortic pulsations. The celiac axis and superior mesenteric artery are commonly noted branches emanating from the anterior aortic surface. The inferior mesenteric artery is usually not recognized sonographically. The origin of the renal arteries is also not appreciated on routine parasagittal scans of the aorta, although the right renal artery is often seen behind the inferior vena cava on oblique views. Longitudinal scanning in the left lateral decubitus position can sometimes delineate the origin of the renal arteries,[2] but

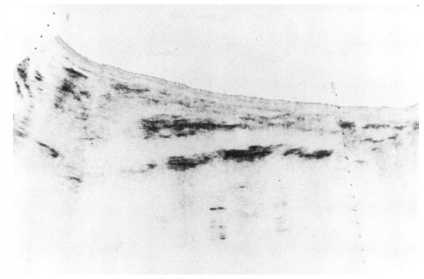

Figure 18-1.   A longitudinal scan demonstrates the normal aorta.

ultrasound is not the study of choice for detecting renal artery stenosis. Computed tomography is the preferred study for precisely determining the position of the renal arteries in relation to aortic aneurysm, and arteriography is the procedure of choice for assessing renal artery blood flow.

Anatomic variation of the origin of the major aortic branches may be detected by ultrasound, including replaced origin of the right hepatic artery from the superior mesenteric artery (Fig. 18-2). This variation, which occurs in approximately 14 percent of individuals, is best seen on transverse scans. A small vessel will be noted to originate from the right side of the superior mesenteric artery. With real-time imaging, this artery may be followed along a course parallel and immediately *dorsal* to the portal vein. By comparison, the normal right hepatic artery originates from the common hepatic artery and lies *ventral* to the portal vein. Occasionally, unusual variations are noted, such as a common origin of the celiac artery and the superior mesenteric artery. One can also appreciate tortuosity of the splanchnic vessels. Large aneurysms of the splanchnic arteries, particularly those lying near the midline, can compress or distort the aorta and must be differentiated from aortic aneurysms.[3]

Ultrasound scanning is of distinct importance for distinguishing between a normal and aneurysmal aorta in patients suspected clinically of having an aneurysm. Thin patients in whom the aorta lies close to the anterior abdominal wall often have an easily palpated distal aorta, and prominent pulsations palpated in such individuals may be confused with an aneurysm. Obese patients may have diffuse pulsations also suggestive of an aneurysm. In both cases, ultrasound can rapidly make the distinction between the normal and aneurysmal aorta.

however, and to ensure precise measurement, the following technical points should be observed:

1. The sonographer must first review preceding studies to determine the previous maximum diameter and to find the location of the greatest dilatation.
2. Care must be taken to use similar planes of section in measuring the aneurysm during the current study. Real-time scanning is extremely helpful for ensuring accurate measurement, since it allows easy identification of the point of maximum aortic widening.
3. Ideally, transverse images used for measurement should be at right angles to the aortic axis. Since the aneurysmal aorta usually is tortuous, the orientation of such images are often oblique to the body axis.
4. The scans from which measurements are taken should demonstrate the wall as clearly as possible. Since aneurysms may be largest in their transverse dimension, it is particularly important to define clearly the lateral surfaces of the aneurysm as seen on transverse scans. If the lateral surfaces are not well seen from an anterior transducer location, improved definition may be accomplished by pressing the transducer into the abdomen either to the right or left of the aneurysm and aiming the sound beam directly at the lateral surface.
5. The largest cross-sectional diameter should always be used for recording the size of the aneurysm, regardless of whether it is an anteroposterior or transverse measurement.
6. The full thickness of the arterial wall must be included in all measurements (outer surface to outer surface); otherwise, significant underestimation of aortic size may occur.

Arteriography tends to underestimate the size of aneurysms because only the functional lumen is depicted. Large aneurysms often contain a great amount of circumferential thrombus, which is seen on sonograms as echogenic material distinct from the functional lumen (Fig. 18-5). On inspection of the surgical specimen, this circumferential thrombus is firm and gritty organized material that has been deposited over a long time. Ultrasound may also demonstrate atheromatous plaque in "normal" and aneurysmal aortas. Tissue characterization of atheromatous plaques using high-resolution ultrasound in vivo demonstrates that plaque with densely calcified foci is highly echogenic and associated with acoustic shadowing, while ulcers produce marked surface irregularities or excavations.[13] In vivo, the functional lumen of an aneurysm tends to be centrally located, since laminar flow produces the greatest velocity down the center of the aortic lumen. Curiously, fresh clot within the artery cannot be detected with static ultrasound images.[14]. When the aorta is occluded, lack of pulsations on real-time examination may lead one to suspect this diagnosis.

Aortic calcifications may be identified radiographically in only about 55 percent of aneurysms. These lie within the vessel wall; hence, ultrasound measurements correspond well with those based on radiographically visible calcifications, when radiographic magnification is taken into consideration.[15] Since ultrasound is not invasive, does not employ ionizing radiation, and is relative inexpensive, it is the ideal tool to determine the natural history of abdominal aortic aneurysm in a particular patient. The rate of aneurysmal

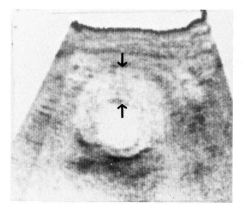

Figure 18-5. Circumferential thrombus (arrows) is demonstrated in this transverse sonogram of an abdominal aortic aneurysm.

enlargement increases in proportion to the size of the aneurysm. Chan and colleagues[16] noted the following average growth rates: "For aneurysms measuring 3–6 cm in largest transverse diameter, the mean expansion rate averaged 0.4 cm/year. The expansion rate increased to 0.64 cm/year for aneurysms greater than 6 cm in diameter." In general, smaller aneurysms will demonstrate little or no change when scanned at 6-month intervals; however, the rate of progression varies greatly among aneurysms, and a specific aortic aneurysm may progress with small increases in size while another enlarges rapidly. The lateral wall pressure of a hollow viscus increases directly with the radius of curvature; hence, rapid increase to a large diameter (≥ 6 cm) is an important signal of increasing stress, decreasing wall resistance, and impending aortic rupture.

Once an abdominal aortic aneurysm has been identified, ultrasound is of further value in determining whether iliac extension is present. Sonographic detection of an iliac aneurysm is especially important because such lesions are usually not detectable on physical examination. A large but occult iliac aneurysm may be more dangerous than a small but clinically obvious aortic aneurysm. Therefore, it is a good policy to examine routinely the iliac arteries in the course of every sonographic study of the abdominal aorta. The technique for such examination is described below. Patients with iliac aneurysm, claudication, or other indications of peripheral vascular disease usually require arteriography before surgical aneurysm repair, since the choice of vascular prostheses in such cases hinges on the extent of arteriosclerotic involvement.

An ultrasound examination for abdominal aortic aneurysm should include inspection of the kidneys to detect renal atrophy or hydronephrosis. Renal function is an important indicator of how well the patient will do after surgery. Both proximal and distal abdominal aortic aneurysms may extend to involve the renal arteries. Although ultrasound can sometimes detect the origin of the renal arteries, routine identification of these vessels is not possible; nonetheless, one can usually estimate the distance between the neck of the aneurysm and the renal arteries by locating the origin of the superior mesenteric artery. This vessel arises from the aorta within 1 cm above the renal arteries; hence, a distal aortic aneurysm that extends proximally to the level of the superior mesenteric artery may well involve the renal arteries, while one that begins well below the superior mesenteric artery probably will not. Computed tomography remains the ideal noninvasive method for assessing whether the renal arteries are involved in the aneurysmal process.[17,18] If multiple or low-lying renal arteries are suspected, or renal atrophy is observed, angiography may be needed, since it is the only currently used technique capable of directly assessing renal artery flow. The role of magnetic resonance imaging in evaluating flow in abdominal vessels remains to be determined.

Proximal abdominal aortic aneurysms (i.e., those centered above the renal arteries) are almost always extensions of thoracic aortic aneurysms (Fig. 18-6). Proximal aneurysms tend to distort the relationship of the celiac and superior mesenteric arteries (commonly splaying these vessels). An isolated proximal atherosclerotic aneurysm is distinctly unusual, but traumatic aortic aneurysms, in contrast, may occur anywhere along the course of the aorta. These are false aneurysms; that is, they are not contained by all three arterial wall components.

In some patients thought to have an aortic aneurysm on physical examination, sonography instead demonstrates a mass that surrounds the aorta or displaces it anteriorly off of the spine. Masses that mimic aortic aneurysms include retroperitoneal tumors, lymphoma, other sources of adenopathy, retroperitoneal fibrosis,[19] and horseshoe kidney (Fig. 18-7). Such masses transmit the aortic pulse and thereby become indistinguishable from aortic aneurysm on physical examination.[10]

Abdominal Aortic Rupture

Which aneurysms are likely to rupture? Size is the best correlate. An abdominal aortic aneurysm that exceeds 7 cm in diameter has a 76 percent risk of rupture within 5 years, whereas an aneurysm smaller than 6 cm in diameter has a 16 percent chance of rupture during the same period, and an aneurysm smaller than 5 cm has only a 5-percent risk of rupture during the ensuing 5 years.[20] Since the surgical mortality for an abdominal aortic aneurysm before rupture is only about 4 percent,[20] patients with aortic aneurysms—particularly those with aneurysms larger than 6 cm—should be considered for surgical intervention. The physiologic rather than the chronologic age of the patient should be considered in deciding whether surgery is indicated. Surgical treatment definitely prolongs life expectancy.

Aortic rupture is a devastating complication of abdominal aortic aneurysm associated with a mortality that approaches 100 percent in the untreated patient and 50 percent in those who are taken to surgery for aneurysmectomy.[21] Because of the catastrophic nature of aortic rupture, few patients have preoperative sonography.[22,23] The abdominal aorta usually ruptures into the retroperitoneum 1–2 cm distal to the renal arteries.[24] Because this rupture is associated with massive bleeding in the para-aortic and adjacent retroperitoneal area and because the resultant hematoma cannot be totally evacuated at surgery, patients examined sonographically in the postsurgical period typically have relatively large hypoechoic collections around the aortic graft and in the retroperitoneum.[24] The

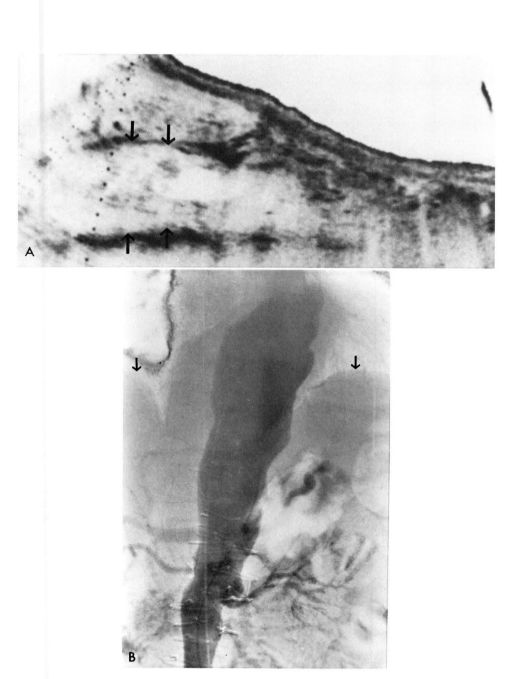

Figure 18-6. (A) A longitudinal sonogram demonstrates a huge, proximal abdominal aortic aneurysm (arrows) filled with thrombus. (B) Aortography in the same patient demonstrates that the aneurysm extends into the abdomen from the thorax. The arrows point to the diaphragm.

429

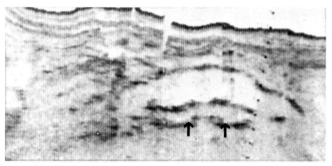

Figure 18-7.   A longitudinal sonogram demonstrates elevation of the aorta off the spine by interposed adenopathy (arrows).

hematoma in these cases may transmit pulsations from the adjacent pulsatile aortic graft, but real-time observation will demonstrate absence of intrinsic pulsations, thereby excluding the diagnosis of false aneurysm formation. The hematoma will resolve with time.

Aortic Dissection

A dissecting abdominal aortic aneurysm is not a true aneurysm but, rather, a propagatng hematoma that initially extends within the media of the aorta and eventually ruptures back into the intimally lined aortic lumen. The great majority of aortic dissections begin in the thoracic aorta, and only 2 percent of aortic dissections are confined to the abdominal aorta.[25] The descending thoracic aorta is the most commonly involved segment, but dissection may also arise in the ascending aorta.[26] In the thorax, ultrasound is of no value in defining the aortic abnormality except in areas visible through cardiac structures or where the dilated aorta abuts the thoracic wall. In other regions, intervening air-filled lung scatters and deflects the sonic beam.

In the abdomen, real-time assessment of the aorta may immediately identify the presence of a dissection by the curious and dramatic flapping of the media–intimal aortic interface that has become separated from the parent media–adventitia[25,27] (Fig. 18-8). Real-time imaging also allows the examiner to assess the extent of the dissection distally by determining where the aortic wall returns to normal. On static imaging, the media–intima flap may assume a zigzag appearance within the lumen because the flap is moving back and forth while the scan is made. When a patient enters the hospital with crushing epigastric pain, ultrasound is an extremely expeditious way to confirm the clinical suspicion of abdominal aortic dissection. Aortography, as well as computed tomography, then may be used to define the total extent of the process, including thoracic extension and major branch involvement. The most common fatal event in dissection is through-and-through rupture of the aorta, but this tends to be in the thoracic aorta and, with the exception of extravasation into the pericardial sac, cannot be detected by ultrasound.

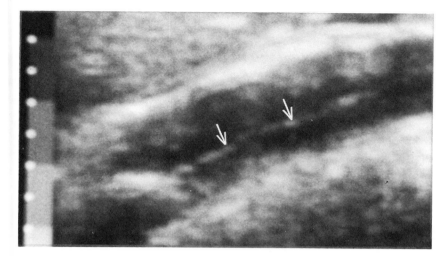

Figure 18-8. The distinct intima–media interface (arrows) of an aortic dissection is seen on this real-time, longitudinal sonogram.

Aortic dissection is almost always associated with systemic hypertension. More rarely, aortic dissection has been associated with pregnancy, Marfan's syndrome, congenital bicuspid aortic valve, and aortic isthmus coarctations. Spontaneous aortic dissection may also occur, and the cause of this disorder is unknown.[25] Trauma is a rare cause of aortic dissection that is most likely to occur iatrogenically from cannulation of the femoral artery for cardiopulmonary bypass or from femoral insertion of an intra-aortic balloon counterpulsation device. In our experience with a case of spontaneous dissection in the abdominal aorta, much more dramatic flapping of the media–intima aortic interface was observed than in a case of traumatic aortic dissection produced by a counterpulsation device. In the latter case, a clear separation was identified in the posterior aortic wall of the distal aorta, but the flap was rather rigid on real-time examination.

Aortic Occlusions

Our experience with four cases of aortic occlusion below the renal arteries[28] concurred with the study of Anderson and colleagues[3]; the aorta in all cases had a normal appearance on static images. The occluded aortic lumen was not echo-filled, as one might have expected. Real-time imaging was remarkable, however, in that the proximal aorta in all four patients pulsated normally, while the distal aorta was pulseless. The use of real-time aortic imaging is emphasized by this experience. Were it not for real-time imaging, these cases of occlusion would not have been diagnosed. For this and other reasons, we feel that all aortic studies should include real-time examination. Duplex Doppler examination would be an effective means of confirming aortic occlusion, but this technique was not available during examination of the patients described above.

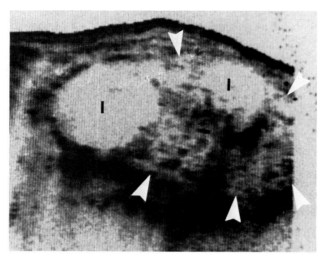

Figure 18-12. Iliac artery aneurysms (I) are demonstrated on this transverse sonogram. The left iliac aneurysm has ruptured, producing the mass effect (arrowheads) seen about the aneurysm. The dot-to-dot distance is 1 cm (I, iliac aneurysm).

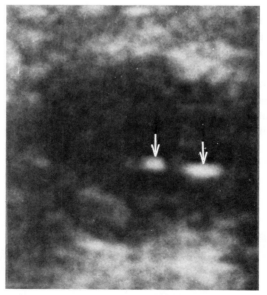

Figure 18-13. A 5-French catheter (arrows) is seen within the lumen of a distal abdominal aortic aneurysm on this longitudinal real-time sonogram obtained during arteriography.

Iliac Occlusive Disease

Occluded and patent iliac arteries have a similar appearance on static images. Failure to identify pulsations may be the only finding in occlusion; therefore, iliac artery pulsations should always be scrutinized with real-time imaging. In thin patients, it may be possible to test the compressibility of the iliac artery as it emerges from the pelvis above the inquinal ligament. If the arterial walls can be apposed by pressure with the transducer, patency is verified, as discussed in Chapter 16. A duplex ultrasound unit is possibly the ideal device for making a decision about iliac occlusion noninvasively, because duplex instruments may simultaneously image the vessel and detect the presence of flow.[36]

A number of Doppler methods may be used to quantify iliac artery occlusive disease, as discussed in Chapter 14. Quantitative Doppler methods are capable of detecting significant aortoiliac disease with an accuracy of 90–96 percent.[37] Using a 5-MHz continuous-wave Doppler unit combined with real-time spectral analysis on 175 aortofemoral graft segments in vivo, Johnson and associates[38] showed that the pulsatility index (the peak-to-peak height of the wave form divided by the mean value) was 95 percent sensitive and specific in detecting hemodynamically significant aortoiliac disease. Significant disease reduced the pulsatility index to <5.5. Qualitative assessment of the frequency-analyzed Doppler waveform also provides an accurate assessment of aortoiliac disease.[39] For example, Doppler blood flow velocity recordings are damped distal to significant arterial stenosis. Deeply penetrating duplex instruments may be capable of directly detecting flow abnormalities resulting from iliac stenosis, including increased velocity and turbulence. Such findings may be used to measure directly the severity of stenotic lesions in a manner analogous to carotid diagnosis. The accuracy and diagnostic value of direct duplex interrogation of iliac vessels has not been assessed.

Although Doppler, B-mode, and duplex methods may be valuable for detecting aortoiliac occlusion and for assessing its severity, arteriography remains the final arbiter for surgical planning.

CATHETER LOCATION

The 5-French catheter, which is 1.67 mm in diameter, is commonly used for arteriography. We have demonstrated in vitro and in vivo (during arteriography) that ultrasound can identify this catheter (Fig. 18-13) in the aorta, the axillary artery, the brachial artery, and the iliac artery.[29] In a single case, we have used ultrasound to monitor the portion of a catheter placed in the popliteal artery for infusion therapy of a well-defined, echogenic arterial embolus.[29,30]

Occasionally, a catheter will break off during angiography, particularly during its removal through a rigid vascular prosthesis. In these instances, real-time ultrasound may be the study of choice to determine whether the catheter fragment still lies within the vessel at the site of introduction or has embolized to a distal site. If located at the site of introduction, the catheter is subject to local surgical removal.[31]

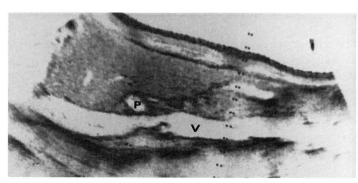

Figure 18-14. Longitudinal sonogram demonstrating the normal portal vein (P) as it crosses the inferior vena cava (V).

PORTAL VEIN SONOGRAPHY

Normal Portal Vein Anatomy

The main portal vein is almost universally visualized in B-mode sonography of the right upper quadrant.[40] The main portal vein lies immediately ventral and nearly perpendicular to the vena cava (Fig. 18-14). Ranging in size from 10.3 to less than 13 mm,[41,42] the main portal vein courses with the hepatic artery and the bile duct into the liver, where it divides into the right and left branches (Fig. 18-15). The portal vein serves as an orienting landmark used for identification of upper abdominal anatomic structures such as the extrahepatic bile ducts and the pancreas.[43,44]

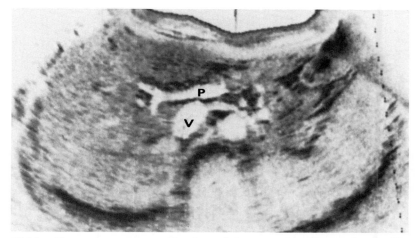

Figure 18-15. Transverse sonographic view of the normal main portal vein (P) and the right portal vein, which divides into the anterior and posterior branches. Note that the main portal vein is located immediately anterior to the inferior vena cava (V).

Portal Hypertension and Portal Occlusion

With real-time sonography, the main portal vein may be seen to increase significantly in size during inspiration and then decrease in size during expiration.[45] The main portal vein may also increase in size by as much as 50 percent within 30 minutes after a large meal.[37]

When the respiratory response of the portal vein is damped or absent, portal hypertension is a viable diagnosis.[45] Also, when the portal vein cannot be visualized sonographically, occlusion must be considered. Portal vein thrombosis may occur secondary to tumor compression or invasion. Hepatoma, pancreatic and gastric carcinoma, and lymphoma are particularly prone to cause portal vein occlusion. Other etiologies of portal vein thrombosis include inflammation (Fig. 18-16), cirrhosis, trauma, and blood dyscrasia.[47] When the portal vein is thrombosed, multiple serpiginous collateral veins develop along the course of the main portal vein, a condition termed *cavernous transformation of the portal vein*.[40,48,49] Cavernous transformation is characterized sonographically by failure of visualization of the extrahepatic portal vein, demonstration of increased echogenicity in the region of the porta hepatis, and visualization of multiple serpiginous vascular channels around the thrombosed portal vein.

In adults, cavernous transformation of the portal vein results from chronic portal vein obstruction secondary to a variety of etiologies that include alcoholic

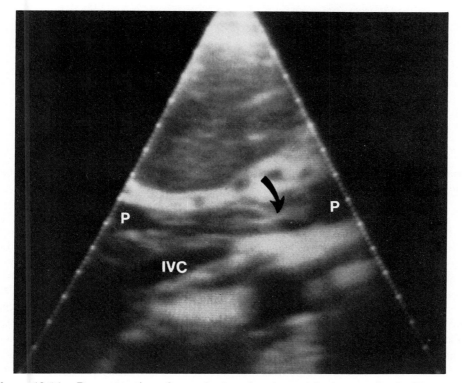

Figure 18-16. Demonstration of a septic thrombus (arrow) in the portal vein (P) secondary to appendicitis in a transverse oblique sonogram (IVC, inferior vena cava).

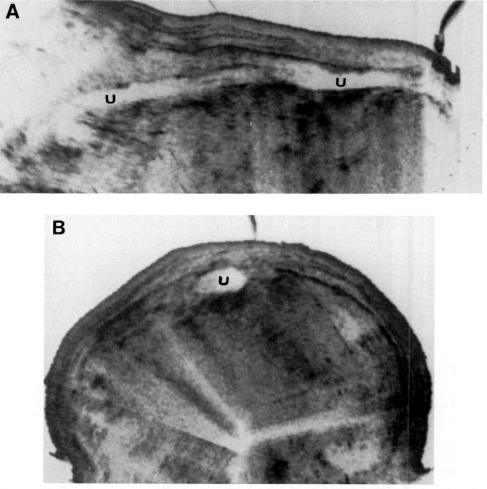

Figure 18-17. A patent umbilical vein (U) is demonstrated on longitudinal (A) and transverse (B) sonograms.

cirrhosis, pancreatitis, and pancreatic carcinoma. A pulsed-Doppler examination defines a spectral waveform that is peculiar to the hepatic portal system, that is, a continuous venous flow of relatively low frequency with mild turbulence that clearly differentiates it from the systemic arterial flow.[50] Van Gansbeke and co-workers[51] found cavernomatous transformation of the portal vein to occur in 19 percent of 21 adults with portal vein thrombosis. More frequently, hyperechoic thrombus was present in the lumen of the portal vein (57 percent), while portal collateral circulation occurred in 48 percent and enlargement of the thrombosed segment of portal vein was evident in 38 percent.

With the development of portal hypertension (usually due to hepatic cirrhosis), a recanalized paraumbilical vein is commonly noted as a sonolucent superficial vascular channel that runs from the umbilicus to the left portal vein[52–56]

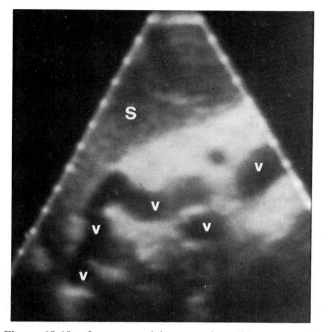

Figure 18-18.   Large, serpiginous varices (V) are seen in the vicinity of the spleen (S) on this longitudinal section.

(Fig. 18-17). Other portosystemic venous collaterals may be identified by sonography in patients with portal hypertension, including the coronary gastroesophageal veins that feed gastroesophageal varices, splenorenal veins that course from the splenic hilar area through the pancreatic and retroperitoneal veins to the left renal vein, and gastrorenal veins. The hemorrhoidal vein, as well as other intestinal veins from the mesentery, may also form collateral circuits between the portal and systemic venous systems[57–59] (Fig. 18-18). McCormick and colleagues[60] demonstrated that blood flow patterns in esophageal varices monitored by Doppler ultrasound are both cephalad and caudad toward the stomach. B-mode ultrasound has been reported to detect coronary collateral veins in 85 percent of patients with portal hypertension, the patient umbilical vein in 100 percent, and short gastric veins in 10 percent.[61,62] If doubt exists whether an enlarged vascular structure is an ectatic hepatic artery, an obstructed bile duct, or a portal collateral vein, duplex sonography may be used to identify the vessel on the basis of flow patterns.[63,64]

Portocaval Shunts

The primary therapy for portal hypertension is surgery. Portocaval shunts may be created to drain the portal vein into the inferior vena cava, while mesocaval shunts drain the superior mesenteric vein into the inferior vena cava. These shunts are difficult to demonstrate with B-mode sonography but may be rysms: sonographic and CT diagnosis. Am J Roentgenol 138:154–156, 1982

22. McGregor JC, Pollock JG, Anton HC: Ultrasonography and possible ruptured abdominal aortic aneurysms. Br Med J 3(5975):78–79, 1975

23. Chisolm AJ, Sprayregen S: Angiographic manifestations of ruptured abdominal aortic aneurysms. Am J Roentgenol 127:769–773, 1979

24. Gooding GAW: Ruptured abdominal aorta: Postoperative ultrasound appearance. Radiology 145:781–783, 1982

25. Roberts WC: Aortic dissection: Anatomy, consequences and causes. Am Heart J 101(2):195–214, 1981

26. Conrad MR, Davis GM, Green CE, et al.: Real-time ultrasound in the diagnosis of acute dissecting aneurysm of the abdominal aorta. Am J Roentgenol 132:115–116, 1979

27. Kumari SS, Pillari G, Mandon V, et al.: Occult aortic dissection: Diagnosis by ultrasound. Br J Radiol 53:1093–1095, 1980

28. Gooding GAW, Effeney DJ: Static and real-time B-mode sonography of arterial occlusions. Am J Roentgenol 139:949–952, 1982

29. Gooding GAW, Bank WO: Ultrasound visualization of the five-French catheter. Radiology 144:647–648, 1982

30. Gooding GAW, Sollenberger RA: Ultrasound localization of an indwelling arterial catheter and adjacent arterial embolus during a therapeutic infusion. J Ultrasound Med 3:191–192, 1984

31. Woo VL, Gerber AM, Scheible W, et al.: Real-time ultrasound guidance for percutaneous transluminal retrieval of nonopaque intravascular catheter fragment. Am J Roentgenol 133:760–761, 1979

32. Gooding GAW: Ultrasonography of the iliac arteries. Radiology 135:161–163, 1980

33. Gooding GAW: Aneurysms of the abdominal aorta, iliac and femoral arteries. Seminars in Ultrasound 3(2):170–179, 1982

34. Marcus R, Edell SL: Sonographic evaluation of iliac artery aneurysms. Am J Surg 140:666–670, 1980

35. David RP, Neiman HL, Yao JST, et al.: Ultrasound scan in diagnosis of peripheral aneurysms. Arch Surg 112:55–58, 1977

36. Strandness DE Jr: The use of ultrasound in the evaluation of peripheral vascular disease. Prog Cardiovasc Dis 20:403–422, 1978

37. Johnston KW, Kassam M, Koers J, et al.: Comparative study of four methods for quantifying Doppler ultrasound waveforms

from the femoral artery. Ultrasound Med Biol 10(1):1–12, 1984

38. Johnston KW, Kassam M, Cobbold RSC: Relationship between Doppler pulsatility index and direct femoral pressure measurements in the diagnosis of aortoiliac occlusive disease. Ultrasound Med Biol 9(3):271–281, 1983

39. Walton L, Martin TRP, Collins M: Prospective assessment of the aorto-iliac segment by visual interpretation of frequency analyzed Doppler waveforms—a comparison with arteriography. Ultrasound Med Biol 10(1):27–32, 1984

40. Merritt CRB: Ultrasonographic demonstration of portal vein thrombosis. Radiology 133:425–427, 1979

41. Weinreb J, Kumari S, Phillips G, Pochaczevsky R: Portal vein measurements by real-time sonography. Am J Roentgenol 139:497–499, 1982

42. Subramanyam BR, Balthazar EJ, Raghavendra BN, Lefleur RS: Sonographic evaluation of patients with portal hypertension. Am J Gastroenterol 78(6):369–373, 1983

43. Filly RA, Laing FC: Anatomic variation of protal venous anatomy in the porta hepatis: Ultrasonographic evaluation. J Clin Ultrasound 6:83–89, 1978

44. Carlsen EN, Filly RA: Newer ultrasonographic anatomy in the upper abdomen: I. The portal and hepatic venous anatomy. J Clin Ultrasound 4(2):85–90, 1975

45. Bolondi L, Gandolfi L, Arienti V, et al.: Ultrasonography in the diagnosis of portal hypertension: diminished response of portal vessels to respiration. Radiology 142:167–172, 1982

46. Bellamy EA, Bossi MC, Cosgrove DO: Ultrasound demonstration of changes in the normal portal venous system following a meal. Br J Radiol 57(674):147–149, 1984

47. Hill MC, Sanders RC: Sonography of the upper abdominal venous system, in Sanders RC, Hill MC (eds): Ultrasound Annual 1983, New York, Raven Press, 1983, pp 271–313

48. Kauzlaric D, Petrovic M, Barmeir E: Sonography of cavernous transformation of the portal vein. Am J Roentgenol 142:383–384, 1984

49. Marx M, Scheible W: Cavernous transformation of the portal vein. J Ultrasound Med 1:167–169, 1982

50. Weltin G, Taylor KJW, Carter AR, Taylor RR. Duplex Doppler: Identification of cav-

ernous transformation of the portal vein. Am J Roentgenol 144:999–1001, 1985

51. Gansbeke DV, Avni EF, Delcour C, et al.: Sonographic features of portal vein thrombosis. Am J Roentgenol 144:749–752, 1985

52. LaFortuna ML, Constantin A, Breton G, et al.: The recanalized umbilical vein in portal hypertension: A myth. Am J Roentgenol 144:549–553, 1985

53. Glazer GM, Laing FC, Brown TW, Gooding GAW: Sonographic demonstration of portal hypertension: The patent umbilical vein. Radiology 136:161–163, 1980

54. Aagaard J, Jensen LI, Sorensen TIA, et al.: Recanalized umbilical vein in portal hypertension. Am J Roentgenol 139:1107–1109, 1982

55. Fakhry J, Gosink BB, Leopold GR: Recanalized umbilical vein due to portal vein occlusion: Documentation by sonography. Am J Roentgenol 137:410–412, 1981

56. Saddekni S, Hutchinson D, Cooperberg PL: The sonographically patent umbilical vein in portal hypertension. Radiology 145:441–443, 1982

57. Juttner HU, Jenney JM, Ralls PW, et al.: Ultrasound demonstration of portosystemic collaterals in cirrhosis and portal hypertension. Radiology 142:459–463, 1982

58. Kane RA, Katz SG: The spectrum of sonographic findings in portal hypertension: A subject review and new observations. Radiology 142:453–458, 1982

59. Dach JL, Hill MC, Pelaez JC, et al.: Sonography of hypertensive portal venous system: Correlation with arterial portography. Am J Roentgenol 137:511–517, 1981

60. McCormack TT, Rose JD, Smith PM, Johnson AG: Perforating veins and blood flow in oesophageal varices. Lancet 2(8365-8366):1442–1444, 1983

61. Dokmeci AK, Kimura K, Matsutani S, et al.: Collateral veins in portal hypertension: Demonstration by sonography. Am J Roentgenol 137:1173–1177, 1981

62. Subramanyam BR, Balthazar EJ, Madamba MR, et al.: Sonography of portosystemic venous collaterals in portal hypertension. Radiology 146:161–166, 1983

63. Huey H, Cooperberg PL, Bogoch A: Diagnosis of giant varix of the coronary vein by pulsed-Doppler sonography. Am J Roentgenol 143:77–78, 1984

64. Berland LL, Lawson TL, Foley WD: Porta hepatis: Sonographic discrimination of bile ducts from arteries with pulsed Doppler with new anatomic criteria. Am J Roentgenol 138(5):833–840, 1982

65. Forsberg L, Holmin T: Pulsed Doppler and B-mode ultrasound features of interposition meso-caval and porta-caval shunts. Acta Radiol 24:353–357, 1983

66. Bender MD, Ockner RK: Ascites, in Sleisenger MH, Fordtran JS (eds): Gastrointestinal Disease (ed 3), Philadelphia, WB Saunders, 1983, pp 335–355

INTRAOPERATIVE AND POSTOPERATIVE VASCULAR DIAGNOSIS

During the interval since the publication of the first edition of this textbook, increased attention has been devoted to postoperative and intraoperative assessment of vascular repair procedures. Postoperative B-mode evaluation of vascular prosthetic grafts is an area of particular confusion for most sonographers and sonologists, but in Chapter 19, Dr. Gooding nicely ameliorates this state of confusion through succinct description of the normal and abnormal ultrasound findings in patients with prosthetic grafts. Chapters 20 and 21 are concerned with intraoperative evaluation of vascular surgery results. Dr. Zierler (Chapter 20) describes Doppler intraoperative techniques, while Dr. Sigel and colleagues (Chapter 21) outline the use of B-mode ultrasound. Both these methods appear to assess accurately the results of vascular procedures, and it appears that each technique may eliminate the need for intraoperative arteriography. The editor wonders, however, whether duplex examination would offer additional advantage by combining both techniques. It does not appear that duplex sonography has been used for intraoperative vascular studies, primarily because of lack of small, superficially focused scanheads. Perhaps the new, more compact probes now available will be used for intraoperative evaluation, and it will be interesting to note the results of duplex intraoperative methods.

Gretchen A.W. Gooding, M.D.

19

B-Mode and Duplex Evaluation of Vascular Prosthetic Grafts

SCANNING TECHNIQUE

The same technique recommended for scanning the native aorta is used for scanning the aortic grafts. Longitudinal and transverse scans are used for imaging the aorta, and oblique planes are used for the iliac branches. Real time ultrasound is essential for determining whether pulsatility exists and is more convenient than static imaging for following the course of the graft limbs, especially when they deviate from the normal vessel position. The femoral anastomasis may be imaged in longitudinal and transverse planes using a high-resolution (7.5- or 10-MHz) instrument designed for superficial imaging. Because of the superficial location of the femoral artery, linear array instruments are especially effective.

GRAFT MATERIALS AND METHODS OF ANASTOMOSIS

Knitted Dacron, which is porous, is the most common material for aortoiliac and aortofemoral grafts. Nonporous woven grafts are used for repair of ruptured aneurysms to decrease blood loss and operating time.[1] Autologous saphenous vein segments are used for femoropopliteal grafts and for replacement of small arteries.

End-to-end anastomosis is usually used to unite the proximal end of the graft to the abdominal aorta (Fig. 19-1). Occasionally, an end-to-side aortic anastomosis is employed. With this configuration, the end of the prosthetic graft is united to the side of the aorta. The aorta below that point is closed with sutures. The distal (iliac and femoral) anastomosis is usually of the end-to-side variety, regardless of the graft type or the configuration of the proximal anastomosis (Figs. 19-2 and 19-3).

The end-to-end graft typically has a slightly dilated configuration at the

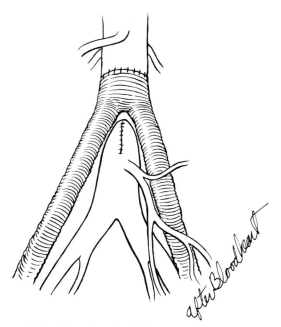

Figure 19-1. Drawing depicting an end-to-end anastomosis of an aortofemoral graft to the distal aorta. (From Wylie EJ, Stoney RJ and Ehrenfeld WK (eds): Manual of Vascular Surgery, Volume I. New York, Springer-Verlag, 1980. With permission.)

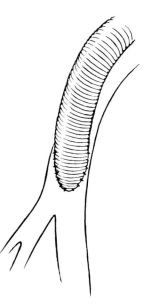

Figure 19-2. Drawing demonstrating the distal end-to-side anastomosis of an aortofemoral graft to the common femoral artery.

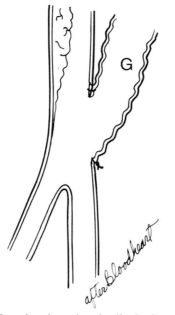

Figure 19-3. Drawing in a longitudinal plane showing a distal end-to-side anastomosis of an aortofemoral graft (G) to the common femoral artery. Anastomosis is located just proximal to the bifurcation of the common femoral artery into superficial and deep branches. (From Wylie EJ, Stoney RJ and Ehrenfeld WK (eds): Manual of Vascular Surgery, Volume I. New York, Springer-Verlag, 1980. With permission.)

proximal (aortic) anastomosis (Fig. 19-4). In the case of the end-to-side graft, ultrasound demonstrates the vascular prosthesis emanating from the anterior wall of the distal aorta (Fig. 19-5). One cross-section distal to the end-to-side anastomosis, one can identify both a native aorta and the graft immediately ventral to it. The graft on ultrasound has a relatively smooth, well-demarcated wall that is easier to image than the native vessel because of strong specular reflections that emanate from the graft surface.[2] Duplex examination of arterial grafts demonstrates flow through the lumen in addition to imaging the graft wall.[3,4]

Aortic aneurysms are typically repaired by incising the aneurysm, implanting the graft, and then wrapping the residual aneurysmal sac around the implant as a stabilizing force. Bleeding in the immediate postoperative period tends to produce a hematoma that is interposed between the graft and the encircled aortic wall and results in a characteristic lumen-within-a-lumen appearance.

Aortoiliac Graft

Aortoiliac and aortofemoral grafts are commonly used to correct atherosclerotic occlusive disease. The aortoiliac graft appears on ultrasound as a tube with either an end-to-side or an end-to-end proximal anastomosis to the aorta. The

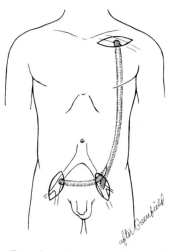

Figure 19-11. Drawing demonstrating axillofemoral and femorofemoral vascular prosthetic grafts. (From Crane C, Warren R (eds): Procedures in Vascular Surgery. Boston, Little, Brown & Co., 1976. With permission. Drawing by Harriette R. Greenfield.)

may also be used if an adequate saphenous vein is not available, but patency rates are better with vein grafts than with prostheses. Femoral-popliteal grafts are best imaged with high-resolution, real-time, superficial structure scanners. Transverse and longitudinal scans of the proximal femoropopliteal graft are obtained with the patient in a supine position. The distal portion of the graft and its anastomosis with the popliteal artery are revealed with the patient in a prone position, scanning at the level of the popliteal fossa. The 5-year patency rate for autologous femoropopliteal grafts is 78 percent, but the patency rate is directly proportional to the quality of runoff from the popliteal artery and inversely related to the degree of presurgical ischemia.[1]

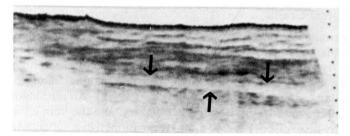

Figure 19-12. The normal appearance of a femoropopliteal graft as shown in longitudinal section.

VASCULAR PROSTHETIC GRAFT COMPLICATIONS

Graft Occlusion

Grafts may occlude for a variety of reasons, including (1) technical error, (2) embolization, (3) trauma, (4) progression of the arteriosclerotic process, (5) heavy smoking, (6) poor runoff, and (7) primary acute or chronic thrombosis without predisposing cause. An additional etiology for graft occlusion, especially for femoropopliteal grafts, appears to be kinking of the graft near its anastomotic site. Duplex scans of arterial grafts at the hip and knee joints frequently show kinking with flexion, which might be a causative factor in acute occlusion. This mechanism may be particularly important in occlusions occurring following long periods of immobility, such as a prolonged journey by airplane.[8]

Although graft occlusion is usually suspected clinically, it may sometimes be difficult for the clinician to determine whether pulsation emanates from the graft or from the native vessel. Typically, graft limb occlusion is confirmed by angiography; however, ultrasound may be used effectively to screen for occlusion in suspicious cases, and the ultrasonographer will occasionally encounter patients with unsuspected graft occlusion in the routine caseload of an elderly population. Graft occlusion may appear in one of three ways on standard units not equipped with pulsed Doppler:

1. In the most common presentation, the static examination of the graft appears normal, but the real-time examination fails to detect any pulsatility within the graft.
2. Less commonly, the occluded limb cannot be detected by ultrasound. This may stem from long-term changes within the graft, filling it with hyperechoic material that blends with the surrounding soft tissues.
3. Finally, using a high-resolution transducer, the occluding material may actually be seen within the lumen of the graft but in our experience, intraluminal thromus cannot be imaged routinely.

The best way to confirm graft occlusion is to employ a duplex instrument to directly interrogate flow within the graft. Doppler flow signals will be absent in the occluded graft.

Graft Dilatation

Uncommonly, some vascular grafts may progressively dilate over the years.[10] False-positive diagnosis of occlusion is possible in some patients who have very large graft limbs that have expanded with time if duplex methods are not used. Pulsations in such grafts are very subtle and are difficult to detected with real-time imaging.

False Aneurysm

False aneurysms are basically pulsating hematomas. In a study of 4000 patients with prosthetic grafts, Aagaard and co-workers[11] reported a 6-percent incidence of graft–anastomosis false aneurysm. Sonographically, a false aneurysm may easily be recognized as an intrinsically pulsating, sonolucent mass adjacent to

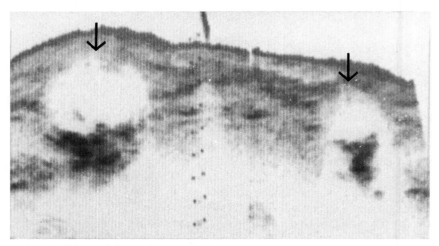

Figure 19-13. Bilateral femoral artery aneurysms (arrows) are seen in a transverse scan.

or communicating with an artery. False aneurysms in patients with vascular prosthetic grafts occur at the anastomotic sites, particularly at the femoral anastomosis[12,13] (Fig. 19-13). A number of reasons are postulated for this occurrence. In the past, silk sutures were used that degenerated with time, with resulting disruption of the anastomosis,[14] but the synthetic suture material now used resists deterioration. In some instances, aneurysms arise from technical error, including inadequate incorporation of the vessels, incomplete suturing, or excessive tension at the suture site. When technical problems occur, the anastomosis may fail acutely or may degenerate over time. Graft infection and hematoma also are recognized precursors of false aneurysm formation.

Proximal false aneurysm of the aorta tends to be silent clinically but is associated with a high mortality (50–80 percent) because of sudden rupture. These aneurysms are easily recognized on ultrasound as a periaortic mass with intrinsic pulsation. Traumatic aneurysm may occur in a patient who has a prosthetic graft, but in contradistiction to anastomotic aneurysms, these occur anywhere along the length of the prosthesis. Intrinsic defects in the graft wall also may produce false aneurysms, but such defects are exceedingly rare.

Perigraft Fluid

When postoperative ileus has cleared following aortic, aortoiliac, or aortofemoral graft implantations (usually 7–10 days), the graft can ordinarily be well delineated proximally. It is not abnormal at this time to visualize fluid around the graft; nonetheless, this fluid is cause for concern and should be closely followed,[3,15] since fluid from a hematoma, seroma, lymphocele, or abscess cannot be differentiated by its ultrasonic appearance alone. In general, the fluid collections appear as relatively hypoechoic regions with discrete margination and enhanced echoes posteriorly. Fluid may collect focally, either at the proximal or distal anastomosis, or may be seen tracking along the graft (Fig. 19-14). Small amounts of fluid in the first 10 days after an implantation usually regress without further

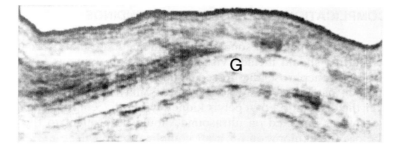

Figure 19-14.   Fluid is noted tracking along the length of an aortofemoral graft limb (G). In this case, the fluid represented an abscess surrounding the graft.

complications. Fluid collections that increase in size or that become symptomatic—that is, with pain, swelling, and focal redness—suggest further complications. False aneurysms can be distinguished from hematomas or other fluid collection by the presence of intrinsic pulsatility in an aneurysm, as seen on real-time imaging.

The hematoma surrounding a graft is an excellent culture medium, and, as a result, infection complicates approximately 1–3 percent of graft implantations.[1] When clinically indicated, the fine-needle aspiration technique may be used under ultrasonic guidance to yield material for culture and to exclude abscess, the most serious of graft complications. Radionuclide imaging with [117]indium-labeled white blood cells is another method used to confirm the presence of prosthetic infection.[16] When a graft becomes infected, it must be removed and the infection must be aggressively treated, since graft infection is associated with a 40-percent mortality.[1] Extra-anatomic bypass is usually required to carry the blood peripherally following graft removal.

Aortoduodenal Fistula

Aortoduodenal fistula is a lethal complication of graft implantation. Although aortoduodenal fistula may occur spontaneously, this catastrophe most often is associated with a vascular prosthesis. The most common location of aortoduodenal fistula is between the infrarenal portion of the abdominal aorta and the third portion of the duodenum, probably because of the proximity of the aorta and the duodenum in this area and the relative immobility of this portion of the duodenum. There are no reported cases of this entity on ultrasound that this author is aware of, but one patient examined after surgery had a large hematoma around the proximal aortic anastomosis and, in addition, fluid tracking along the right limb of an aortofemoral graft. The patient subsequently developed an aortoduodenal fistula and died of massive gastrointestinal bleeding. It would seem that a proximal fluid collection around the aorta may be the first indication of the development of an aortoenteric fistula and should be viewed with suspicion, particularly in those patients who demonstrate episodic gastrointestinal bleeding.

Doppler ultrasound is a safe and effective method for evaluating the immediate results of arterial reconstruction. Prompt recognition and correction of technical errors should ensure the best possible functional result and minimize the perioperative complications of vascular surgery. When used intraoperatively, Doppler ultrasound provides an immediate assessment of blood flow without any additional puncture of manipulation of the vessels being examined. The intraoperative Doppler method has been successfully used in a variety of clinical circumstances: (1) to predict the eventual result of arterial surgery in terms of symptomatic relief or graft failure, (2) to assess the viability of ischemic intestine, (3) to detect errors related to surgical technique, and (4) to select patients for operative arteriography.

DOPPLER INSTRUMENTATION

Detection of blood flow with ultrasound is based on the Doppler effect as discussed in Chapter 2. Most Doppler instruments operate with transmitting frequencies in the range of 3–10 MHz. Higher frequencies (8–10 MHz) are preferred for intraoperative applications, and a 20-MHz direction-sensitive pulsed Doppler has been developed specifically for intraoperative use.[13] This instrument, combined with a spectrum analyzer, has been used for both animal model and patient studies.[13–18] The probe for this instrument consists of a small ultrasonic transducer mounted on the end of a 16-gauge needle, and the sample volume is approximately 0.2 mm^3. This tiny sample volume permits assessment of center-stream flow patterns in small vessels such as the internal carotid and tibial arteries.

The attenuation of ultrasound in tissue is proportional to the transmitting frequency, so higher frequences are best suited for examining structures at close range. Doppler transducers used intraoperatively must be focused in the near field, since the transducer is usually placed in direct contact with the vessel.

Pulsed Doppler systems are well suited for sophisticated signal processing methods such as spectral analysis and have been used primarily for the diagnosis of carotid artery disease.[14,19] Continuous-wave instruments are generally preferred for intraoperative use, since they are easier to use than pulsed systems and are quite satisfactory for qualitative evaluation of flow patterns. Continuous-wave Doppler signals are suitable for auditory analysis and generating analog waveforms, as discussed below.

Doppler probes for intraoperative use may be gas-sterilized. Only the probe and its connecting wire are brought into the operative field; all other Doppler hardware and any associated recording equipment are placed on a cart that can be positioned near the operating table.

DOPPLER METHODS

Technique

When an arterial reconstruction has been completed, a qualitative assessment can be rapidly performed using a sterile continuous-wave Doppler probe and auditory analysis.[20] The Doppler probe is applied directly to the external surface of the exposed vessels. Acoustic coupling is achieved with a small amount of blood or saline solution. Since the Doppler frequency shift is proportional to the incident angle of the ultrasound beam (θ), a constant angle should be maintained during the examination. Experience has shown that optimal Doppler signals are obtained when the beam angle is approximately 60°.[13,17]

Doppler Signal Analysis

The Doppler shift in vascular examinations is in the range of several hundred to several thousand cycles per second. This signal can be amplified to provide an audio output, and the pitch (or frequency) of the audible signal is directly proportional to blood velocity. Auditory analysis by the person performing the examination is the simplest type of Doppler signal interpretation. By listening to the quality of the sound, an experienced examiner can differentiate between normal and abnormal flow patterns. The harsh, high-frequency signal associated with severe arterial stenosis is readily distinguished from a smooth laminar flow signal. Although the auditory approach is rapid and requires inexpensive equipment, it is purely qualitative and subjective. Thus, auditory analysis may not detect subtle flow disturbances associated with minor disease and technical errors.

Several methods have been developed to extract more quantitative information from the Doppler signal. The most commonly used technique is to record the Doppler signals with a zero crossing frequency meter, as described in Chapter 2. The resulting analog waveform represents the change in Doppler shift frequency with respect to time. Forward and reverse velocity components are indicated by positive and negative deflections relative to a zero baseline (Fig. 20-1). Although this method is subject to errors and artifacts, as described in Chapter 2, the analog representation of the Doppler signal is suitable for qualitative or quantitative analysis.[12,21] For example, discriminant analysis and pulsatility index are two quantitative approaches for analyzing the Doppler analog waveform.[22,23]

Spectral analysis is a method for processing Doppler signals that avoids the inherent limitations of the analog waveform. As discussed in Chapter 3, the frequency spectrum is typically presented graphically, with frequency on the vertical axis, time on the horizontal axis, and amplitude indicated by the intensity of the gray scale (Fig. 20-2). At present, the most commonly used technique for spectral analysis is the digital fast Fourier transform.[14]

Pulsed-wave Doppler signals are best used for spectral analysis, since the signal may be obtained from discrete locations in the arterial flow profile such as the center-stream. Spectral analysis of continuous-wave Doppler signals is complicated by superimposed vessels and minor flow disturbances that are normally present near the arterial wall.

Normal Postoperative Doppler Signals

Following a technically satisfactory arterial anastomosis or endarterectomy, multiphasic flow patterns of typical extremity or carotid flow should be evident in the reconstructed vessels. With experience, the surgeon can easily recognize these normal pulsatile patterns. Animal model studies of center-stream flow patterns distal to graft-to-artery anastomoses have shown minor spectral broad-

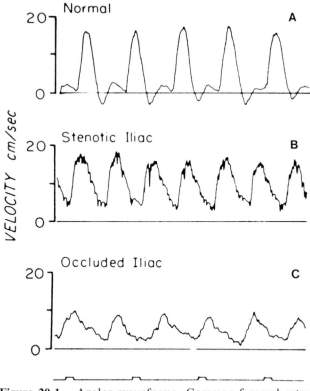

Figure 20-1. Analog waveforms. Common femoral artery analog waveforms obtained with a continuous-wave Doppler and zero crossing meter. The normal waveform is triphasic with a small reverse flow component. Iliac artery disease results in a monophasic, damped waveform. Flow velocity is proportional to Doppler frequency. (From Strandness DE, Sumner DS: Hemodynamics for Surgeons, New York, Grune & Stratton, 1975. With permission.)

ening in late systole and early diastole due to turbulence at the anastomotic site. The surgeon will learn that this mild degree of flow disturbance is acceptable and can be recognized in both the audible Doppler signal and the Doppler frequency spectrum.

Abnormal Doppler Signals

The use of spectral analysis for intraoperative detection of arterial lesions is based on the observation that certain arterial abnormalities give rise to characteristic flow patterns, as discussed in Chapter 3. For the intraoperative diagnosis of arterial lesions, the principal spectral abnormalities observed are (1) altered pulsatility above or below a severe obstruction, (2) increased flow velocity in the area of narrowing, (3) spectral broadening due to turbulent flow in an area of wall

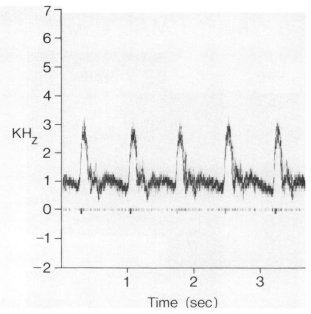

Figure 20-2. Spectrum from a normal common carotid artery. Doppler shift frequency (KHz) is on the vertical axis, time is on the horizontal axis, and amplitude is indicated by shades of gray.

irregularity or downstream from a stenosis, and (4) absence of Doppler signals in an occluded vessel.

The flow pattern distal to a stenotic lesion is monophasic and low-pitched and reaches the peak frequency slowly. Within an arterial stenosis, harsh, high-pitched, "continuous" Doppler signals are produced by increased flow velocity and turbulence. If no flow signal is found or an abrupt "water hammer" pulse is noted, arterial occlusion is present.

By moving the Doppler probe over the exposed vessels, it is possible to determine the flow contributions of the proximal arteries, the reconstructed segment, and the major outflow branches. This assessment is facilitated by momentary compression and release of the vessels under evaluation. Particular attention should be given to anastomoses and endarterectomy endpoints where localized abnormal flow patterns may indicate a technical error. In general, if the Doppler signals sound similar proximal and distal to an anastomosis or endarterectomy site, it is unlikely that a significant technical error is present.

As previously mentioned, a more quantitative assessment of the arterial reconstruction can be performed using a pulsed Doppler and spectrum analyzer. A series of animal model studies has been performed using a 20-MHz pulsed Doppler system and spectral analysis.[15] In this work, it was shown that minor stenoses of only 10–15 percent diameter reduction produced significant spectral broadening in late systole and early diastole. As the severity of stenosis increased, spectral broadening occurred earlier in systole, and with high-grade, pressure-reducing stenoses, spectral broadening occupied the entire cardiac cycle. In-

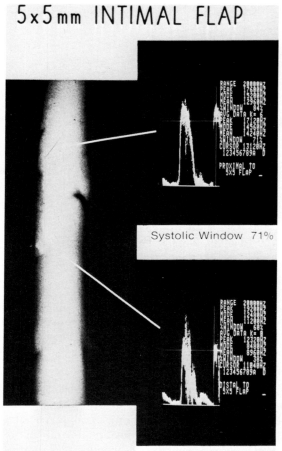

Figure 20-3. Spectra proximal and distal to a 5- × 5-mm intimal flap in the canine aorta. The center-stream pulsed Doppler spectra show an increase in spectral width just distal to the flap. The systolic window is inversely proportional to spectral width.

creases in flow velocity, as indicated by increased spectral frequencies, have also been associated with experimental and clinical stenoses.[14] A similar study was done to evaluate the accuracy of pulsed Doppler spectral analysis in detecting simulated technical errors such as intimal flaps and intraluminal thrombi.[17] Large intimal flaps (5 × 5 mm) and thrombi produced a significant increase in center-stream spectral width, while smaller flaps and intimal defects were not reliably detected by spectral analysis (Figs. 20-3 & 20-4). Common to all these model studies was the important observation that the flow disturbances created by minor stenoses, anastomoses, and simulated technical errors were localized within several vessel diameters distal to the lesion. Thus, the method requires a precise

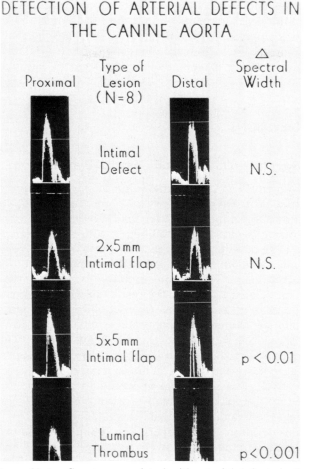

Figure 20-4. Spectra associated with arterial defects in the canine aorta. Intimal flap (5 × 5 mm) and luminal thrombus produced significant center-stream increases in spectral width distal to the defects.

examination of the reconstructed vessel that can best be accomplished by direct contact between the Doppler probe and artery.

The ankle systolic blood pressure, measured with a pneumatic cuff and Doppler flow detector, has also been used to assess the immediate results of arterial surgery.[24,26] With this method, the Doppler instrument serves as a sensitive electronic stethoscope to detect flow in the posterior tibial or dorsalis pedis arteries. The required equipment can be used either in or out of the sterile field, depending on the location of the operative incisions. Dividing the ankle pressure by the arm pressure provides an ankle/arm systolic pressure index suitable for comparison of serial studies.[12] Although noninvasive pressure measurement has been extremely helpful in the preoperative and postoperative evaluation of patients with arterial disease, its value for intraoperative assessment is limited. Because significant changes in pressure only occur with major arterial obstruction, pressure measurements will not be sensitive to the minor gradients caused by some technical errors. In addition, changes in the ankle systolic pressure do not indicate the location of the responsible arterial lesions. For these reasons, the direct Doppler examination is preferred for intraoperative assessment.

CLINICAL APPLICATIONS

Intraoperative Doppler Following Aortofemoral Bypass

Garrett and co-workers studied the value of intraoperative ankle pressure measurement during aortofemoral bypass for predicting which patients would be relieved of symptoms.[25] An increase in ankle/arm index of 0.1 or more measured immediately following bypass correlated highly with symptomatic relief. On the other hand, no change or a decrease in the ankle/arm index correlated with a lack of symptomatic improvement and also indicated the presence of a technical error or the need for additional arterial reconstruction.

Keitzer and associates compared the results of 35 elective aortic operations that included a qualitative, continuous-wave Doppler assessment and 22 similar procedures in which the Doppler was not used.[27] In the former group, five patients required nine reoperations to manage vascular complications, while in the latter group 15 reoperations were needed in seven patients. The reoperation rate was significantly lower in the group having an intraoperative Doppler assessment. The use of intraoperative assessment also appeared to affect mortality; only one patient subjected to Doppler examination died postoperatively, while seven patients not having the examination died.

A major consideration during operations on the abdominal aorta is the adequacy of blood flow to the small bowel and colon. Although bowel ischemia is an infrequent complication of aortic surgery, the mortality and morbidity of the condition are extremely high.[28] The colon, particularly the sigmoid portion, is more commonly involved than the small bowel. Bowel ischemia can be avoided by intraoperative recognition of inadequate arterial supply and appropriate mesenteric revascularization. In most cases, reimplantation of a patent inferior mesenteric artery will be sufficient; rarely, a graft will be required to increase flow in the superior mesenteric artery or celiac axis.

Clinical assessment of intestinal viability is based on a subjective evaluation of color, peristalsis, and palpable pulsations in the mesenteric vessels. More precise information on intestinal perfusion may be obtained using a sterile continuous-wave Doppler probe.[29,31] Normally, arterial flow signals should be audible when the Doppler probe is lightly applied to the antimesenteric surface of the bowel. During aortic surgery, the blood supply to the sigmoid colon should be assessed before and after temporary occlusion of the inferior mesenteric artery. When this maneuver causes a marked diminution or absence of flow in the colonic wall, the inferior mesenteric artery must be preserved or reimplanted into a graft. If flow signals are maintained with the inferior mesenteric artery occluded, then collateral circulation is adequate and the artery may be ligated if necessary.

Intraoperative Doppler Following Femoropopliteal and Femorotibial Bypass

Barnes and Garrett used a sterile continuouse-wave Doppler probe to assess 31 femoropopliteal bypass procedures.[26] The qualitative interpretation of the Doppler flow signals was compared with the results of operative contrast arteriography, and no technical errors were identified by either method. In a similar study, Keitzer and co-workers[27] performed 24 femoropopliteal bypasses with intraoperative Doppler assessment and 14 femoropopliteal bypasses in which Doppler was not used. Two patients in the former group required three reoperations for vascular complications, while in the latter group six patients required 13 reoperations. A significant difference was found between the two groups in favor of intraoperative Doppler assessment.

The 20-MHz pulsed Doppler system and spectrum analyzer have also been used to assess bypass grafts in the leg.[17] Center-stream spectra were recorded proximal and distal to anastomotic sites in 17 femoropopliteal and seven femorotibial bypass grafts. Maximum graft flow velocity was calculated using the Doppler equation and the peak systolic frequency obtained from the spectrum. The maximum graft velocity was significantly higher in femoropopliteal grafts than femorotibial grafts (Fig. 20-5). Four bypass grafts occluded in the early postoperative period. The mean maximum graft velocity of the failed grafts was significantly less than that of the successful grafts, and only the failed grafts had maximum graft velocities of less than 65 cm/sec. These observations support the concept that low-flow velocity contributes to early graft thrombosis.

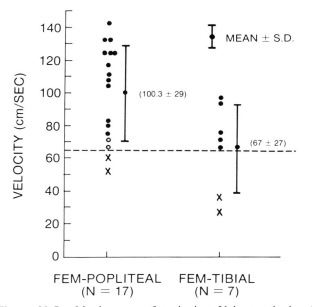

Figure 20-5. Maximum graft velocity. Values calculated using the Doppler equation and peak spectral frequency. Differences between mean values were significant ($P < 0.05$).

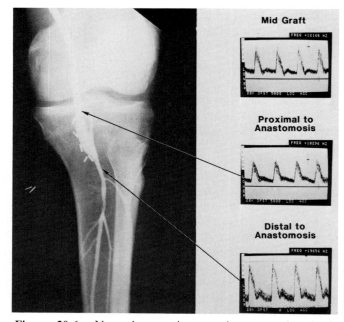

Figure 20-6. Normal operative arteriogram and pulsed Doppler spectra. Arteriogram shows a technically satisfactory vein graft to artery anastomosis. The pulsed Doppler spectra show only minimal flow disturbances within the graft and across the anastomotic site. (From Bandyk DF, Zierler RE, Thiele BL: Detection of technical error during arterial surgery by pulsed Doppler spectral analysis. Arch Surg 119:421, 1984. With permission.)

In a related study, pulsed Doppler spectral analysis and operative contrast arteriography were used to evaluate 20 femoropopliteal and 10 femorotibial bypass grafts. Center-stream spectra were evaluated for localized increases in peak systolic frequency and spectral width. Arteriographic lesions considered significant were intimal flaps larger than 2 mm, stenoses greater than 30 percent diameter reduction, and any intraluminal defects consistent with thrombus. A normal operative arteriogram and the corresponding pulsed Doppler spectra are shown in Figure 20-6. Significant spectral abnormalities were noted in five of the 30 bypass grafts. In these cases, operative arteriography identified defects requiring immediate correction in three grafts (one graft kink, two greater than 30 percent stenoses), while the remaining two grafts contained only minor defects (one spasm, one less than 20 percent stenosis). No other significant defects were noted, and none of the grafts thrombosed within 1 month after surgery. When the operative arteriogram was used as a standard for comparison, the pulsed Doppler method detected significant technical errors with a sensitivity of 100 percent, specificity of 93 percent, negative predictive value of 100 percent, positive predictive value of 60 percent, and overall accuracy of 93 percent. The relatively low-positive predictive value (high false-positive rate) can be attributed to the ability of pulsed Doppler spectral analysis to detect flow disturbances associated with minor arterial lesions.

Intraoperative Doppler Following Carotid Endarterectomy

Audible interpretation of continuous-wave Doppler signals was used by Barnes and Garrett to assess the results of 42 carotid endarterectomies.[26] All the internal carotid signals were considered normal; however, obstructive signals were noted in three external carotid arteries. In these three patients, the external carotid was explored and an intimal flap was removed at the endarterectomy endpoint. A satisfactory result was confirmed by repeat Doppler examination.

Spectral analysis of 20-MHz pulsed Doppler signals and operative contrast arteriography were used to evaluate the technical results of 50 carotid endarterectomies.[13] Center-stream internal carotid spectra were examined for evidence of flow disturbances consistent with technical errors (Fig. 20-7). Comparison of internal carotid spectra before and after endarterectomy showed

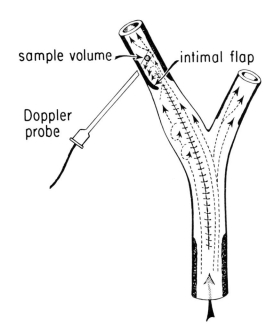

Figure 20-7. Pulsed Doppler assessment of carotid endarterectomy. Downstream from an intimal flap in the internal carotid artery, flow disturbances are identified by spectral analysis of the Doppler signal. The Doppler sample volume is positioned in the center of the flow stream. (From Zierler RE, Bandyk DF, Thiele BL: Intraoperative assessment of carotid endarterectomy. J Vasc Surg 1:73, 1984. With permission.)

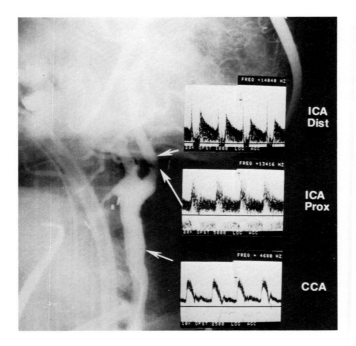

Figure 20-8. Operative arteriogram and pulsed Doppler spectra associated with a technical error. Internal carotid spectra are abnormal, and a constriction is present at the tip of the middle arrow. (ICA Dist, distal internal carotid; ICA Prox, proximal internal carotid; CCA, common carotid artery.) (From Zierler RE, Bandyk DF, Thiele BL: Intraoperative assessment of carotid endarterectomy. J Vasc Surg 1:73, 1984. With permission.)

improvement of the flow pattern in the majority of cases. Major flow disturbances were observed in seven internal carotid arteries, and in two of these cases operative arteriography showed defects that required immediate repair. No other technical errors were noted, and there were no perioperative strokes or transient neurologic deficits in the patients studied. Figure 20-8 shows the operative arteriogram and spectra from a patient with a constriction in the internal carotid artery following endarterectomy. The internal carotid spectra are markedly abnormal, with increased peak systolic frequencies and spectral broadening. Doppler examination after repair by vein patch angioplasty shows significant improvement with only minor flow disturbances in the internal carotid artery; the operative arteriogram confirms a satisfactory technical result (Fig. 20-9). This experience with pulsed Doppler assessment of carotid endarterectomy is similar to that described previously for femoropopliteal and femorotibial bypass grafts. The method is extremely sensitive, and the absence of false-negative results yields a high negative predictive value.

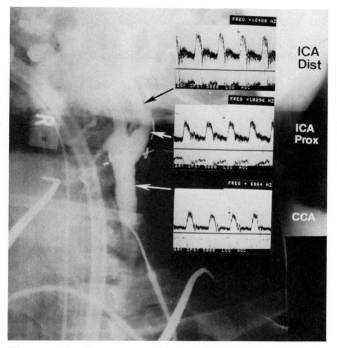

Figure 20-9. Repeat examination after vein patch angioplasty. Minor flow disturbances are present in the internal carotid artery, and the arteriogram confirms a satisfactory technical result. (From Zierler RE, Bandyk DF, Thiele BL: Intraoperative assessment of carotid endarterectomy. J Vasc Surg 1:73, 1984. With permission.)

SUMMARY

Doppler ultrasound provides a safe and effective method for assessing the immediate results of arterial surgery. The continuous-wave Doppler examination is simple and can be performed rapidly, while pulsed Doppler ultrasound is more suitable for detailed studies of arterial flow patterns. With either type of Doppler instrument there will be a learning curve, and further improvements in diagnostic accuracy can be expected as experience is gained.

Because the flow disturbances associated with arterial defects are confined to the involved vessel segments, the value of direct intraoperative Doppler assessment is limited to those vascular structures in the operative field. If examination of proximal or distal vessels is necessary, operative arteriography should be performed. In addition, the Doppler methods cannot identify the morphologic features of technical errors. Detection of flow disturbances that are not associated with significant technical errors results in a loss of specificity and a high false-positive rate. Residual minor flow disturbances, such as spectral broadening in late systole or early diastole, have been observed in reconstructions with satisfactory operative arteriograms. It is likely that these abnormal flow patterns are related to alterations in vessel geometry and wall properties produced by arterial surgery. The influence of these postoperative flow disturbances on progression of arterial disease and graft failure requires further study.

Intraoperative Doppler assessment could be used to select patients for operative arteriography. In this approach, only those patients most likely to benefit from operative arteriography would be subjected to the more invasive procedure.

Because reoperative vascular surgery is associated with significant morbidity and mortality, every reasonable effort should be made to achieve the best possible result during the initial procedure. Therefore, the routine use of intraoperative assessment methods is justified if they are safe and lead to the correction of technical errors that could cause failure of arterial reconstructions.

R. Eugene Zierler, M.D.
Assistant Professor of Surgery
University of Washington
School of Medicine, and
Chief, Vascular Surgery Section
Seattle Veterans Administration Medical Center
1660 South Columbian Way
Seattle, Washington 98108

D. Eugene Strandness, Jr., M.D.
Professor of Surgery
University of Washington
School of Medicine
RF 25
Seattle, Washington 98195

REFERENCES

1. LiCalzi LK, Stansel HC: Failure of autogenous reversed saphenous vein femoropopliteal graft in — pathophysiology and prevention. Surgery 91:352–358, 1982
2. Collins GJ, Rich NM, Anderson CA, et al.: Stroke associated with carotid endarterectomy. Am J Surg 135:221–25, 1978
3. Towne JB, Bernhard VM: Neurologic deficit following carotid endarterectomy. Surg Gynecol Obstet 154:849–852, 1982
4. Sproul G, Pinto JM, Turner MJ: Reoperation for early complications of arterial surgery. Arch Surg 104:814–816, 1972
5. Plecha FR, Pories WJ: Intraoperative angiography in the immediate assessment of arterial reconstruction. Arch Surg 105:902–907, 1972
6. Blaisdell FW, Lim R, Hall AD: Technical result of carotid endarterectomy—arteriographic assessment. Am J Surg 114:239–246, 1967
7. Courbier R, Jausseran JM, Reggi M: Detecting complications of direct arterial surgery—the role of intraoperative arteriography. Arch Surg 112:1115–1118, 1977
8. Sigel B, Coelho JCU, Flanigan DP, et al.: Ultrasonic imaging during vascular surgery. Arch Surg 117:764–767, 1982
9. Lane RJ, Appleberg M: Real-time intraoperative angiosonography after carotid endarterectomy. Surgery 92:5–9, 1982
10. Hobson RW, Rich NM, Write CW, et al.: Operative assessment of carotid endarterectomy—internal carotid arterial back pressure, carotid arterial blood flow, and carotid arteriography. Am Surg 41:603–610, 1975
11. Dean RH, Yao JST, Stanton PE, et al.: Prognostic indicators in femoropopliteal reconstruction. Arch Surg 110:1287–1293, 1975

12. Zierler RE, Strandness DE: Ultrasonic technique of lower extremity arterial diagnosis, in Zwiebel WJ (ed): Introduction to Vascular Ultrasonography, New York, Grune & Stratton, 1982, pp 251–272

13. Zierler RE, Bandyk DF, Thiele BL: Intraoperative assessment of carotid endarterectomy. J Vasc Surg 1:73–83, 1984

14. Zierler RE, Roederer GO, Strandness DE: The use of frequency spectral analysis in carotid artery surgery, in Bergan JJ, Yao JST (eds): Cerebrovascular Insufficiency, New York, Grune & Stratton, 1983, pp 137–163

15. Thiele BL, Hutchison KJ, Greene FM, et al.: Pulsed Doppler waveform patterns produced by smooth stenosis in the dog thoracic aorta, in Taylor DM, Stevens AL (eds): Blood Flow Theory and Practice, New York, Academic Press, 1983, pp 85–104

16. Bandyk DF, Zierler RE, Berni GA, et al.: Pulsed Doppler velocity patterns produced by arterial anastomoses. Ultrasound Med Bio 9:79–87, 1983

17. Bandyk DF, Zierler RE, Thiele BL: Detection of technical error during arterial surgery by pulsed Doppler spectral analysis. Arch Surg 119:421–428, 1984

18. Zierler RE, Bandyk DF, Berni GA, et al.: Intraoperative pulsed Doppler assessment of carotid endarterectomy. Ultrasound Med Bio 9:65–71, 1983

19. Fell G, Phillips DJ, Chikos PM, et al.: Ultrasonic duplex scanning for disease of the carotid artery. Circulation 64:1191–1195, 1981

20. Mozerksy DJ, Summer DS, Barnes RW, et al.: Intraoperative use of a sterile ultrasonic flow probe. Surg Gynecol Obstet 136:279–280, 1973

21. Johnston KW, Marozzo BC, Cobbold RSC: Errors and artifacts of Doppler flowmeters and their solution. Arch Surg 112:1335–1342, 1977

22. Rutherford RB, Hiatt WR, Kreutzer EW: The use of velocity wave form analysis in the diagnosis of carotid artery occlusive disease. Surgery 82:695–702, 1977

23. Thiele BL, Bandyk DF, Zierler RE, et al.: A systematic approach to the assessment of aortoiliac disease. Arch Surg 118:477–481, 1983

24. Williams LR, Flanigan DP, Schuler JJ, et al.: Intraoperative assessment of limb revascularization by Doppler-derived segmental blood pressure measurements. Am J Surg 144:578–579, 1982

25. Garrett WV, Slaymaker EE, Heintz SE, et al.: Intraoperative prediction of symptomatic result of aortofemoral bypass from changes in ankle pressure index. Surgery 82:504–509, 1977

26. Barnes RW, Garrett WV: Intraoperative assessment of arterial reconstruction by Doppler ultrasound. Surg Gynecol Obstet 146:896–900, 1978

27. Keitzer WF, Lichti EL, Brossart FA, et al.: Use of the Doppler ultrasonic flowmeter during arterial vascular surgery. Arch Surg 105:308–312, 1972

28. Ernst CB: Presentation of intestinal ischemia following abdominal aortic reconstruction. Surgery 93:102–106, 1983

29. Hobson RW, Wright CB, O'Donnell, et al.: Determination of intestinal viability by Doppler ultrasound. Arch Surg 114:165–168, 1979

30. Cooperman M, Martin EW, Carey LC: Evaluation of ischemic intestine by Doppler ultrasound. Am J Surg 139:73–77, 1980

31. Lee BY, Trainor FS, Kavner D, et al.: Intraoperative assessment of intestinal viability with Doppler ultrasound. Surg Gynecol Obstet 149:671–675, 1979

Bernard Sigel, M.D., Junji Machi, M.D., Ph.D.
D. Preston Flanigan, M.D., James J. Schuler, M.D.

21

Intraoperative B-Mode Ultrasound Techniques for Arterial Evaluation

INDICATIONS

There are two main indications for using real-time ultrasonic imaging during vascular surgery. The first is to localize pathologic conditions precisely after a vessel is exposed but before it is opened. The second indication is to detect vascular defects after a reconstructive operation has been completed and flow has been restored but before the incision has been closed. Preoperative arteriography usually provides detailed and accurate information about the location and distribution of atheromatous lesions within arteries. Such preoperative studies significantly contribute to the decision to operate and to the choice of operative procedure most suitable for the patient. Preoperative arteriography, however, may not completely visualize the lumen beyond an occlusion in the absence of retrograde filling of the distal portion of the vessel; therefore, the extent of the occluded segment may not be revealed with arteriography. In these situations, operative ultrasonography may accurately determine the exact extent of occlusive disease. Such information may be very useful in confirming preoperative intentions and determining specifically where to perform an arteriotomy for graft placement.

By far the most common indication for the use of ultrasonic imaging during vascular operations is immediately after reconstruction. The rationale for this use is to be certain that significant defects resulting from the operation have not inadvertently been left behind. Defects such as strictures, thrombi, and intimal flaps may initially be too small to produce discernible hemodynamic effects. Thus, they may not be apparent on inspection, palpation, or Doppler ultrasound studies of the velocity profiles or distal pressure. Yet, the ideal time to find and correct significant operative defects is during the initial operation, immediately after the surgeon has completed an endarterectomy, anastomosis, or another procedure. Operative ultrasound imaging is performed as soon as the clamps have been

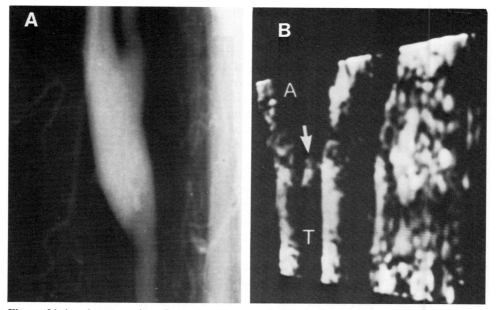

Figure 21-4. A composite of an operative arteriogram and a sonogram demonstrating a vein graft–tibial anastomosis. The arteriogram did not show any vascular defect, while the sonogram detected a 2-mm intimal flap (arrow) in the tibial artery (T). The artery was re-explored and the flap was found and corrected. (A, anastomosis.) (From Sigel B, Flanagan DP, Schuler JJ, et al.: Imaging ultrasound in the intraoperative diagnosis of vascular defects. J Ultrasound Med 2:337–343, 1983. With permission.)

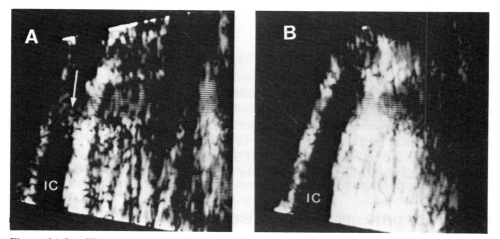

Figure 21-5. The sonogram on the left shows a 4- × 5-mm thrombus (arrow) detected in an internal carotid (IC) after endarterectomy. This thrombus was considered to be clinically significant and was removed. The sonogram on the right shows the normal appearance of the same vessel following removal of the thrombus. (From Sigel B: Operative Ultrasonography, Philadelphia, Lea & Febiger, 1982. With permission.)

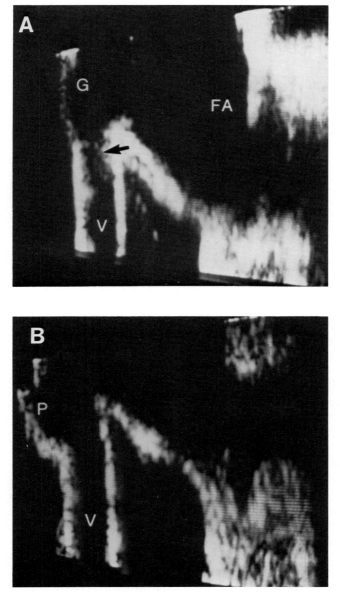

Figure 21-6. The upper sonogram, obtained following a femoral–popliteal bypass operation, indicates a stricture at an anastomosis of the vein graft (G, V) to the femoral artery (FA). This stricture was repaired by placing a venous patch (P) over the stenotic portion (bottom sonogram). (From Sigel B: Operative Ultrasonography, Philadelphia, Lea & Febiger, 1982. With permission.)

Table 21-1

Comparative Accuracies of Operative Ultrasonography and
Arteriography

	Ultrasonography (%)	Arteriography (%)
Sensitivity	92.3	92.3
Specificity	97.5	93.8
Efficiency	96.8	93.5
Predictability of a negative test	98.7	98.7
Predictability of a positive test	85.7	70.6

operations, vascular defects were considered clinically insignificant and vessels were not reexplored. In 10 percent of operations, however, vessels were reexplored. Thus, most defects were not considered significant enough to warrant the risk of reexploration. Most of the defects that were not reexplored were intimal flaps of 2 mm or smaller, usually located in a noncritical artery. Reexplored defects also were commonly intimal flaps but larger and more frequently located within small-caliber vessels considered to be critical for regional flow.[6]

The outcome of operative procedures in this series was essentially the same for patients without defects, those with insignificant defects, and those with serious operative defects requiring revision. The fact that equivalent surgical success rates were observed in patients without defects and those with "insignificant" defects suggests that the decisions not to reexplore "insignificant" defects probably were justified. The fact that the reexplored patients in whom a defect was found and corrected did as well as patients without defects suggests that revision was useful. We reach this conclusion because many of the reexplored defects were severe enough to create potential for serious thromboocclusive complications in the early postoperative period.

Our observations are based mainly on clinical evaluation, but we also assessed the accuracy of operative ultrasonic imaging by comparison with operative contrast arteriography. Operative arteriography was performed with static, single-plane radiographs either to detect vascular defects or to evaluate the circulation in the distal arterial tree. Table 21-1 indicates the result of arteriographic comparison at the reconstructed sites (mostly in the lower extremities). For detecting defects of all types, ultrasound was comparable to arteriography in in sensitivity, specificity, efficacy, and negative predictive value. In terms of positive predictive value, ultrasound provided better results than arteriography.[1-6]

The extreme sensitivity of ultrasound in diagnosing vascular defects after reconstruction raises the issue of whether ultrasound imaging may be too sensitive for this application. We believe this high level of sensitivity is readily managed by our ability to judge precisely the significance of a defect (by its relative size and location) in relation to the clinical situation of the patient. Thus, while sensitivity is high, specificity is also high, and the specificity of the technique allows us to grade the significance of positive findings.

LIMITATIONS AND BENEFITS OF B-MODE ULTRASONIC EVALUATION DURING VASCULAR OPERATIONS

There are three basic limitations of B-mode ultrasound as used in vascular surgery. The first two limitations are generic to all ultrasound applications; namely, a prolonged learning period is required for performing and interpreting ultrasound studies, and furthermore, the relative newness of the technique as compared with radiography is a cause of anxiety for some surgeons. Such problems are readily soluble if the surgeon is patient enough to develop the requisite experience, and especially if working relations can be established with radiologists and ultrasonographers. The third limitation of B-mode ultrasound during vascular operation relates to the area that can be studied. Ultrasound can assess only that portion of the vascular system that is in the operative field. Radiographic arteriography, on the other hand, can provide information about the arterial bed distal to the operative site. Thus, ultrasound is applicable primarily for gathering information about the blood vessels within the operative field, and, except for some Doppler techniques, assessment of the distal arterial circulation requires radiographic arteriography.

The general advantages of ultrasound in comparison to radiography primarily relate to the ease with which B-mode sonography may be used to direct visualization of defects with B-mode imaging and to the elimination of contrast injections. Doppler or B-mode scanning in real-time imaging permits unhurried study of a vessel to define thoroughly the presence and extent of a defect. With B-mode imaging, vascular defects may be visualized directly with ultrasound rather than indirectly as filling defects on an arteriogram. Direct visualization enhances detection and assessment of abnormalities. Elimination of the need for contrast injection removes risk normally associated with arteriography, including contrast reaction and air embolism. Avoidance of these risks is particularly important in carotid surgery where serious complications of contrast studies have been reported.[9,10]

SUMMARY

Intraoperative B-mode sonography is reliable and cost-effective alternative to radiographic imaging for detecting postreconstruction vascular defects. We believe that the wide applications of B-mode imaging for this purpose can reduce early complications associated with undetected vascular defects that are best corrected at the initial operation. This is especially true for smaller caliber critical arterial sites such as the carotid arteries and the popliteal branches in the lower extremity. We feel that operative ultrasonography should become an integral and routine part of vascular reconstructive surgery.

Bernard Sigel, M.D.
Professor and Chairman
Department of Surgery
The Medical College of Pennsylvania
3300 Henry Avenue
Philadelphia, Pennsylvania 19129

Junji Machi, M.D., Ph.D.
First Department of Surgery
Kurume University School of Medicine
Kurume, Japan

D. Preston Flanigan, M.D.
Associate Professor of Surgery
Chief, Division of Vascular Surgery
University of Illinois at Chicago
P.O. Box 6998
Chicago, Illinois 60680

James J. Schuler, M.D.
Assistant Professor of Surgery
Division of Vascular Surgery
University of Illinois at Chicago
P.O. Box 6998
Chicago, Illinois 60680

REFERENCES

1. Sigel B, Coelho JCU. Flanigan DP, et al.: Ultrasonic imaging during vascular surgery. Arch Surg 117:764–767, 1982

2. Sigel B, Coelho JCU, Flanigan DP, et al.: Comparison of B-mode real-time ultrasound scanning with arteriography in detecting vascular defects during surgery. Radiology 145:777–780, 1982

3. Sigel B, Coelho JCU, Flanigan DP, et al.: Detection of vascular defects during operation by imaging ultrasound. Ann Surg 196:473–480, 1982

4. Sigel B, Coelho JCU, Machi J, et al.: The application of real-time ultrasound imaging during surgical procedures. Surg Gynecol Obstet 157:33–37, 1983

5. Sigel B, Flanigan DP, Schuler JJ, et al.: Imaging ultrasound in the intraoperative diagnosis of vascular defects. J Ultrasound Med 2:337–343, 1983

6. Schuler JJ, Machi J, Ramos J, et al.: The role of intraoperative ultrasonography in vascular surgery. Bruit 8:234–238, 1984

7. Coelho JCU, Sigel B, Flanigan DP, et al.: Detection of arterial defects by real-time ultrasound scanning during vascular sugery: An experimental study. J Surg Res 30: 535–543, 1981

8. Coelho JCU, Sigel B, Flanigan DP, et al.: An experimental evaluation of arteriography and imaging ultrasonography in detecting arterial defects at operation. J Surg Res 32:130–137, 1982

9. Andersen CA, Collins GJ, Jr, Rich NM: Routine operative arteriography during carotid endarterectomy: A reassessment. Surgery 83:67–73, 1978

10. Collins GJ, Jr, Rich NM, Andersen CA, et al.: Stroke associated with carotid endarterectomy. Am J Surg 135:221–225, 1978

11. Sigel B: Operative Ultrasonography, Philadelphia, Lea & Febiger, 1982

Index